CREATIVE LONG-TERM CARE ADMINISTRATION

Fourth Edition

CREATIVE LONG-TERM CARE ADMINISTRATION

Edited by

GEORGE KENNETH GORDON, Ed.D.

Associate Professor Emeritus and former Coordinator
Center for Long-Term Care Administration
School of Public Health
University of Minnesota
Minneapolis, Minnesota

LESLIE A. GRANT, Ph.D.

Associate Professor and Director
Center for Aging Services Management
Carlson School of Management
University of Minnesota
Minneapolis, Minnesota

RUTH STRYKER, M.A., R.N.

Associate Professor Emerita
Center for Long-Term Care Administration
School of Public Health
University of Minnesota
Minneapolis, Minnesota

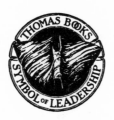

CHARLES C THOMAS • PUBLISHER, LTD.
Springfield • Illinois • U.S.A.

Published and Distributed Throughout the World by

CHARLES C THOMAS • PUBLISHER, LTD.
2600 South First Street
Springfield, Illinois 62704

© *2003 by* CHARLES C THOMAS • PUBLISHER, LTD.

ISBN 0-398-07350-3 (hard)
ISBN 0-398-07351-1 (paper)

Library of Congress Catalog Card Number: 2002027100

With THOMAS BOOKS *careful attention is given to all details of manufacturing
and design. It is the Publisher's desire to present books that are satisfactory as to their
physical qualities and artistic possibilities and appropriate for their particular use.*
THOMAS BOOKS *will be true to those laws of quality that assure a good name
and good will.*

Printed in the United States of America
SR-R-3

Library of Congress Cataloging-in-Publication Data

Creative long-term care administration / edited by George Kenneth Gordon, Leslie A.
Grant, Ruth Stryker.--4th ed.
    p. ; cm.
    Includes bibliographical references and index.
    ISBN 0-398-07350-3 (hard) -- ISBN 0-398-07351-1 (paper)
    1. Long-term care facilities--Administration. I. Gordon, George Kenneth. II. Grant,
Leslie A. III. Stryker, Ruth Perin.
    [DNLM: 1. Long-Term Care--organization & administration. 2. Nursing Homes--organ-
ization & administration. 3. Skilled Nursing Facilities--organization & administration. WT
31 C912 2003]
RA999.A35 C74 2003
362.1′6--dc21

                                                                    2002027100

CONTRIBUTORS

BARBARA PORTNOY BARRON, MHA, LNHA

Team Elite General Manager
Marriott Senior Living Services
Atlanta, Georgia

WAYNE CARON, PH.D., L.M.F.T.

Lecturer, Department of Family Social Science
University of Minnesota
St. Paul, Minnesota

KAREN S. FELDT, PH.D., R.N., GNP

Associate Professor, Center for Nursing Research of Elders
School of Nursing, University of Minnesota
Minneapolis, Minnesota

GEORGE KENNETH GORDON, ED.D.

Associate Professor Emeritus and former Coordinator
Center for Long-Term Care Administration
School of Public Health, University of Minnesota
Minneapolis, Minnesota

LESLIE A. GRANT, PH.D.

Associate Professor and Director
Center for Aging Services Management
Carlson School of Management, University of Minnesota
Minneapolis, Minnesota

WILLIAM F. HENRY, PH.D.

President, ForeSight Strategy Associates
St. Paul, Minnesota
Lecturer on Governance and Co-Director
Independent Study Health Care Administration Program
University of Minnesota
Minneapolis, Minnesota

SHAWN MAI, MDIV

Director of Pastoral Care
Walker Methodist Senior Services
Minneapolis, Minnesota

MICHELE MICKLEWRIGHT, DMIN, BCC

St. Croix Chaplaincy Association
Stillwater, Minnesota

CHRISTINE MUELLER, PH.D., R.N.

Associate Professor, Center for Nursing Research of Elders
School of Nursing, University of Minnesota
Minneapolis, Minnesota

SANDRA J. POTTHOFF, PH.D.

Associate Professor, Department of Health Care Management
Carlson School of Management, University of Minnesota
Minneapolis, Minnesota

JAMES R. REINARDY, PH.D., MSW.

Associate Professor, Director of Graduate Studies
School of Social Work
University of Minnesota
St. Paul, Minnesota

RUTH STRYKER, MA, R.N.

Associate Professor Emerita
Center for Long-Term Care Administration
School of Public Health, University of Minnesota
Minneapolis, Minnesota

CARLA E.S. TABOURNE, PH.D., CTRS

Associate Professor and Graduate Faculty
School of Kinesiology and Leisure Studies
University of Minnesota
Minneapolis, Minnesota

We dedicate this book with fond memories and highest regards to the more than three decades of students who have become our esteemed colleagues.

PREFACE

During the last 30 years, we have had the privilege of having long-term care administrators from all over the United States study with us at the University of Minnesota. These men and women have been creative, perceptive, and often quite adroit in applying academic knowledge to their administrative practice. They have also been generous in teaching us to understand which areas of practice might need and benefit from academic inquiry. This reciprocal teaching-learning relationship has always guided the selection and development of content for this book.

Prior editions of *Creative Long-Term Care Administration* (1983, 1988, and 1994) have been used as textbooks for both undergraduate and graduate courses. They have also been popular as a basic resource for an array of other long-term care practitioners and professions, as well as housing managers, board members, and owners.

This, the fourth edition, has been revised extensively. There is, for example, the fundamental updating throughout to reflect structural and regulatory changes which have been occurring in the field as well as the introduction of recent research findings, evolving ideas, and new practices. In addition, there are new perspectives introduced by nine new chapter authors plus three entirely new chapters: monitoring clinical outcomes, spiritual care, and using information technology. Finally, we particularly welcome the seasoned scholarship and visionary leadership provided by Dr. Leslie Grant as third editor of this fourth edition.

George Kenneth Gordon
Ruth Stryker

CONTENTS

Part IV
OPTIMIZING HEALTH CARE OUTCOMES

Part V
CREATING A SUPPORTIVE LIVING ENVIRONMENT

Part VI
CREATING A BETTER FUTURE

CREATIVE LONG-TERM CARE ADMINISTRATION

Part I

THE EVOLUTION OF
LONG-TERM CARE

Chapter 1

THE HISTORY OF CARE OF THE AGED

RUTH STRYKER

Every society develops ways of dealing with its marginal citizens—those who consume more than they produce and who, to that extent, are dependent upon society for support. They are usually referred to as "the poor" or "those on welfare." Historically, the poor included the chemically dependent (inebriates), the developmentally disabled (imbeciles), the mentally ill (lunatics), the disabled (cripples), criminals and the aged. The labels used to identify these groups in the past (as indicated in parentheses) contrast with those used today and reflect gradual social and attitudinal changes which have mainly taken place during the past three decades.

Cultural attitudes, expediency and both the capability and willingness of a society dictate how it will deal with its unproductive members. Nomadic tribes often left them behind to die, and Eskimos commonly put them on an ice floe. During the Greco-Roman era, medical attention was given only to those who could be cured, thus abandoning the disabled and aged to prevent a drain on resources. European societies tended to group "all of the poor" by isolating them in some kind of spartan housing arrangement. Primary, financial responsibility, while always mixed, has shifted across the centuries from the family to the church and philanthropy and, more recently, to the public through taxes with attempts to increase family responsibility.

Cultural attitudes toward nonproductive members of society have also varied. Helper motivations differ. For example, the Roman privileged class cared for "unfortunates" in order to achieve a sense of individual virtue. In contrast, Maimonides, the twelfth century Jewish physician and philosopher, declared that a recipient of benefactions should be spared a sense of shame and that assistance should enable persons to help themselves—a modern day rehabilitation philosophy! The contrast in motivation of the "helper" is startling—one for the benefit of the benefactor, the other for the benefit of the recipient. One might note that human nature does not seem to change; both the self-right-eous and the altruist are among us today.

In addition, there is often conflict between individual and collective will-ingness to help the poor. While some families are willing and able to care for one another, others cannot or will not. Because some children feel it is their right to inherit family money, they accept annual parental gifts without any expectation of using them to postpone welfare eligibility for their parents. Others feel no right to spend money they themselves did not earn and will use it for their parents. Some taxpayers are concerned about welfare cheats while others are concerned about the needy. Nursing home residents, their families, our employees and the taxpayers of this country hold these views also. In long-term care, we deal with value systems and motivations that dif-fer from our own on a daily basis. You might say, "so does everyone else." True, but compared to business and other health care settings, it has a far greater impact on the financial structure, the community image, staff morale and self-esteem of residents. These almost schizophrenic aspects of modern society challenge the development of more progressive methods of caring for the aged.

HISTORY OF NURSING HOMES

Saint Helena (250–330 AD) established what is probably one of the first homes for the aged (gerokomion). She was a wealthy, intelligent, Christian convert and mother of Constantine the Great. Like other early Christian "nurses" who devoted their lives to the sick and needy, she gave direct care herself. For many centuries, individual benefactors, benevolence societies, and religious groups remained responsible for care of the poor and led the development of early hospitals. Indeed, early English law prohibited govern-ment sponsored help because it "encouraged idleness."

Major changes occurred during the Renaissance (1500–1700 AD) through-out Europe. Books became more available to universities, Da Vinci made his anatomical drawings, Leeuwenhoek invented the microscope, and medical, pharmacy, and nursing schools were established.

During the Reformation, the British Parliament attempted to suppress the influence of the church through dissolution of monasteries and hospitals run by the church. As a result, "low" women took over the care of the sick in hos-pitals, bringing a dark period of history for health care. It was at this time that care of the poor became a societal rather than a religious responsibility. The English Poor Law of 1601 explicated how this would be done. If possible, par-ents, grandparents, and children of "every poor, old, blind, lame, and impotent person or other person not able to work" were required to support such relatives. An overseer set able-bodied paupers to work and provided relief for those without relatives and unable to work. This system of "relief" was brought to New England by the colonists.

In America, some paupers were auctioned off to families either for care or work. This inhumane practice declined after the revolution and was replaced by contracting with one person to care for all the poor in one town. Because these privately owned almshouses made a profit (usually from the work of the "inmates," as they were known), towns frequently decided to run their own almshouses, which were sometimes called poorhouses, poor farms or work houses. Poverty and illness were viewed as signs of a character defect, moral weakness or punishment for sin. Therefore, some minimal gratitude for care was expected. Inmates were thus expected to contribute to their keep through work. Quarters were spartan and were expected to cost as little as possible. Privileges for leaving the premises were directly related to "good" behavior and the number of years of residence in a particular area.

During the early 1900s, privately owned "boarding homes" became available to the more affluent aged, and church-sponsored homes for the aged emerged. A certain number of deserving citizens who had fallen on hard times were often allowed to "spend their last days" at many of these homes through the donations of benefactors. A few institutions introduced a nurse to care for the bodily needs of those who required it, but only personal and custodial care were envisioned.

At the same time, able bodied workers were drawn from the poor houses. Convicts were sent to prisons. Orphanages were built to prevent exploitation of children without parents. Hospitals were established for the mentally ill and mentally retarded. Special homes were built for the blind and the deaf. Gradually, only the poor aged remained in the poor houses.

When the first Social Security Act was passed in 1935, conditions in county poor farms had become deplorable. The Act specifically denied anyone living in a public institution from receiving assistance payments. While the intent of this regulation was to force closure of county poor houses, it did not work out that way in many instances. Some counties leased the poor farm to a private individual, thus, it was no longer a public institution technically, so "inmates" could stay and still receive their payments. Residents who feared they could not find a better situation stayed where they were, but others left and found a private boarding house. Indeed, this exit to the community enabled some owners to maintain large homes by taking in "paid guests" during the depression. Ultimately it also gave impetus to the start of many proprietary nursing homes.

Throughout the next 30 years, the number of aged continued to increase and many homes for the aged became nursing homes. The latter increased from 1270 in 1929, 7000 in 1954, 11,981 in 1965 to about 17,000 in 2000. During this period, hospitals became technologically more sophisticated, medical and hospital insurance became available to the majority of people, education of health professionals became more complex and new health professions emerged. Prior to 1965, there was little or no relationship between hospitals and nursing homes. Hospitals had grown out of medical sciences and health care; nursing homes had grown from the welfare system and various private housing arrangements. Their missions differed, and their historical roots were not the same.

Legislation

Hospitals and nursing homes were barely on speaking terms in 1965 when Congress passed Medicare and Medicaid, which were enacted because of the need for improved health care of the elderly. Initially, this legislation had both positive and negative effects on the aged and residents of nursing homes. The positive effects included (1) improved medical care for the elderly, both outpatient care and hospitalization; (2) mandated working relationships between hospitals and nursing homes; and (3) improved medical supervision and therapies for nursing home residents. It also brought confusion. First, the concept of "extended care" actually meant time-limited, post-hospital treatment as opposed to continued care of the physically and mentally impaired aged. This was a great disappointment to many people. Secondly, the legislation was based on the hospital/medical model which emphasizes disease rather than functional competence, treatment rather than quality of living and regulation of residents as a group rather than consideration of individuals. Third, and perhaps the greatest problem, was the emphasis on physical rather than emotional and mental needs.

This legislation also mandated a two-tier system for classifying nursing home residents: intermediate care (ICF) and skilled care (SNF). While staffing and service standards for these two levels differed, residents who needed skilled care were often declared to need only intermediate care in states where Medicaid costs were kept to a minimum. For example, at one time, 98 percent of Oklahoma's nursing home beds *were classified* intermediate care (ICF) and 90 percent of Connecticut's beds were classified skilled care (SNF). Obviously, the nursing home residents of these two states *could not have* differed to that extent.

Twenty years after the enactment of Medicaid and Medicare, major new nursing home legislation was passed in the form of OBRA '87 (the Omnibus Budget Reconciliation Act of 1987). This act amended both Medicare and Medicaid under the heading of Nursing Home Reform. The major areas of the Act included (1) resident assessment and care planning using the MDS (minimum data set) to record care needs on an ongoing basis, (2) use of alternative measures to the use of physical restraints, (3) restricting the use of psychotropic drugs, (4) enumeration of ten basic rights of residents, and (5) improvement of quality of care through quality assurance measurements. It also required that nursing assistants attend a state-approved training course before employment.

In addition, OBRA '87 attempted to redress the maldistribution of ICF and SNF beds among states. All Medicaid certified nursing homes are designated nursing facilities (NF) and Medicare certified facilities are designated skilled nursing facilities (SNF). Homes may have both certifications and all homes are licensed by the state also. A state surveyor conducts both federal and state surveys to assure compliance with regulations.

A new reimbursement system gradually emerged from this legislation. Residents are first assessed according to their dependencies and needs. Next, these needs are classified into a resource utilization group (RUG). Reimbursement is then determined by a formula based on the RUG in which an individual's score falls.

The Balanced Budget Act of 1997 (BBA '97) changed Medicare reimbursement for all classes of providers. Before BBA '97, hospitals could discharge a patient to a long-term care facility before the average length of stay (ALOS) for the person's diagnostic related group (DRG), but the hospital received the full reimbursement for the DRG. Organizations receiving the patient (SNF's and home health agencies) then billed on a fee-for-service basis. In the past, there were also instances of different providers billing Medicare Part A and Part B for the same services.

BBA '97 set up ten DRG groups subject to a new transfer rule. If someone in one of these groups leaves a hospital a day short of his or her ALOS, it is treated as a transfer and the hospital is paid on a per diem rate rather than the full DRG payment. In effect, hospitals are penalized for early transfers. For long-term care facilities, the SNF cost-based Medicare Part A reimbursement system is replaced by a prospective payment system (PPS). This system bundles all costs into a single per diem payment based on the patient's acuity as measured by a comprehensive patient assessment (MDS). This is then categorized into a RUG-III group, each with a specific payment level. The actual per diem PPS payment is then determined. This payment system is heavily dependent on the quality of the assessment of patients. See Chapter 15 for details.

Finally, BBA '97 introduced Consolidated Billing (CB). This is intended to prevent double billing to Medicare Part A and Part B by making the SNF responsible for billing all ancillary services and supplies. The SNF then pays the service providers, rather than having each provider do its own billing to Medicare.

LONG-TERM CARE TODAY

The Number of Elders

Older Americans in the United States numbered 3.1 million in 1900 and almost 35 million in 2000. During this same time period, the 65+ age group increased from 4 percent of the total population to 12.6 percent with a corresponding increase in life expectancy at birth from 48 years to 77 years of age. Worldwide, the number of persons age 65 has tripled over the past 50 years to 420 million. The more startling demographic shift, however, is occurring in the 85+ age group which now numbers over 4 million (2000), more than the total number of persons 65+ in 1900! With the aging of baby boomers, these numbers will continue to escalate.

These dramatic population increases represent changes in the elderly themselves. The aging process is being delayed, as evidenced by the increasingly later onset of chronic diseases and available advances in medical treatment of many chronic problems. Other differences include the fact that each *new* cohort of elderly is better educated, more affluent, healthier, and more active than the previous cohort.

With greater availability of home health care services and a wide array of innovative housing arrangements, the age of persons entering nursing homes is older. Of all nursing home residents, 13.5 percent are 65–74 years of age, 36.1 percent are 75–84 years of age, and 50.4 percent are over 85 years of age. Today's nursing home residents require more complex care as indicated by the following indicators: 83.3 percent have three or more dependencies requiring assistance, 47.7 percent have dementia, and 37.6 percent have both bladder and bowel incontinence.

Because of the changes in our societal composition, federal and state governments are making every effort to contain the growth and cost of publicly supported health care. As a result, all health care sectors have experienced a major shift to greater severity of client illnesses.

Long-Term Care Services

Long-term care services include almost any service one's imagination could conjure up. As a result, there are many definitions of long-term care. However, most authorities agree that long-term care encompasses an array of health, personal, and social services for persons who lack one or more functional abilities for self-care. Short-term or continuous service may be required, and it can take place in the home, a variety of housing arrangements or a nursing home.

Home care includes a wide range of services. Homemaker services relate to nonmedical services such as cleaning, shopping, cooking, other household chores, and helping with transportation. Home health care, refers to health-related services, usually provided by a nurse or a supervised home health aide. These services consist of bathing, monitoring a specific health condition, giving insulin injections, assisting with rehabilitation exercises, etc. Services often overlap between agencies and services also vary among agencies.

Respite care is a temporary service provided to give family caregivers an opportunity to vacation and rest. It is often provided by a nursing home with clients staying short periods of time while receiving physical assessments and rehabilitative services during the stay.

Adult day care centers may be sponsored by a nursing home, hospital, or church. Some adult day care centers provide therapies (usually physical, occupational or speech). Others are mainly recreational. Transportation may be included in the service and one meal is ordinarily provided. Occasionally, one may find a center that specializes in one condition, such as Alzheimer's Disease.

As the twenty-first century begins, traditional roles and expectations of all health care sectors are changing. Financial constraints have driven many of these changes. Competition and reassessment of organizational missions increase opportunities for creative managers and provide many new options for the elderly.

Hospitals mainly provide care to acutely ill inpatients while many former inpatient services take place in outpatient, same-day surgery and emergency departments. Some hospitals also operate postacute services and long-term care facilities.

At the same time, nursing homes are changing. Multi-institutional corporations control 47% of all certified nursing facilities. Many include senior housing. Most organizations provide more than one level of care. In addition, many have specialty units serving AIDS, coma, or Alzheimer's patients. Sub-acute units serve those needing post-surgical and rehabilitative care. The latter groups were formerly cared for in hospitals. These programs greatly increase the technology of nursing home care, making a hybrid organization which is more complex to manage.

In the mid-1980s, assisted living organizations emerged. Assisted living became popular for a variety of reasons. First, the architectural and interior design provided a home-like atmosphere. Individual living spaces looked more like a beautiful apartment rather than the typical nursing home room which was usually shared with another person. Most of these new buildings provided a defined living room area with a small kitchen and a separate bedroom. The units were completely private unless the resident wished to have a spouse or relative live there also.

Assisted living organizations provide two or three meals a day in a separate dining room. They also provide limited maid services and 24-hour monitoring in case of an emergency. Nursing, social, and therapy services are available on a cost basis with charges frequently in as small as 15-minute segments.

Owners and administrators continue to favor this kind of long-term care organization because they do not fall under the tight regulations imposed on nursing homes. In addition, they do not have to deal with the complicated restrictions of Medicaid and Medicare because few services are eligible in this type of housing. As a result, assisted living organizations mainly serve private pay residents.

There is no doubt that this is the pleasantest kind of environment for most older people. However, when one part of a system changes, it naturally changes other parts of the system. Many residents using assisted living facilities are very similar to those who used to be cared for in nursing homes at the ICF level. Now, nursing homes have become the place where Medicaid patients reside, where very ill patients (mainly those with severe dementia) go for care, and often where post-hospital rehabilitation is provided on a short-term basis, care that is often eligible for Medicare support.

At the time of admission, nursing home services are paid for by Medicare (29.7%), Medicaid (38.2%) and private pay (28.2%). With so much of a home's revenue coming from government reimbursement, there is little room in the budget to increase employee compensation. On the other hand, HCFA's comprehensive 1998 nursing home report to congress expressed concern about the level of staffing in nursing homes. To address the escalating costs of care, there is an effort to shift costs from the federal government to states, individuals, families, and long-term care insurance. There are also efforts to shift long-term care dollars to community-based services as opposed to institutional services. These problems are far from settled. It should be noted that the Health Care Financing Administration (HCFA) has recently changed its name to the Centers for Medicare and Medicaid Services.

To address quality of institutional care, many demonstration projects are aimed at more consumer-directed care and home-like environments. The Eden Alternative (discussed further in Chapters 7 and 23) has laid out ten principles of beliefs and values aimed to ward off loneliness, helplessness, and boredom in a more sociable setting. The Lazarus project emphasizes empowerment of both residents and employees. The Lyngblomsten Service House (in St. Paul, Minnesota) replicates a Swedish model where residents are cared for in small clusters and each cluster of residents has only one caregiver (the universal caregiver) who gives total care—cooking, bathing, house-keeping, giving medications, etc. (discussed further in Chapter 11). This flexibility results in a more coordinated and quicker response to a person's needs.

The term "nursing home" conjures up negative perceptions for many people. A natural dread of becoming mentally and/or physically disabled, well publicized nursing home problems, and a lay person's inability to assess quality contribute to this phenomenon. Recognizing this problem, the term, nursing home, is used less frequently. Many homes have changed their names to health care center, and several professional associations have dropped "nursing home" from their names. However, long-term care insurance is mainly concerned with nursing home care, licensure boards still use the term, as do the yellow pages of telephone books, and the term is heard in everyday conversation.

The long-term care administrator of the twenty-first century frequently oversees a campus of elderly persons with widely divergent needs. The basic goal is to provide the least restrictive environment for each individual and to provide as many choices as possible. For example, a person with arthritis may only need a cleaning service at home while a person in the final stage of Alzheimer's disease may need 24-hour supervision in a nursing home.

PROFESSIONAL KNOWLEDGE AND ADMINISTRATOR LICENSURE

Today's long-term care organizations evolved from almshouses, county poor farms, homes for the friendless and a host of small, religious, secular and charitable living arrangements. The goal of these organizations was to meet survival needs and little else. Superintendents of such facilities were either self-appointed or selected because of their ability to farm, nurse, administer "justice" or prepare inmates to "meet their maker." If he or she kept the place marginally clean, kept expenses down and did not allow any untoward incidents, nothing more was expected. Paid little, some were humane while others were not. Housekeeping, cooking, maintenance and other work was done by inmates so little staff was necessary. Professional staff was unheard of with the exception of an occasional nurse who (at best) had served a hospital apprenticeship or a clergyman to pastor their souls.

In 1903, when the word "gerontology" first appeared in the *Oxford English Dictionary,* it said, "see thanatology." It was not until 1945 that "gerontology" was even defined in Webster's dictionary. Gerontological knowledge and research were unheard of. There was no established body of knowledge available to persons working with the elderly. Knowledge of practitioners was no different than that of the general public. Therefore, intuition and common sense were the highest qualifications available in any organization.

Because knowledge and research in the field of aging is so recent, it explains (at least in part) today's wide gap between practice in the care of the elderly and available knowledge. There are very few long-time, knowledgeable practitioners in the field of aging. Few physicians are educated in geriatric medicine even today. The same can be said of nurses. Both medical and nursing students have experience working with the hospitalized elderly, but only recently are they learning how to assess and care for the complex relationship of physiologic, psychosocial, nutritional and environmental problems in other settings. Education of social workers, physical therapists, recreational therapists and other professionals frequently have had similar deficits. Many skilled health care professionals in the field of geriatrics are knowledgeable because personal interest and curiosity drives them to study available research and literature and to seek special educational programs.

There are, of course, other problems. Some people are more motivated by curing than by effecting gradual improvement or small but vital increments in function to improve quality of life. Others are uncomfortable with physical disability, mental confusion and the prospect of death. In addition, the public, families and many health care workers tend to attribute disabilities and behaviors of the elderly to the "aging process" rather than to physical disease, emotional problems, depression, nutrition or the environment. The result is most unfortunate, as many problems of the elderly go untreated, both in the community and in institutions.

Long-term care administrators have had similar problems related to education. Prior to the 1970s, only a handful of colleges or universities provided any educational programming for nursing home administrators. These programs were scattered across the United States and were unavailable to the vast majority of persons in the field. As a result, nursing home administrators had to rely upon themselves (personal experience, trial and error, commitment and intuition) and occasional educational meetings of trade or professional associations.

When licensure of nursing home administrators was federally mandated in 1971, it was very difficult to implement the recommended educational requirements for a variety of reasons. First, few higher educational institutions had monies to develop an entirely new curriculum. Few faculty persons had the time or knowledge to search the literature and select appropriate content from such diverse fields as psychology, medicine, gerontology, business, architecture, etc. Second, practicing administrators did not initiate this law. Indeed, this law was unique in three ways: (1) it was the first and (to date) only *federally* mandated health occupation licensure law; (2) because it evolved from external pressure to upgrade nursing homes receiving federal dollars, it had little support from practitioners in the field; and (3) it had no grandfather clause to accommodate established practitioners–all practitioners were required to take an examination after completing a specified number of class hours of education.

While licensure was federally mandated, each state was allowed to develop its own licensure law. As a result, nursing home administrator licensure laws differ greatly among the states. Some require minimal education beyond high school; some require a baccalaureate degree. This, of course, makes reciprocity for licensure among states very difficult and sometimes impossible. Not only does the amount of formal education vary, but the knowledge and skills of preceptors for internships (three to 12 months long) are diverse. This results in kaleidoscopic beliefs, knowledge and skills even among new administrators and a great variance in norms for practice. The latter is further intensified by the perspective of each administrator's previous work experience, such as hospital administration, mortuary science, public school teaching, social work, the ministry, accounting, pharmacy, business, nursing and many blue-collar and white-collar occupations.

Annual continuing education requirements for licensure are not standard among states either. While continuing education is crucial for keeping administrators abreast of new laws and providing opportunities to share ideas, it is usually not possible to provide depth of content for individual learning needs.

Today, very few long-term care administrators have been educated in their field of practice, and most were educated *after* they entered the field, a direct reversal of practice in almost every established profession. Some observers have noted that the consequence has been a "show and tell" quality to professional education because there was no other way of passing on long-term care administrative practice. Until very recently, most new entrants to the field of nursing home administration have had no way of distinguishing untested, personal opinion from thoughtful analysis of tested knowledge and research in the long-term care setting.

The limited amount of research-based knowledge in this field has made it particularly vulnerable to outside criticism. Today, however, new knowledge from research in many disciplines seems to be emerging almost daily. Educational programs for long-term care administrators are currently based on selected content from gerontology, business, hospital administration, and other fields. Greater testing of the applicability of these disciplines and exposure to other sciences related to the special problems of long-term care is generating new knowledge that will further delineate the field. Today's administrators are beginning to have resources that can help them to take new initiatives that will change the image of a nursing home by changing the organization. The administrative challenge is to develop a truly therapeutic care environment with emphasis on quality of life, determined individually with and for residents.

SUMMARY

Long-term care administrators and managers of residential living often must deal with a subtle antipathy toward their organizations. This antipathy comes from a variety of sources, some obvious and some illusive. Historical and societal biases regarding aging and illness are held by staff, families, administrators, government surveyors, and even residents themselves. In order to understand the work environment and to be able to reduce the effects of such biases on elderly clientele, administrators need to know the history of the field, the impact of federal and state legislation, the make-up of one's local work force, the scope of long-term care, and the kinds of workers who are drawn to the field. This is the foundation for entering any administrative career in a long-term care setting today.

The superintendent of a county poor farm was basically helpless because of societal attitudes and lack of resources; the long-term care administrator today has the possibility of an exciting future. At last, educational programs for health care professionals are turning their attention to the aging clientele. Research is starting to sort out opinions from facts. Sheer numbers of aged are forcing both personal and public attention to the aged. At no time in its history have there been greater resources, greater opportunities for learning and more need for the contribution of knowledgeable leaders with fresh ideas and creativity.

REFERENCES

Bishop, C. (1999). Where are the missing elders? The decline in nursing home use, 1985–1995. *Health Affairs, 18*(4), 146.

Chevremont, N.K. (1999). *The Eden alternative,* www.edenmidwest.com/eden-paper.html

Cohen, M.A. (1998). Emerging trends in the finance and delivery of long-term care: Public and private opportunities and challenges. *The Gerontologist, 38*(1), 80.

Dolan, J. (1968). *History of nursing.* Philadelphia: W.B. Saunders.

Gabrel, C. Characteristics of elderly nursing home current residents and discharges: Data from the 1997 National Nursing Home Survey. Centers for Disease Control and Prevention. *Advance Data, No. 312,* April 25, 2000.

Grant, L.A. Lyngblomsten service house demonstration. *Research in practice.* Carlson School of Management. University of Minnesota, August 2001.

Grant, L.A. Staffing and administrative issues in special care units. *Alzheimer's Quarterly,* Summer, 2001.

Kari, N., & P. Michels. (1991). The Lazarus Project: The politics of empowerment. *American Journal of Occupational Therapy, 45*(8), 719.

Krauss, N., & Altman, B. (1996). *Characteristics of nursing home residents.* www.meps.ahcpr.gov/papers/99-0006.htt.

McClure, E. (1968). *More than a roof.* St. Paul, MN: Minnesota Historical Society.

Morford, T.G. (1988). Nursing home regulation: History and expectations. *Health Care Financing. Review,* Annual Supplement.

Olson, J.K. (2001). Is this really a nursing home? Innovative models focus on enhancing quality of life. *Contemporary Long-Term Care,* p. 19, June.

Rhoades, J., Potter, D.E.B., & Krauss, N. (1996). *Nursing homes–Structure and selected characteristics.* www.meps.ahcpr.gov/papers/98006.htt

Shore, H. (1977). *History of education for long-term care administration.* Paper presented at Faculty Institute in LTC Administration, AUPHA, New Orleans, February 8.

Turnbull, G. (2000). Understanding the Balanced Budget Act of 1997. *Ostomy Wound Management, 46*(1) 40.

U.S. Census Bureau. *Statistical Abstract of the United States: 2000* (120th ed.). Washington, DC.

Vaca, K. et al. (1998). Review of nursing home regulations. *Medsurg Nursing, 7*(3) 165, June.

The World Almanac and the Book of Facts. (2002). *Vital Statistics.* New York: World Almanac.

Zinn, J.S., Brannon, D., & Mor, V. (1995). Organizing for nursing home quality. *Quality Management in Health Care, 3*(4) 37.

Chapter 2

CHARACTERISTICS OF THE LONG-TERM CARE MODEL

RUTH STRYKER

Medicare and Medicaid legislation thrust an unwilling nursing home industry into the health care system in the 1960s. The answer to concern about the quality of health care provided in nursing homes was to make them more hospital-like. However, the remedy lacked an understanding of the nature of chronic care compared to acute care. Even today, some policymakers, boards, owners, administrators, and even health care professionals are unable to articulate the major components of long-term care. Because many health care professionals receive predominantly hospital-based educations, they may unwittingly bring counterproductive practices to their elderly clients. For these reasons, it is imperative to identify the major features of existing care models, some of which were carefully designed to avoid the medical model.

MAJOR AREAS OF DIFFERENCE

General Comments. The medical/hospital model is driven by high technology, physician directed, and designed for persons with immediate health care needs. Treatment of disease is the principal goal. The long-term care model is driven by psychosocial disciplines, directed by an interdisciplinary team, and designed for persons with chronic physical and mental functional deficits. Quality of life is the major goal. The residential/hospitality/hotel model is driven by marketing data on client desires, client directed, and designed for persons with minimal care needs. Security, independence, and comfortable living arrangements are major goals.

Clearly, as a person becomes less competent by virtue of disease, an increasing number of health and support services may be required. However, the individual's sense of self-direction and self-esteem must be protected throughout any transition across settings.

When health care is delivered in a residential setting, it incorporates client-driven decision-making as much as possible in order to maintain the highest possible psychological and physical functioning. The hospital care system is inappropriate for chronic conditions. Provision of maintenance health care, attention to a quality living environment, and client and family decision-making characterize both the long-term care and residential care models. Assisted living is a hybrid between these two models. Today's long-term care organizations are expected to provide an increasing amount of health care such as post-surgical and rehabilitative care but they must not lose sight of their psychosocial goals.

In any event, the manager or administrator in any of these settings must be especially attuned to the care environment. Indeed, the environment (both physical and psychosocial) has a direct impact on the welfare and outcomes of residents. It should be therapeutic with respect to enhancing a person's self esteem and quality of life.

Scientific Knowledge. Hospital care is heavily rooted in biomedical and technological sciences while long-term care is more heavily rooted in the psychosocial sciences. The major problems of hospital patients are physical, while the major problems of older persons are social, economic, and emotional. The physical problems of the frail elderly are usually chronic, long-standing and under medical control. The nursing home deals with the more severe affective, cognitive, social and mental disorders. Supervised or supportive housing deals with similar but less severe psychological problems accompanied by less severe physical problems.

Goals of Care. The main purpose of a hospital is to diagnose, treat and discharge its patients as quickly and efficiently as possible. The main purpose of a long-term care organization is to provide a secure psychosocial environment that promotes the highest physical and mental function for an improved quality of life. Rehabilitation and maintenance of physical and mental function must, of course, go hand in hand to accomplish this goal, but it is provided in a residential setting. In essence, the primary objective of a hospital is to provide a treatment environment; the primary objective of a nursing home is to provide maintenance and rehabilitation in a psychosocially healthful living environment. Health care is less intensive in the hospitality model which has a greater emphasis on personal care services (cleaning, nutrition, shopping, transportation, etc.).

Diagnoses/Client Problem. A patient usually comes to a hospital with a primary physical diagnosis or complaint and organizational energies are focused on that primary problem. The long-term care client is far more complex. He or she has two or more chronic diseases, which may be fairly well controlled and of long duration, a variety of sensory deficits such as diminished hearing, vision and tactile sense, age-related conditions such as loss of stamina and energy, loss of mobility caused by stiff and aching joints and muscles, and a host of psychological and mental conditions. In addition, there may be depression over loss of friends, spouse, children, home and diminished income. Even with loss of memory and confusion, an overlying depression can exacerbate mental symptoms.

All too frequently a depression goes untreated and can even be increased by living in an emotionally sterile or insensitive environment. Because the aged person lives in a long-term care organization with multiple chronic physical diseases, sensory losses, age-related symptoms and behavioral problems, a medical diagnosis has limited value in planning care. Therefore, functional diagnoses become mandatory. Knowing that an elderly person has arthritis gives guidance for directing treatment goals, but it tells nothing about needed support services. Data on medical diagnoses of nursing home residents rarely provide any clear picture of the multiplicity and complexity of actual problems or needs that confront personnel. Functional assessment is equally important for those who live in the hospitality model.

Therapeutic Expectations. For most hospital patients, the aim is to cure a disease or at least return home and resume normal activity. For most long-term care residents, however, there are few specific therapeutic aims except for goals in physical and mental function: This needs to be replaced by more scientifically-based programs and services that attempt to control or reduce the mental and physical effects of aging, to improve or at least maintain function and to enrich life at home or in a nursing home when discharge is not a truly viable option.

It is this author's contention that an unknown number of elderly can improve and live at a lesser level of care if this objective is taken more seriously by physicians and personnel in all types of health care organizations. Whether an aged person remains at home with depression from feeling like a burden to family over a period of time or enters an institutional environment devoid of social, intellectual, physical or other appropriate stimulation, the effect is the same; namely, the aged person is deprived of assessment and therapy. Lack of goals and expectations by health care professionals compound the aged person's sense of helplessness and hopelessness.

Most hospital patients and staff expect a positive outcome. Most long-term care patients, however, expect a negative outcome. This can become a self-fulfilling prophecy. When patients, families, physicians and staff think everything is "downhill from here on," nothing is done to try to make it otherwise. Fortunately for those who live in nursing homes where staff know better, quality of life is enhanced physically, socially, emotionally and mentally even when discharge is inadvisable. This, of course, includes terminally ill residents whose environment encompasses some of the qualities of the hospice movement.

The Client's Role. The hospital patient's role is to submit to appropriate care this includes permitting dependence and giving up a certain degree of personal freedom in order to obtain appropriate outcomes. The long-term client's role is to participate in his or her own care, maintain individuality, live close to prized belongings, make choices about the daily routine, activities, their timing and to reject any activities that might increase dependence. However, if a frail elderly person is expected to take on the more traditional dependent role of a hospital patient, self-esteem is lowered and functional abilities are reduced. While temporary dependence can help to achieve positive therapeutic outcomes in acute care, a decision-free environment can actually cause negative outcomes and dependence in a long-term care environment.

The Caregiver's Role. The hospital caregiver's role is clearly to direct and give care. The long-term caregiver's role has not been so clearly defined. However, staff surely must (1) encourage self-direction, (2) create a flexible environment, (3) promote choices, (4) be a friend to clients, (5) help persons to help themselves in order to improve self-esteem and competency, (6) encourage individuality, (7) allow emotional expression, (8) promote affectional ties, and (9) support the family, or in some instances, serve as surrogate families. Rather than giving care, care is expedited in long-term care and residential settings.

This requires professional staff to give up much of their control in order to give residents more control over their lives. This requires a breakdown of the staff-resident caste line (Bowker). Situational factors affecting morale of institutionalized aged show that resident control of daily activities is a strong contributor to morale. In Tobin and Leiberman's research, passivity was found to be the only predictor of morbidity and mortality among persons going to nursing homes. They identified a heightened sense of mastery for residents. Perception of choice regarding admission predicts resident well-being. Staff must have an understanding that too much control creates a sense of anonymity, lowers self-esteem, and produces apathy, a sense of powerlessness, and increased helplessness. In practice, this requires developing a tolerance for individual decision-making even if it is not thought to be "good" for the individual. Residents had rights prior to admission, and they need to have as many as possible after admission.

Care System. The hospital has basically a closed system for patients. Most major decisions are made by the physician from the decision to admit to the day of discharge. Other disciplines support and contribute to that care throughout the stay. Long-term care, however, is basically a more open system because there is a greatly altered distribution of power in decisions about care. First of all, residents have a greater "say." Nurses, social workers, families, administrators and other therapists work to increase client decision-making and initiatives about care including opening the resident's life to the community. Even entry to the system differs. While the physician must approve a long-term care admission, it is the family and resident who decide if institutionalization is required, select the facility and arrange for admission, usually working with a social worker and nurse. The hospitality model is of course completely open to client decisions.

Medical Staff. In a hospital, there is an organized medical staff that is influential by virtue of their acknowledged expertise. They visit and monitor hospital care daily. This is not necessary in long-term care. Physicians usually see their patients once a month and work indirectly with a team of other persons who work directly with needs that are not in the physician's province of expertise. Physicians usually desire less input and are not organized as a staff, especially if they have little training or special interest in geriatric care. The multiplicity of problems of the aged requires a greater sharing of expertise with other persons and professions than in a hospital. In all models, it is critical that a full medical evaluation be done, however.

Nursing Staff. A hospital staff is comprised of about three professional staff to one nonprofessional staff. For the most part, staff are educated in acute care and feel confident in their ability to deliver the care that is expected of them. Long-term care organizations have about one-third fewer staff per bed and have a ratio of three nonprofessionals to one professional staff person. Therefore, nurses (often without a geriatric or management background) must supervise a greater number of nonprofessionals, and they have fewer peers and other support people to call upon. The combination of greater responsibility, fewer professional backup persons and less education in their field of practice presents formidable challenges for the professional nurse. This is often true for home care providers also.

The source of personnel gratification differs with models. In the hospital and residential models, the patient or resident and family usually express appreciation for the help, care, and comfort provided. In long-term care, families may be upset and residents may be angry or confused. As a result, the organization needs to be active in providing staff appreciation and recognition more often.

Family Impact. The impact of families on the care of hospital patients is quite minimal. Their role is to receive medical and other information about their relative and to support the patient. In the long-term care setting, however, the family is very much involved in several aspects. First, the family initially selects the nursing home in most instances. After admission, they can become a very important part of the treatment system by providing information, some direct care and access to the external environment, other family members and the community. Family participation also requires some relinquishing of authority by personnel. Finally, families often need to receive help to deal with their grief, guilt, anger, and depression. In the home or hospitality setting, families provide many support services, to the elderly person directly.

Resident Impact. The social and psychological impact of the patient on organizational function is usually minimal or occasional in the hospital. In the residential or long-term care setting, however, the resident greatly influences (for better or worse) the behavior of other residents, staff and the general operation of programs and services. Encouraging greater control by residents is crucial. However, like any community, a wide variety of behaviors will be exhibited, and individualized interventions may be necessary when disruptive behavior occurs. The housing manager will find this a frequent area of concern and responsibility.

Architectural Design. Hospitals are designed around the provision of services and the most efficient and cost effective use of personnel in delivering those services. Long-term care and housing organizations should be designed around the concept of living and function of residents. Private accommodations are strongly recommended. However, if a double room is designed, a toe-to-toe bed arrangement rather than side-to-side beds provide both residents with greater privacy as well as a window. Furniture can be arranged in a manner that suggests more of a bed-living room rather than merely a bedroom.

Color can increase or decrease confusion as can the amount of glare or dark areas from lighting in halls, living rooms, activity rooms and dining rooms. There are a host of other considerations that can improve self-esteem through greater independence such as the shape of doorknobs, grab bars, the type of window openers, and the height of clothes poles in closets. Nonroom space in long-term care organizations is not used for x-ray, lab, O.R., etc.; it is used for living space, privacy space, reading areas, conversation areas, social space, activities, etc.—features of a residence.

Cost/Reimbursement. The per diem rate of hospitals is five or six times that of nursing homes. Indeed hotel rates are often double that of nursing homes. Some observers think that nursing home care is our best health care bargain. However, because of the obvious difference in length of stay, long-term care becomes very expensive for an individual over a prolonged time.

Payment of services for hospital care comes largely from insurance companies and Medicare while the payment of services for nursing home care comes mainly from private funds or Medicaid. Although long-term care insurance availability is growing, it is owned by few, so the impact on private resources can still overwhelm an individual or family. Home care and hotel models save both public and private dollars when intensive health care and supervision are unnecessary. However, assisted living is mainly paid for by private resources.

Organizational Success. The hospital can be considered an organizational success because its purpose (to diagnose, treat and discharge) is in agreement with the goals of its clients, staff, services and mission statement. Professional staff have been educated in their area of practice. While conflicts may arise about individual situations, they rarely relate to overall purpose and goals. Long-term care residential organizations, on the other hand, often exhibit many contradictions within themselves. Stated goals often conflict with actual care. Because of lack of education in geriatrics, physicians may withdraw from residents, and nurses may emphasize physical care without equal emphasis on rehabilitative and psychosocial care.

Most elderly, even those in nursing homes, consider themselves fairly well, but health caregivers perceive them as ill. In addition, families are likely to expect dependence-oriented care. Apathy on the part of the public, a sense of hopelessness on the part of families, residents and other professionals as well as certain regulatory policies contribute to a state of mixed perceptions and expectations in many long-term care settings. As a result, success is often defined quite differently by each party involved.

ADMINISTRATIVE RESPONSIBILITIES

How do all of these factors influence the performance of the administrator of a long-term care organization? First of all, the administrator must take leadership in formulating a mission statement. A mission statement needs to include a commitment to education and research as well as care. It might include a specific target population, the Lutheran, Catholic or community elderly, or the elderly with particular disabilities, either mental or physical. The creative geriatric center provides parallel services, medical and social care. Seven major components can be identified: (1) medical care, (2) residential and personal care, (3) mental health care, (4) dying care, (5) education programs, (6) research activities and (7) community services. The administrator must also take leadership in educating the board and/or owners of what the real mission and potential accomplishments of the organization can be. Board members or owners must be committed to exploring creative efforts if the organization is to become a dynamic community resource.

Second, the administrator of a residential care organization must have some gerontological knowledge in order to take leadership in the quality of care through environmental intervention. When a hospital administrator resigns, the quality of direct care is not likely to be influenced. However, when a housing manager or an administrator of a long-term care organization leaves, the entire atmosphere of the organization may quickly alter from a therapeutic environment to one that is not or vice versa. Quality of life is highly dependent upon the quality of the psychosocial environment set by the administrator or manager.

A second reason for gerontotogical knowledge relates to the physical design and interior of the building, because it must be planned with knowledge of sensory changes, physical adaptive needs and mental states that are found in many residents. The administrator must also understand that self-esteem and morale of residents are nourished by the attitudes of employees. Clinical knowledge helps to identify which routines, procedures, policies and organizational practices diminish life satisfaction of residents. The employer needs a clear idea of what personal characteristics employees need if they are to enhance residents' quality of life. In summary, this knowledge provides a base for selecting appropriate programs, personnel, architectural design, interior decoration and even furniture, all of which can make the difference between dependence and independence, self-esteem and depression, or satisfaction and despair.

Third, the administrator must have broad and diverse management and interpersonal skills that allow him or her to function with fewer professionals, in an environment with conflicting and sometimes indifferent participants, with fewer trained assistants and department heads, and a somewhat hostile public environment. Most hospitals have a pyramidal organizational structure with several levels of middle management, many with special expertise to support financial, personnel, and planning decisions. By contrast, long-term care organizations have a flat structure with few if any middle management positions. These factors, of course, place a wider variety of responsibilities on the administrator. As a result, the administrator must assume yet another role, that of educator. Staff development, in fact, may become a primary role in many instances.

Finally, in order to be successful in administering services to the elderly, a more than superficial knowledge of change theory is required to lead an organization from the hospital model to a therapeutic long-term care model that constantly asks itself, "Would I like to live here?" John Gardner states in his book, *Self-Renewal,* "Knowledge will be a safe weapon only if it is linked to a deeply rooted conviction that organizations are made for men and not men for organizations. The whole purpose of such knowledge is to design environments conducive to individual fulfillment. . . ." Succeeding chapters will suggest ways of accomplishing this.

REFERENCES

Bowker, L.H. (1982). *Humanizing institutions for the aged.* Lexington, MA: Lexington Books.

Gardner, J. (1963). *Self-renewal.* New York: Harper & Row.

Tobin, S., & Leiberman, M. (1976). *Last home for the aged.* San Francisco, CA: Jossey-Bass.

Part II

DEVELOPING THE ORGANIZATION

Chapter 3

GOVERNING THE LONG-TERM CARE ORGANIZATION

WILLIAM F. HENRY

Governing boards—boards of directors or boards of trustees—perform essential roles in organizations. Without governance, there is no context within which the administrator can function. Despite their importance, however, boards are seldom understood, frequently misused, and often a source of frustration both for those who serve on them and for those who seek to manage the organization they purport to govern. This chapter seeks to outline the function of governance in the organization and to suggest a variety of ways in which the board's work can be more fruitful.

The information in this chapter should be of use to the long-term care administrator in at least two ways: it should foster better working relationships between the administrator and the governing board, and it should enable the administrator to serve as an effective member of other governing boards in the community.

JUST WHAT IS GOVERNANCE?

Governance is the process that links an organization to whatever higher power or authority has the right to decide whether the organization will exist and what it will do. As such, governance is inherently representational—governing bodies act on behalf of some collective of people. Governance includes three key functions:

- Deciding the right thing for the organization to do (usually embodied in statements of purpose, mission and vision, and in strategic plans).

29

- Assuring appropriate management of the organization (usually seen as appointing and overseeing the organization's chief executive and then delegating management of the organization to that person).
- Evaluating the effectiveness of the organization in serving the purpose that the governing body has identified for it.

Governance is probably best understood in the case of a small shop, owned by a single person. That owner develops goals for the shop, holds a sense of what effects the shop will have in the world, decides what the shop will do or sell, monitors the effectiveness of the shop against the goals that he/ she has set for it, and receives the profit—or covers the losses—generated by the shop. It is clear that the owner is accountable for these functions, though they may be performed in a larger context of the many other functions—management, production, client development, accounting, etc.—that the owner must perform to keep the shop successful. In any event, the owner governs the shop.

That same relationship holds for larger for-profit businesses as well: the owners (whether they be a few individuals or other firms, or thousands of stockholders) govern the business, generally through a board of directors that is elected or appointed by the owners, and which is accountable to those owners for the outcomes achieved by the company.

A nonprofit organization is governed on the same principle—a board of directors (or trustees or governors or other designation) governs the organization and is accountable to the owners for the organization's outcomes. However, among the distinctions between for-profit and not-for-profit governance are two that are central to understanding how nonprofit boards function. One of these is the identification of the owners (or stakeholders) of the organization, and the other is the determination of the outcomes to be achieved. In both cases, the work of the for-profit board is made a great deal easier by the situation at hand. First, the owners of a for-profit business are easily identified—they are those people who own legally defined shares in the company, usually identified in lists of stockholders. In contrast, the "owners" of a nonprofit organization are those who have a stake in its outcomes—the clients, employees, donors, and other interested parties. Indeed, one of the steps that nonprofit boards should take is to identify the various stakeholders to whom they might be accountable, and establish a priority among those stakeholders.

The second fundamental distinction between for-profit and nonprofit boards is in the determination of the purpose of the organization. For-profit boards contend with no ambiguity on this point—they exist to develop a profit that is then shared among the owners. Nonprofit organizations, though, do not have such an easily identified purpose. Instead, the boards of nonprofit organizations must identify what the organization's purpose is—why it exists, and what it will seek to achieve. Often that purpose is identified in the non-profit's articles of incorporation or in some other document developed at the time the organization is founded. As will be noted later, there is a very real distinction between the purpose of an organization (*why* it exists) and its mission (*what* it intends to do to achieve that purpose).

Particularly in long-term care, discussions of governance must include government agencies and institutions as well as for-profit and nonprofit organizations. The governance of government agencies serves the same functions as the governance of nonprofit organizations, but is often less easily identified. Many government agencies and institutions are governed by boards of commissioners at the local (county, municipality, special district) level, sometimes with the assistance of advisory boards made up of citizens of the geographic area that is served by the organization. Other government institutions—particularly those that are large organizations serving a national constituency, such as the U.S. Veterans' Administration Health System or national health systems in other countries—are really governed by the legislative bodies of those countries. In those cases, study of the governance of the organization really amounts to study of national health policy issues.

ISSUES IN GOVERNANCE: THE PIT OF DESPAIR

The September 6, 1999 issue of *New Yorker* magazine carried a cartoon by Kim Warp that is all too characteristic of the process followed by many governing boards of long-term care organizations. The cartoon shows eight people seated around a large board table in a palatial room. Two baskets of laundry rest on the table, and a person standing at the head of the table says, "And I'm sure no one will mind if we fold a few clothes while we talk."

Most governing boards spend a good deal of their time "folding clothes," or otherwise engaged in activity that distracts them from the central functions of their role in governing the organization. In his 1990 book entitled *Boards that Make a Difference,* John Carver, one of today's best thinkers about boards, says:

> Board members arrive at the table with dreams. They have vision and values. Yet, by and large, board members do not spend their time exploring, debating, and defining those dreams. Instead, they expend their energy on a host of demonstrably less important, even trivial, items. Instead of impassioned discussion about the change to be produced in their world, board members are ordinarily found passively listening to staff reports. Most of what the majority of boards do either does not need to be done or is a waste of time when done by the board.

In a 1996 piece *(Governance, Unit 11)* written for the ISP Executive Study Program in Health Care Administration at the University of Minnesota, Carver identifies a number of "governance flaws," including "time on the trivial" (where major issues are not addressed because the board spends its time on issues of little import to the organization), "short term bias" (where the principal criteria for items entering the board's agenda is their immediacy), and "reactive stance" (where the board creates little of value to the organization and merely reviews, rehashes or re-does work that others have already completed).

Why is it that boards are so easily sidetracked from the work of governing the long-term care organization? Some of the reasons may be the following:

- BOARD MEMBERS COME FROM SUCCESS IN MANAGEMENT. It is almost always the case that success in managing a business, a professional practice, community volunteer efforts, or ones' own wealth is what gets one noticed as a candidate for service on a governing board. Difficulties arise, however, because it is governance rather than management that must occupy the board.
- GOVERNANCE IS NOT UNDERSTOOD. As noted, board members come to the board from some success in managing something. While the board is there to govern, rather than manage, it is seldom clear to board members just what governance is or how it differs from management.
- THEY DON'T FEEL ACCOUNTABLE FOR GOVERNANCE. In most cases, boards that engage in management rather than governance get by—no one asks why the organization is not better governed because they do not understand what that would mean.
- THEY DON'T KNOW TO WHOM THEY ARE ACCOUNTABLE. In many organizations, the people to whom the board is accountable—that is, the organization's stakeholders—are not sufficiently well identified as to leverage their accountability. And, most of those stakeholders not only do not see themselves as being able to enforce accountability, but they do not know the individuals that serve that supposed accountability as board members.
- THEY ARE BUSY MANAGING. Because most board members come from success in management and because they do not understand what governance is, most boards devolve to a higher order management function.
- THEY ARE BUSY HELPING. Carver says that "the board is not there to help," but instead to represent the interests of stakeholders in governing the organization. However, many boards function as helpers to the CEO and many board members feel they have fulfilled their accountability by being helpful to the CEO or the organization.

- THEY ABDICATE TO PROFESSIONAL STAFF. In fields such as long-term care that are based on expertise, it is often difficult for boards to see that they do not need to understand the technical nature of the organization's business in order to be good governing board members. In such cases, board members sometimes allow the organization's professional staff to make governance decisions which are then ratified with little discussion by the board.
- THEY DON'T TAKE RESPONSIBILITY FOR THEIR OWN DEVELOPMENT. As will be discussed later in this chapter, effective boards take responsibility for the continual improvement of their ability to govern the organization.
- THEY HAVE NOT LEARNED TO LEARN TOGETHER. Learning—in the classical sense of "organizational learning" espoused by Peter Senge—is essential for effective governance by a board. Those that are most effective work at learning together.
- THEY ARE FOCUSED ON THE PRESENT. As shall be shown, the present is the concern of management—the board's concern is the future of the organization. Boards that are focused exclusively on the organization's present—its current financial and strategic performance—cannot possibly govern the organization effectively.
- THEY WON'T DEAL WITH CONFLICT. Each board member brings a unique set of wisdom and judgment—to say nothing of knowledge and experience—to the board table. Effective boards make use of the breadth and depth of this wisdom and judgment by generating and effectively managing conflict among the various perspectives represented among the board members. If there is no conflict among board members, there might just as well be only one board member.

TOWARD A MODEL OF GOVERNANCE: A LADDER OUT OF THE PIT

What seems to be missing in the way most boards approach governance is a fundamental understanding of a technology of governance. We are accustomed to the technology of management and the many schools, journal articles and books that it engenders. By contrast, the technology of governance seems almost a highly classified secret. Without a technology of *governance,* a board has no way to describe what it does, no way to assess its effectiveness, and no way to improve its functioning.

Without a vocabulary and conceptual framework that relate to *governing,* the board will use (by default) the concepts and vocabulary of management, among other things, that is the experience base of most board members. When this happens, things get worse while they seem to be getting better.

One place to start in building a technology of governance is with the fiduciary responsibilities generally attributed to boards. These responsibilities are usually identified as three duties:

The duty of care	requires board members to perform their duties with the reasonable care, diligence, and skill that an ordinarily prudent person would use in similar circumstances.
The duty of loyalty	requires board members to exercise their powers in the interest of the organization, not in their own interest or in the interest of another entity or person.
The duty of mission	requires board members to work to achieve the mission of the organization as defined by the board and limited by the purpose outlined in the bylaws or articles of incorporation.

Another point of departure for a technology of governance is the list of management functions identified by Henri Fayol in the late nineteenth century. These functions–plan, organize, direct, control and evaluate–have come to characterize many management textbooks and curricula in schools of management. In essence, they identify the activities that must be accomplished if an organization is to succeed; they are what our shopmaster must do to make the business succeed. They can also be used to make useful distinctions between management and governance and, thereby, to build a clearer model of what governance is and is not.

This argument begins with a distinction in the first of Fayol's functions, planning. It asserts that there are really two kinds of planning, one describes the *right way* something is to be accomplished, and the other describes the *right thing* to do. This first distinction is diagrammed below:

Decide the right thing to do ⇐ **Plan** ⇒ Decide the right way

Once the right thing to do is determined, and the right way to do it is identified, then the organization goes about organizing, directing and controlling. When it comes time to evaluate the organization's work, another distinction is presented, corresponding to the two forms of planning previously identified. One form of evaluation relates to whether the organization did things the right way and focuses on the outputs and efficiency of the organization. The other–far more difficult–form of evaluation is concerned with whether the organization did the right thing and focuses on its outcomes and its effectiveness. This distinction can be diagrammed as below:

Effectiveness, outcomes ⇐ **Evaluate** ⇒ Efficiency, output

Incorporating these distinctions into Fayol's list yields the following:

Decide the right thing to do ⇐ **Plan** ⇒ Decide the right way

Organize

Direct

Control

Effectiveness, outcomes ⇐ **Evaluate** ⇒ Efficiency, output

The revised list can then be used to identify the three key functions of governance in an organization. They are to identify the right thing for the organization to do, to assure good management, and to assess the effectiveness of the organization. These are described more fully in the following paragraphs.

DECIDING THE RIGHT THING

Boards identify the right thing for the organization to do when they specify its purpose, mission, and strategies. The model shown on page 37 illustrates the board's role in planning. It shows the organization's mission arising from two sources: the organization's purpose and an understanding of current realities. The organization's *purpose* is the answer to the question, "Why does this organization exist?" For our shopkeeper friend, and for companies organized to generate a profit, the answer is straightforward—the purpose is to make money. For nonprofit organizations, however, the answer is more complex and, unfortunately, often obscure or ignored. For those organizations, the purpose is often included in the articles of incorporation or other founding documents. For most nonprofit, long-term care organizations, the purpose usually has something to do with enhancing the lives of people with disabilities or chronic health conditions.

Understanding the purpose of the organization is absolutely critical to effective governance. Boards that do not understand and focus on the organization's purpose cannot hope to achieve the ends for which the organization exists. They usually focus instead on what the organization produces, rather than on what it achieves. The boards of most for-profit organizations do not have difficulty in this area because they have a more immediate sense of their organization's purpose and far more opportunities to measure and discuss it. In contrast, it is not uncommon to find boards of nonprofit organizations that are not aware of the purpose they serve. One indicator of such a situation is a mission statement that is explicit about *what* the organization does, but silent as to *why* it does that. A mission statement that says something like "this organization exists to provide the best care possible to elderly residents of our community," begs the question of "why?" Why does the organization provide such care? Is it to make money? To keep old folks out of their homes? To provide employment for nurses? To enhance the lives of residents? To strengthen the community's health care system?

Understanding the purpose of the organization is also essential to effective strategic planning. As Figure 3.1 shows, the purpose of the organization is the lens through which the board looks to understand the current realities that the organization must address. In organizations where purpose is not understood, the mission becomes the lens through which the board looks at current realities. When that happens, strategic planning focuses on continuous improvement of existing services rather than developing new services. Such an organization risks becoming increasingly proficient at something that is increasingly irrelevant.

In contrast, when boards understand the organization's purpose and use that purpose to view changing realities, they can add or delete services in response to those realities. In the context of modern long-term care, failure to understand purpose means that the organization is destined to forever be what it is today—a nursing home, for example—and that it cannot cease being a nursing home in order to become something else of more value to the community such as a provider of a broad range of senior housing options or a rehabilitation provider.

This is a phenomenon long recognized by people who write about planning in organizations such as Peter Drucker ("The Theory of the Business," *Harvard Business Review,* September–October 1994) and Arie deGeus (*The Living Company,* Harvard Business School Press, 1997). These writers detail the successful strategy transformations in organizations that are clear about their purpose. In one case, related by deGeus, a Swedish company succeeds over eight centuries by moving into and out of radically different businesses. It was able to make those transitions because it has been very clear about why it exists.

Standing at the point of view of the organization's purpose, the board must comprehend the current realities facing the organization—the needs and resources of the community to be served, competing organizations, reimbursement, and other financial factors, etc.—and the changes that are likely to occur in those realities over time. This is not something that occurs quickly or in an afternoon at the annual board retreat. Rather, it is the continuing work of the board and ought to occupy something like 75 percent of its time. Understanding the current realities allows the board to identify what the organization will do to achieve its purpose over time.

From their understanding of both the purpose of the organization and its current realities, the board frames a mission statement that identifies the end in view for the organization and specifies both why the organization exists

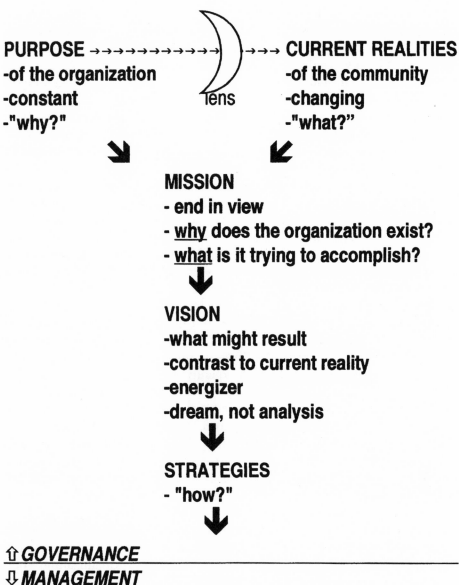

Figure 3.1. Model of the board's role in planning.

and what it intends to do. Because the purpose of the organization does not change, and the current realities change continually, the mission should change at some pace between the two–probably every three to five years– and ought to be reviewed at least annually.

Out of the mission statement flows a vision of how the world would be different if the organization succeeded in achieving its mission. That vision is stated in very concrete terms and describes an ideal state to which the organization will direct its energies. When contrasted with the current realities, the vision not only energizes the organization, but also provides the direction necessary to make it successful in the future. For example, if the board of a nursing home understands its purpose is to enhance the health of people in the community it serves, and if it sees the realities facing that community as changing from encouraging very long-term skilled nursing care to seeking more diversity in senior housing and more concerted efforts at rehabilitation, it will likely form a vision that includes (in part) older people living in a variety of situations, with many opportunities for access to a broad array of support services. That vision, effectively communicated throughout the organization, will lead it to make changes that move it toward the ideal state it describes.

From the contrast between the vision and the current realities, the board develops a handful of strategies that will focus the organization over the next year or two. Those strategies identify how the organization will pursue its mission and usually relate to both the quality of present operations and the evolution of new lines of business. The document generated by the board should be a "good enough" plan–one that is clear in its direction to the organization, but which is not so lengthy as to resist the need for it to change as time requires. A number of authors have written of the need for flexibility in planning (see, for example, the article by Eisenhardt and Brown on "Patching: Restitching Business Portfolios in Dynamic Markets," in *The Harvard Business Review* May–June 1999). At most, the planning document developed by the board should be a couple of pages in length.

That document is then handed off to management who develops the budgets, goals and objectives, staffing plans, marketing plans, etc. that are needed to translate the board's work into effective strategy for the organization. These more detailed plans are reviewed by the board to test their applicability to the more basic purpose, mission, vision, and strategies they have developed.

ASSURING GOOD MANAGEMENT

The board's second function is to make sure that the organization is well managed. For effective boards, that means that they hire a capable chief executive officer, provide that person with the resources and incentives necessary to superior performance, monitor that performance, and make changes as necessary. While that appears to be a straightforward proposition, it is the area in which many boards have a great deal of difficulty. As noted above, most board members come from some experience of their own in managing something. Especially in those cases where governance is not understood, and the board is not effectively engaged in planning on a continuing basis, that predisposition to management leads them to meddle in the management of the organization. While there are rare situations where the board must take on the responsibilities of management (for example, when the CEO position is temporarily vacant), as a general rule, boards should be so busy governing that they do not have the time to manage.

ASSESSING EFFECTIVENESS

The third role of the board is to assess the performance of the organization against the mission and purpose that has been identified. As noted earlier, this assessment focuses on the organization's outcomes, rather than its outputs. This is another critical distinction in understanding governance and one that is particularly important in long-term care. An organization's outputs are those things it produces—for a long-term care facility, outputs could be days of care, meals served, medications administered, people admitted, people discharged, etc. Its outcomes are the effects of those outputs on the purpose and mission for which the organization exists. In the case of a for-profit organization, the question is the amount of profit that is generated by the outputs. For a nonprofit organization, the question is the degree to which the organization's purpose (for example, to enhance the lives of elderly people in the community) and mission (to enhance the lives of elderly people by providing a full range of residential and service options) are achieved.

The board of that nonprofit organization faces a particularly vexing issue in assessing the organization's effectiveness. That issue is the dearth of data available on the organization's effects on its purpose and mission. In a nonprofit organization, there is no single, easily measured index—comparable to profit—that will tell the board how successful the organization is. Instead, the board of such an organization must rely on a variety of information that more or less describes the effects of the organization. Rather than being able to extract a single measure of progress, as is the case in the for-profit, the nonprofit board must base its assessment on judgment and wisdom.

Note that long-term care organizations are reimbursed on the basis of the output they generate, rather than for their outcomes; certifying days of care provided within certain standards, for example, is sufficient to generate payment. Organizational outcomes are not typically part of the formula. As a result, it is possible for long-term care organizations to succeed on the basis of their outputs, without much attention being paid to outcomes. Again, boards of for-profit organizations have an advantage here because the outcomes they seek are more easily measured. On the nonprofit side, if the board does not attend to outcomes, no one will, at least not until the market responds.

IMPLICATIONS OF THE MODEL

This model of governance gives rise to a number of implications which are identified in the paragraphs that follow.

1. **Board members are accountable to owners.** A board member's accountability is first and foremost to the owners of the organization. As noted earlier, in a for-profit organization it is easy to identify the owners because they hold the company's stock. In a nonprofit, the "owners" are those people and other organizations who have a stake in the outcomes generated by the organization. Clearly that encompasses the customers of the organization–or the patients or residents of a long-term care facility. But it also includes the families of those residents, the organizations from which they are referred, the physicians who provide some of their care, the staff of the facility, people who donate to the organization, the community at large, and potentially many others.

    It is especially incumbent on board members to put the interests of the organization they govern before their own interests. This need is the basis for conflict of interest policies on boards, an example of which appears, on the following pages. As in the example, such policies usually require board members to identify potential conflicts that might arise between the organization's interests and their own–for example, these might include owning a business from which the organization buys supplies, marriage to an employee of the organization, or ownership of land immediately adjacent to one of the organization's facilities. When an issue comes before the board that provokes a conflict of interest, affected board members are generally expected to exclude themselves from the portion of the board's discussion that deals with that topic.

    Note that the primary accountability of board members is to the owners of the organization, not to the organization itself. It is that accountability that allows (in fact, requires) board members to change an organization's mission or even to take the organization out of business when it no longer serves the interests of the owners.

2. **Focus on purpose, then on mission.** Board members must focus on the purpose of the organization first and then on its mission. This primacy of purpose keeps the board's attention on the outcomes that are generated, rather than merely on the outputs.

3. **Assure good management.** Because board members come from a background in management and because governance is not widely understood, many boards tend to manage, rather than govern. Effective boards find ways to assure that good management is in place, and spend the bulk of their efforts in governance.

4. **The board is not there as "volunteers" to help.** Long-term care organizations provide many opportunities for productive volunteer work, and many board members engage in that work from time to time. However, it is essential that board members recognize that such volunteer work requires them to wear two hats: one as a board member, and one as a volunteer. In some ways these two roles conflict with each other. While volunteers are there to help the organization, the board is not there to help—instead, it is there to represent the interests of the owners in seeing to it that the organization fulfills its purpose. Further, many boards get caught up in doing good things that help the organization, and mentally substitute those good things for the real work of governance. It seems rational to assert that board members should only think about volunteer service in the long-term care organization after they are certain that they have met their responsibilities in governance.

5. **Ask "so what?" and "what if?"** These are the two critical questions for board members to ask over and over again. The first—so what?—is the question that leads the board away from a discussion of output and toward a discussion of outcomes. It is the question that focuses the board's attention on the difference that the organization is (or is not) making in the world. When told, for instance, that the organization's census is up 20 percent from the same period last year, the board should ask "So what? Does this increase lead to higher or lower profits in for-profit organizations?" or "How does this increase affect our ability to achieve our purpose and mission (in nonprofits)?" When told that revenues are up 12 percent from the previous month, the board must ask "So what?" and when told that the per-day cost of service is down 8 percent, from last year, the board must also ask "So what—what does this increase in efficiency mean for the level of our effectiveness?"

The "what if?" questions are the questions that the board asks in the continuing planning process in which it must engage. This notion comes from the work of Arie deGues, who was vice president of planning for Royal Dutch Shell on the occasion of that company's 100th anniversary. In celebration of that event, Shell surveyed the few other companies throughout the world that had succeeded over 100 years. The results are reported in a wonderful little book entitled *The Living Company*. Among other things, the study found that these companies did not say "this is where we plan to be in 25 years." Instead, they continually asked "What will we do if this happens" and "How will we respond if that happens?" In this fashion, deGues says, they created a "memory of the future"–that is, when one of the events that they had asked about actually occurred, they knew how to respond because they had worked through that contingency earlier.

6. **Be accountable for the future.** Many boards do not have time enough to devote to the future because they are so pre-occupied in monitoring the present operation of the organization; that operation is the responsibility of the chief executive officer and the rest of the management team. Their attention to the company's present operations should free the board to focus on the future (and to ask the "what if?" questions identified above). Boards that must spend the majority of their time monitoring the organization's present operations must ask themselves if the CEO is doing his/her job, and/or whether they really understand their role in governing the organization.

7. **Board-to-board communication.** Especially in nonprofit organizations, boards must be aware of other organizations with similar purposes which serve largely the same set of owners. Since both organizations use the community's resources, board-to-board communication might explore ways in which the two organizations can collaborate in addressing community interests. Clearly, we live in an era of rather intense competition among providers of health–services; collaboration is not always possible and may not be desirable. However, boards should regard it as part of their obligation to the owners (that is, the broader community) to at least understand where opportunities for collaboration might exist, and to include such possibilities in their "what if" considerations.

8. **Board development.** Developing the board's ability to govern the organization is a responsibility that belongs to the board. Yet, in almost all boards, the responsibility (if it is pursued at all) falls to the CEO. Effective boards pursue this responsibility with intention, often creating a board development committee to assist the board. Such a committee might fulfill the following responsibilities:

Develop governance policies:
  On the role of the board
  On the board's relationship to other segments of the organization

Conduct annual board self-assessment:
  Assess performance and satisfaction
  Use as a basis for board education, changes, nominations
  Make longitudinal comparisons

Organize board education:
  Develop annual curriculum for the board that includes:
    Education components of board meetings
    Expectation of attendance at external events
    Focus on key issues relevant to the governance of the organization

Incorporate new member orientation:
  Introduction to the organization and its key issues
  Provide mentors for new members

Oversee board structure and process:
  Agenda format
  Committee and task force structure
  Quality and quantity of information sent to board

Nominations:
  Basic criteria derived from board expectations (see Figure 3.4)
  Strive for diversity of perspectives on the board

9. **Understand the role of the board.** As has been repeatedly noted in this chapter, most board members are unaware of their responsibilities as board members, and boards seldom take the time to explore that topic in any meaningful way. As a consequence, each board member comes to the board with a different view of what their responsibilities are, not knowing that the person across from them holds an entirely different view of what he/she should be doing. One approach to this issue is for the board to negotiate and then adopt a set of board expectations that identify what the board does and how it goes about its work. A sample draft of board expectations is include in Figure 3.4.

10. **Intentionality.** Effective boards are intentional in what they do–they make decisions on issues they hold to be important, are not distracted by lower priority issues, are clear about their roles, pursue information that is appropriate to their work, take conflict of interest seriously, develop and respond to agendas with meaning, etc. At the same time, many boards are victim to circumstances. For the reasons explored in this chapter, they do not understand what they are to do, become lost

in the minutiae of operations, fail to develop an orientation to the future, and devolve into management. When asked, members of these boards might complain about the time that is wasted at board meetings, about the lack of progress made at board meetings, and about how ineffective they feel. In contrast to the way they address issues in other areas of their lives, they do not take active steps to address these issues. Instead, they go along with the dysfunction because they assume that is the only way for a board to behave. It will not come as a surprise to the reader that boards do not have to be victims of the past, and that they can undertake improvements in their functioning if they understand what it is they are expected to do.

11. **Resource development.** It is not enough for the board to determine the future of the organization. It must also develop the resources necessary to achieve that future, lest its vision be merely a cloud passing over the horizon. In some cases, developing those resources is not problematic, either because the volume of required resources is small, or because the organization's operations or the philanthropy available to it are sufficient to generate the needed resources. In many more cases, however, the board must not only plan for the acquisition of those resources, but also participate in their development. That may mean making a meaningful contribution to the annual fund or the capital campaign, asking others in leadership positions in the community to contribute, overseeing a large scale fund-raising effort, or encouraging the purchase of bonds or stock.

12. **Conflict management.** Conflict management is one of the core competencies of effective boards. Because each board member brings a unique set of perspectives and experience to the board meeting, the only way for the board to benefit from that disparate wisdom is for the various points of view represented by board members to be put into conflict. If that does not happen—and it seldom does—then the board is dominated by the one or two strongest members, and loses the intelligence that would come from understanding the other points of view and how those might be combined with others.

The essence of effective conflict management for boards is the form of conversation that takes place at board and committee meetings. Peter Senge has discussed "generative conversation" as that which simultaneously maximizes both inquiry into the views of others and advocacy of one's own beliefs. This sort of conversation is discussed in detail in William Isaacs book, *Dialogue and the Art of Thinking Together* (Currency, 1999). But generative conversation does not just happen—it requires attention and practice, the sort of learning that boards seldom allow themselves the opportunity to undertake.

13. **Governance is learning.** Learning is also a core competency of effective governance; boards that cannot learn together simply cannot engage in the central governance functions of planning and evaluation. The key here is being able to learn *together;* it does little good for one or two members of a board to acquire new knowledge if their fellow board members remain fixed on old ideas Thus, the board should be a learning organization as described by Peter Senge. Years ago, Chris Argyris coined the term "Skilled Incompetence" (*Harvard Business Review*, September 1986) to describe the ways in which people in organizations become locked into invalid assumptions because they refuse to learn new alternatives. That same phenomenon afflicts many boards.

Fred Kofman and Peter Senge ("Communities of Commitment: the Heart of Learning Organizations" from an earlier paper in *Organizational Dynamics*, Autumn, 1993) describe the culture of an effective learning organization that avoids skilled incompetence. Such a culture would do much to advance the ability of a board to learn and to govern. Kofman and Senge describe the culture as based on:

> **Love:** the acceptance of others as legitimate beings, despite their different points of view.
>
> **Humility:** the recognition that any model is a simplification that can be improved.
>
> **Wonder:** seeing changes as opportunities to grow, not as breakdowns.
>
> **Empathy:** the ability to enter into coherent relationships with others.
>
> **Compassion:** accepting that other's behaviors are as valid as our own, despite their arising in a different point of view or belief system.

FIGURE 3.2
CONFLICT OF INTEREST POLICY

XYZ LONG-TERM CARE ORGANIZATION

Board of Directors

Policy Re: Board Members' Conflict of Interest

It is the policy of the board of directors that its members individually and collectively avoid any and all potential conflicts of interest. It is further the policy of the board to avoid even the perception of conflict of interest.

It is the intent of the governing board that this policy shall be implemented and enforced so as to prevent the judgment of a board member from being influenced by an economic or business relationship in which that board member is personally involved.

To accomplish and fulfill this policy, all board members will annually identify all known potential conflicts of interest in which they may be involved. In addition, during delibera-tion or discussion at any board, committee or task force meeting, an individual member will identify a potential conflict of interest and, having so disclosed the potential conflict of interest, not participate in discussion of that issue or in voting on it.

If a member of the board believes that there may be a potential conflict of interest on the part of another member of the board who has not disclosed such potential conflict of interest, he/she is obliged to request review of that potential conflict of interest. The board member who may have a potential conflict of interest can voluntarily refrain from partic-ipation, discussion, and voting. If he/she does not voluntarily remove him/herself from par-ticipation because, in his/her judgment he/she does not have a potential conflict of interest, the organization's legal counsel will provide recommendation on the appropriateness of that board member's continued participation concerning that issue.

Adopted by the board on _____

Board Chair
_____

FIGURE 3.3
CONFLICT OF INTEREST STATEMENT

XYZ LONG-TERM CARE ORGANIZATION

Conflict of Interest Statement

I have read and understand the board's conflict of interest policy. In accordance with that policy, I will (1) disclose any potential conflict of interest relating to the subject matter of a meeting of the board of directors or a committee or task force thereof, (2) withdraw from any such meeting and abstain from voting, and (3) not use my personal influence on the subject matter with my fellow directors.

Further, in accordance with that policy, I am disclosing the following affiliations, director-ships, and other interests which I or members of my immediate family have which I believe could reasonably be anticipated to cause a conflict of interest.

Signature:_____

Date: _____

FIGURE 3.4
STATEMENT OF EXPECTATIONS OF BOARD MEMBERS

EXPECTATIONS OF XYZ BOARD MEMBERS

The XYZ board serves to represent the interests of XYZ stakeholders in the development of the organization and the pursuit of its mission. In that capacity, the board develops the organization's mission and vision, identifies strategies, and evaluates outcomes achieved. The board monitors the strategic and financial performance of the organization, the performance of the CEO, and its own performance as a governing body, to know when and how to make changes.

While the work required of board members will vary both across members and across time, the following expectations are generally held of all board members:

1. The interests of XYZ and its stakeholders are foremost.

2. Participation of board members is key to their contribution—

   A. Board members need to be present and involved in meetings of the board and the committees on which they serve.

   B. Board and committee members need to be actively engaged in discussing issues, sharing perspectives, and raising questions that are essential to good decision-making.

   C. Effective participation derives from continually learning about XYZ and the environment in which it exists. This learning includes those formal opportunities afforded by the board and XYZ, as well as informal opportunities that occur in the course of one's activities.

   D. As a general guideline, members should expect to spend approximately 6 to 8 hours per month in their work on the board and its committees.

3. The XYZ Board is a group of peers—no one member has more standing or power than others, and no individual member has authority in the organization. It is only as a collective that the board has power.

4. Respect for the opinions of each other, and for those with whom the board interacts, is a hallmark of the board's work. Board members seek clarity in presenting their views, and represent a sense of stewardship in all that they do.

5. Board members engage in continual self-assessment of their performance on the board. As needs arise, they seek education and skills necessary to their performance. As a collective, the board conducts an annual self-assessment, and develops changes in its composition, structure and function as needed.

(Continued on next page)

Figure 3.4—*Continued*

6. The board provides opportunities for the education of its members, both as part of the board meetings and retreats, and through access to educational events in other settings. Board members actively engage in this education as part of their responsibility to the board.

7 Board members interact with employees of XYZ—including the top management staff—only through the CEO.

8. The board is responsible for developing the assets needed by the organization to achieve its mission. That responsibility includes supporting the development process, linking the organization to the community as effectively as possible, participating in fund-raising events, and making personal contributions to XYZ.

9. Most of the work of the board is in areas of subjective judgment, where there is seldom enough hard information to make the decisions that are necessary. Board members who are most successful in these decisions are those who are aware of the values they hold, willing to engage in other discussion of those values, and respectful of those values held by others that may differ from their own.

10. The board is composed of individuals with diverse perspectives and experience. The board benefits from the contrasts that this diversity engenders, and seeks to improve the decisions it makes and the actions it takes by understanding the conflicts and resolving the disputes that arise in the discussion of issues and plans. However, while it seeks to engage in productive dispute resolution and decision making, when the board comes to consensus, members are expected to support the resulting decision, no matter what their position was originally in the discussion.

GOVERNING CHAOS: A TWIST ON THE MODEL

Much has been written recently about chaos and complex adaptive systems. In particular, the report of the Institute of Medicine—*Crossing the Quality Chasm: A New Health System for the 21st-Century*—views health care organizations as complex adaptive systems and uses that concept to develop new models of care. The book argues that:

Health care is *complex* because of the great number of interconnections within and among small care systems:

and

Health care systems are *adaptive* because, unlike mechanical systems, they are omposed of individuals–patients and clinicians who have the capacity to learn and change as a result of experience. Their actions in delivering health care are not always predictable, and tend to change both their local and larger environments.

In her book. *Leadership and the New Science: Learning about Organization from an Orderly Universe* (Berrett-Koehler, 1992), Margaret Wheatley notes the differences between the old model of organizations as machines and the new view of complex adaptive systems, or "quantum" or "organic" organizations. The machine model seeks control, predictability, and efficiency, and is best understood as a closed system. In contrast, a quantum organization is organic, responsive to the environment that surrounds it, and creative. It is best viewed as an open system.

Machine systems operate at the edge of equilibrium, always seeking to minimize disturbances, change, and variations. Organic systems operate on the edge of chaos, far from equilibrium, and not quite chaos. These distinctions are important for understanding what it means to lead—or govern—each type of organization. In mechanistic organizations, leadership is limited to a few operatives in a command and control hierarchy. In contrast, quantum organizations seek to promote the richest possible environment in which self-organizing can occur. The central difference is that in mechanistic organizations, there is assumed to be someone at the top of the pyramid who knows what should be done. In a quantum organization, the metaphor is that of a sphere rather than a pyramid, and the task of leadership is not to tell others what to do, but to facilitate their discovery of what to do.

Wheatley offers the following principles of complexity science as central to the understanding of how quantum organizations succeed:

1. View your system through the lens of complexity—stop waiting for the world to get less complex, it won't. (An illustration of this point is found in the sign that adorned the desk of 3M's manager of orthopedic products: "It's orthopedic surgery, it's *supposed* to be complicated.")
2. Build a good-enough vision—do not spend endless hours crafting a 350 page plan that will be obsolete two months before it is distributed.
3. When life is far from certain, lead from the edge of chaos, not equilibrium.
4. Uncover and work with paradox and tension.
5. Pursue multiple actions at the fringes, letting direction arise.
6. Listen to the shadow system—the gossip in the halls, the word on the street.
7. Adapt by "patching."
8. Mix cooperation and competition—it's not one or the other.

If this is the description of the modern long-term care organization, what should such an organization's governance look like? It seems likely that the board of such an organization has several functions, in addition to those outlined at the outset of this chapter. They are:

1. Establishing context: the self-organizing that characterizes quantum organizations requires a clear identity, a context for taking action. Boards seeking to establish context for their organizations will do the following:

   a. Clarify a shared vision: identify purpose and mission, strategies, short and long-term goals.

   b. Enrich the culture: serve as living examples of the organization's culture—board members' presence in the organization (awards dinners, fund-raisers, celebrations, etc.) is important, their pronouncements carry almost the same weight as their presence.

   c. Develop alignment: bring the organization together around a shared purpose, explicit strategy, value principles. The breadth of perspective that the board brings to the organization is critical in this regard. However, if the board itself has not aligned its own perspectives and interests, it will be difficult for it to govern.

   d. Promote understanding: from the external, community perspective that the board represents, interpret information and add meaning to what occurs in the organization.

2. Disturbing the system: living systems are most vital/creative when they are experiencing disturbance. Because the board brings into the organization a unique set of perspectives, it can help the organization avoid the stultifying effects of untested assumptions. In his article on "The Theory of the Business" (*Harvard Business Review,* September–October 1994), Peter Drucker notes that failing to test the assumptions on which a business is based is a major cause of failure. Board actions might include the following:

   a. Create compelling goals: goals that are audacious, inspiring, and unifying (see Jim Collins "Turning Goals into Results: The Power of Catalytic Mechanisms," *Harvard Business Review,* July–August 1999).

   b. Ensure the flow of information throughout the organization: in particular provide "so what" feedback and attend to what is being ignored or distorted in the organization.

   c. Promote diversity of opinion: demonstrate that the board values different viewpoints and that it sees conflict as opportunity.

   d. Hold anxiety: change is difficult for most people. A key role of the board is to continue to function effectively while holding the same anxieties that everyone else in the organization feels. Calm and positive responses to change by the board demonstrate that this is both possible and expected.

3. Cultivating the organization: Self-organizing requires autonomy, clear identity and openness in the organization. Boards seeking to encourage

that environment in their organization can model it through the following:

a. Promote ownership: encourage people in the organization to be self-accountable for success, communicate and model the importance of commitment, create conditions that empower the board and the executives.

b. Nurture relationships within the organization and with external entities: focus on the long-term health of these relationships. Some would argue that such relationships are the essence of the organization's success.

c. Encourage learning in the organization: recognize the value of innovation, support and fund learning, tolerate risk and not knowing, and model learning in the board's experience.

d. Nourish the human spirit: believe that people will self-organize for success and provide meaning to what people in the organization do.

QUASI GOVERNANCE–THE ROLE OF THE
LOCAL ADVISORY BOARD

In large, centrally-governed, multi-site organizations, the local advisory board can be a central link between the organization and the community, and the critical link between the organization and community leaders. It serves to translate the community's current realities (needs, resources, opportunities, threats) into the organization's planning, and to translate the organization's current realities–especially its needs for support and resources–into positive responses on the part of the community.

The advisory board usually has no formal power relative to the governance of the organization–that power belongs to the central governing board. However, given the breadth of their responsibilities, it is unreasonable to expect the central governing board to effectively plan for and develop the local organization as an entity of importance to both the corporation and the local community. In essence, the advisory board can fulfill a *quasi-governance* role by advocating for the community in planning for the local organization, and then advocating for the local organization in planning for the larger corporation.

The advisory board is able to assert this role because of the influence it holds. That influence drives from (a) the personal power of its members in the community, (b) their expertise in both the evolution of the local organization and the interests of the community, and (c) their ability to develop resources–especially financial support and good will–for the local organization.

In particular, the advisory board is indispensable to the local organization if it plans to do significant fund-raising and/or a capital campaign. In a large organization, the central governing board of the corporation is simply not in a position to present a request to the community from an informed governance-level perspective on the local organization. But the only way in which the advisory board can achieve that position is to combine its influence in the community with a thorough knowledge–and "ownership"–of the local organization's plans. Their ability to develop the needed level of credibility depends on their involvement in–and some level of their accountability for–the local organization's planning.

The local advisory board should present a useful conflict between the interests of the local community and the strategic interests of the corporation. In this context, the advisory board should be one of the central places in which these two sets of interests are juxtaposed, discussed, and ultimately balanced. Managing this sort of conflict requires a good deal of skill in both the advisory board and management–skills in advocacy, listening, negotiation, and dialogue that do not come easily to many leaders.

Unfortunately, many advisory boards avoid these conflicts and function as *management* advisory boards–they hear reports on the local organization's present *and* developing programs, and offer counsel on operations. If they are to take on the more difficult, quasi-governance accountability described here, a significant shift in their role–and self image–is needed. That role requires that the advisory board minimize its involvement in the management issues of the *present,* and focus instead on the *future* of the local organization and the connection between that future and the community.

An organization interested in this approach to its local advisory boards may want to consider the following recommendations:

- Clearly identify the expectations that the board should hold of itself (possibly a modification of the draft set presented earlier).
- Enlist the board in developing 3-year goals for its work and in revising them annually; this is an opportunity for an annual board retreat that has real meaning for the advisory board and for the organization. That retreat might also be attended by senior management of the corporation and/or members of the corporate governing board.
- Identify two levels of criteria for recruiting advisory board members:
  1. Use board expectations as base–these define the culture of the board and the basic qualities to look for in board members.
  2. Identify board's needs for diversity of perspective, and develop criteria on basis of needed diversity (for example, in age, gender, ethnicity,

area of residence, profession, etc.). These will change from year to year depending on the composition of the board.

- Identify what information the board does and does not need: focus on governance information; avoid management reports; etc.
- Provide staff support for the board, preferably support that reports directly to the local CEO.
- Structure the board's agenda in three segments:
action items,
information,
education.
- Develop a limited number of board committees.
- Develop and implement an education curriculum for the board, focusing on the future of the local organization and the community it serves.

CONCLUSION

This chapter has taken the reader on a journey through the common difficulties of governing boards, a model of effective governance that seeks to avoid these difficulties, a number of suggestions for effective governance, a short discussion of what it means to govern a complex adaptive organization, and some thoughts on the role of the advisory board. Traveling this journey should better prepare the long-term care administrator to manage in the governance context established by a board, foster the growth of the organization's governing body, and serve in governing capacities in other organizations in the community.

Governance is often misunderstood and, as a result, limiting to an organization's future. As this chapter argues, though, the real function of governance is to extend the organization and to create its future. As such, real governance is a wonderful asset to the organization, those who work in it, its clients, and the community it serves.

REFERENCES

Argyis, C. (1986). Skilled incompetence. *The Harvard Business Review,* September.

Carver, J. (1990). *Boards that make a difference.* San Francisco, CA: Jossey-Bass.

Carver, J. (1996). Governance, Unit II written for the ISP Executive Study Program in Health Care Administration at the University of Minnesota.

Collins, J. (1999). Turning goals into results: The power of catalytic mechanisms. *Harvard Business Review,* July–August.

deGeus, A. (1997). *The living company.* Harvard Business School Press.

Drucker, P. (1994). The theory of the business. The *Harvard Business Review,* September–October.

Eisenhardt, K.M., & Brown, S. L. (1999). Patching: Restitching business portfolios in dynamic markets. *The Harvard Business Review,* May–June.

Fayol, H. (1916). *Industrial and general administration.* Paris: Dunod.

Institute of Medicine. (2001). *Crossing the quality chasm: A new health system for the 21st century.* Washington, DC: National Academy Press.

Kofman, F., & Senge, P. (1993). Communities of commitment: The heart of learning organizations, from an earlier paper in *Organizational Dynamics,* Autumn.

Warp, K. (1999). *New Yorker* cartoon, September 6.

Wheatley, M. (1992). *Leadership and the new science: Learning about organization from an orderly universe.* San Francisco, CA: Barrett- Koehler.

RECOMMENDED READINGS

Courtney, H., Kirkland, J., & Viguerie. (1997). Strategy under uncertainty. *The Harvard Business Review.* November–December.

deGeus, A. (1988). Planning as learning *The Harvard Business Review,* March–April.

Goodspeed, S.W. *Community stewardship: Applying the five principles of contemporary governance.* American Hospital Association Press.

Henry, W. F. (1999). Idiopathic health systems: A more powerful way to look at health resources. *Second Opinion,* September.

Isaacs, W. (1999). *Dialogue and the art of thinking together.* Currency Doubleday.

Kindig, D.A. (1997). *Purchasing population health: Paying for results.* The University of Michigan Press.

Kotter, J. (1990). What leaders really do. *The Harvard Business Review,* May–June.

McKnight, J.(1995). *The careless society: Community and its counterfeits.* New York: Basic Books.

Orlikoff, J.E. (1997). Seven deadly sins of ineffective governance. *Health Care Forum Journal,* July–August.

Orlikoff, J.E. (1998). Seven practices of super boards. *Association Management,* January.

Pointer, D.D., & Ewell, C.M. (1994). *Really governing: How health system hospital boards can make more of a difference.* Delmar Publishers.

Pointer, D.D., & Orlikoff, J.E. (1999). *Board work: Governing health care organizations.* San Francisco, CA: Jossey-Bass.

Senge, P. M. (1990). The leader's new work: Building learning organizations. *Sloan Management Review,* Fall.

Taylor, C., and Holland, T.P. (1996). The new work of the nonprofit board. *The Harvard Business Review,* September–October.

Wheatley, M. (1997). Leadership at the edge of chaos. *Strategy and Leadership,* September.

Chapter 4

EXECUTIVE LEADERSHIP

GEORGE KENNETH GORDON

The term "executive" has become increasingly popular over the last few decades. Most people are aware of time-worn expressions such as executive wash room, executive suite, and executive dining room. More recently, the world of advertising has blossomed with terms such as executive home sites, executive automobiles, and executive car care. In these popular usages, it is apparent that the term executive has the connotations of prestige, high status, privilege, and special treatment.

This popular meaning of the term executive is unfortunate because the executive function in organizations is critically important to their effectiveness. Nevertheless, the popular meaning of the term executive is so pervasive and potent that it is very difficult to lay it aside. It tends to get in the way when we attempt to understand what the executive function is in organization.

This problem is further compounded by the fact that the executive function is not well defined in the literature of formal organizations. A quick scan of the indexes of standard management textbooks, for example, you will typically find that the only listing of the word executive is for a section on "executive compensation" but the word executive, itself, is not defined.

Despite the ambiguities in defining the word executive, however, a number of keen observers and researchers have focused their attention specifically on the top senior managers of organizations who usually, though not always, carry the title of chief executive officer (CEO). The publications that come out of these inquiries are mostly descriptive. They describe the activities, behaviors, and operating procedures through which the CEO carries out her or his role. One generalization that comes out of these studies is that it is hard to generalize about CEO's and how they perform their roles as executives. The CEO's include a wide array of personality types, demonstrate a diverse

56

array of operating procedures, and differ substantially in choosing the organizational issues to which they devote their energies.

TRANSFORMATIVE LEADERSHIP

Nevertheless, there are some recurring themes in the literature on the executive which are worthy of careful consideration. One such theme has to do with the way the executive provides leadership for the organization. This stream of literature has been especially influenced by James MacGregor Burns who contends that leadership is the most widely studied and least understood of human phenomena.

Burns says that most of what we find in textbooks regarding leadership and leadership theory has to do with one particular kind of leadership which he calls transactional leadership. He identifies this kind of leadership in terms of the face-to-face interpersonal influence process between a leader and a follower or work group. Most of this kind of leadership is explained theoretically in terms of transactions or exchanges between leaders and followers.

Burns and his colleagues contend that this understanding of leadership has been developed on the basis of research conducted largely by psychologists studying the supervisory-subordinate relationships in formal organizations. The leadership theories derived from this research may indeed be very helpful for the new supervisor, but Burns contends that the executive does a minimum of direct supervision of people who perform the daily work of the organization. This in no way should be construed as a denigration of the importance of effective supervision (Chapter 5 elaborates the importance of supervisory management for organizational performance). It is, quite simply, a recognition of differential task requirements at different levels in the management system. Nor does this exclude the supervisor from performing transformative leadership. It is a matter of priorities, balance, and the way various positions are defined in the management system.

Burns contends that there is another kind of leadership which he calls transformative leadership. It is this kind of leadership, he suggests, that people have in mind when they talk about our nation's need for leadership. It is the kind of leadership which we associate with names like Ghandi and Martin Luther King, or Churchill and Roosevelt. These are people who exercised tremendous leadership influence over millions of people quite apart from ever meeting them on a face-to-face basis.

In his analysis of this other kind of leadership, Burns says that one of the characteristics of transformative leaders is their capacity to listen to their followers and thereby to identify and understand their deep human needs, aspirations, and hopes for the future. These leaders are able to meld and transform what they learn into a clearly articulated vision of a preferred alternative future and a plan of action through which that vision may be realized. Thereby, such leaders draw people to that vision and the people enlist themselves and their energies toward helping to make the vision a reality. This also has the effect of transforming the follower into an enabled and empowered person with a focus for accomplishment.

Burns says that it is this kind of leadership which we think of when we talk of the need for organizational leadership as compared with supervision. It is part of the function of the executive.

Burns also suggests that every organization, no matter how large or small, has a need for organizational leadership. It is a requirement of the family unit and the corner grocery just as well as it is of the Fortune 500 companies. Obviously there are differences among organizations in the magnitude of the requirement for leadership and the resources that must be devoted to providing leadership. But without the required leadership, the organization, no matter how large or small, is essentially adrift and its effectiveness is compromised. Executive leadership provides focus and direction.

RECURRING THEMES

The foregoing is a very brief attempt to state the core of the Burns formulation regarding transformative leadership. Since Burns published his classic treatment of the subject in 1978, the concept of transformative leadership has been elaborated in various ways and has become a major theme in the literature on executive leadership in organizations.

Futurizing

Another theme has to do with "futurizing" for the organization. This obviously has close affinity with Burns' concept of the transformative leader as envisioning the preferred alternative future. But the futurizing function is worthy of more specific elaboration.

After his retirement as CEO of Blue Cross/Blue Shield, Walt McNerney once pointed out that Blue Cross/Blue Shield were then initiating changes in benefits and new insurance programs which the company had started developing five years before McNerney retired as CEO (see Chapter 3 on Henri Fayol's framework for managing such future-oriented projects). The point McNerney was making is that in a company that size, the leadership has to be thinking and planning at least five years into the future in order to anticipate what will be needed, develop new products, communicate the upcoming changes throughout the organization, and negotiate the acceptability of changes and new programs with the array of stakeholders involved. He added that though five years lead time is indeed a long time in which there is a great risk that circumstances may change considerably, he thought that corporations such as Blue Cross/Blue Shield may soon require as much as ten-year futurizing in order to maintain their positions in their businesses.

Speaking of the same futurizing function and the potential for bad decisions, Peter Drucker has suggested that this is why corporate executives are paid so well. It is the futurity and the irreversibility of their decisions and the courage required to make such decisions that drives the executive compensation systems. Executive leadership requires courage.

Futurizing for the organization should not be thought of as an idling away of time. A former CEO of Sears Roebuck says that during his tenure as CEO, he disciplined himself to think about the organization for two hours every day. Out of ten years of that discipline, he claimed that he had made two critically important decisions regarding the future business of the company.

Goal Setting and Strategy Formation

Futurizing is also the key to setting goals and strategy for the organization which constitute another theme in the literature of executive leadership. The disciplined analysis of the future requires identification of and working through the multiple contingencies facing the organization as well as the identification of new opportunities. This is the discipline which provides the basis for goal setting and strategy formation.

The clarity of future goals and strategy for their achievement has a direct effect on day-by-day operations. Decisions are always made with respect to keeping the organization constantly positioned and repositioned for a variety of contingencies posed by changes in the operating environment while still maintaining the course toward achieving the desired alternative future for the organization. Thus, goal setting and strategy formation provide a framework to guide daily decision making.

Communication

Communication constitutes another theme in the executive leadership literature. The vision of the future of the organization, the goals and strategies, must be clearly articulated and communicated if they are to serve the purposes presented above. Executives see to it that this communication function is fulfilled. They refine their communication skills and become adept at per-

suasion, negotiation, and team building. There is some research support for
the proposition that as organizations grow in size, the executive devotes more
energies to developing the people side of the organization and communication skills become increasingly important.

Affirming Values

A part of the communication function is the affirmation and clarification of
the value commitments and culture of the organization. This values affirmation function is another theme of the current literature of executive leadership. In this respect, there is extensive literature on how the executive
imprints her or his own personality on the organization. Across time, the
entire organization and each of its component parts increasingly reflect the
value commitments and character of the executive.

For one thing, employees who do not agree with the values of the executive
"select themselves out" of the organization over time. In addition, their replace-
ments are likely to be people who fit more comfortably with the evolving value
commitments of the organization. Therefore, as the personal philosophy, value
commitments, and ethics of the executive are incorporated into the organization, there are changes in personnel, program policy, and operating procedures
which leave their distinctive mark on the organization. One effect of this
process is the consolidation of internal consensus regarding the nature of the
organization and how the daily work of the organization is carried out.

External Relations

Another theme in the executive leadership literature has to do with the
executive's attention to the external environment of the organization and the
cultivation of external communication linkages. Obviously, this theme has
distinct relations to several of the other themes, especially futurizing for the
organization.

However, the development of external relationships embraces much more
than support for the futurizing. One of the functions served is that of public
relations. That is, keeping people in the larger environment accurately
informed about the organization and its work. This serves the important function of cultivating constituencies and garnering their support for the organization and its reason for being. Without the support of external constituencies, the
organization may become alienated and encounter antagonism and resistance
with respect to issues such as access to resources and manpower recruitment.

With respect to these last mentioned issues, it is important to note that the
external communication linkages must be established and cultivated long

before a specific need arises. Walt McNerney and his comments on Blue Cross/Blue Shield illustrate the point very well. Every time the company initiates a change in insurance policies or programs, that change must be negotiated with each of the state commissioners of insurance, the labor unions, the employers, and the health care providers. This constitutes an immense network of communication channels and that network must be developed and cultivated long before it is needed to initiate any one specific change. There is a certain investment of executive resources which is required to sustain the external communication linkages of every organization and that is part of the cost of effective organizational performance.

CONSTITUENCIES

Walt McNerney's comments, reported in the preceding paragraph, point to a web of constituencies which reside in the external environment beyond the boundaries of the long-term care organization. Cultivating linkages and identifying mutual interests with these constituencies is important for the viability of the long-term care organization. Both the executive and the board have important roles to play in cultivating contacts with these outside constituents. It is important, however, not to lose sight of the fact that there are internal constituencies with which the executive dare not lose touch. The following are of particular importance.

Governing Board and/or Owner

The governing board or owner is the administrator's "boss" and employer. Their jobs differ (the board decides WHAT the organization will do and the administrator decides HOW to accomplish what is to be done), however the administrator works collaboratively with the board or owner making suggestions on what might be done and asking advice on how a particular project might be implemented. Individual board members or the board as a whole may also serve as a resource to the administrator. For example, the administrator might seek legal, financial, or personnel expertise either from the board or from a recommended source in the community.

Surveyors

There is, by definition and intent, an adversarial relationship between the surveyors and the long-term care facility and its personnel. Surveyors visit a facility to scrutinize how federal and state laws and regulations are being followed. This is the surveyor's job. The administrator and managerial staff do not want to aggravate the procedure. On the other hand, the surveyor and the administrator cannot be collaborating colleagues. This could present a conflict of interest, undermine the survey process, and easily issue in unethical practices.

Both parties walk a fine line with respect to engendering tension in the survey process. Inept social interaction can quickly escalate into abrasive exchanges. Personalities aside, the administrator and department heads must accept the survey process as a given and behave in a professional manner to learn what can be gained from the process. This will smooth the process considerably.

Physicians and Professional Consultants

The administrator is responsible for the quality of medical and consultant services. Therefore, the goal is to find persons who have knowledge of current practices and who wish to apply their expertise to creative improvements to the quality of care and the efficacy and efficiency in resource utilization.

Managers and Department Heads

Good working relationships with other management staff, of course, begins with picking the right people. Respecting their opinions and listening carefully to their problems as well as their ideas are all critical to their effectiveness and job satisfaction. The perceptive administrator will recognize that there are multiple leaders, both formal and informal, in the organization and that these persons need to be cultivated and appreciated.

General Staff

In a large organization the administrator may not be able to be acquainted with every staff member; even simply knowing their names may not be possible. However, acknowledging staff in the everyday work environment is important to morale. In small organizations, the administrator will know each employee by name and have at least some personal acquaintance. In any size organization, empowering capable employees and recognizing good work supports a work environment of mutual respect and appreciation.

Families

Families are usually the first customers of a nursing facility because they frequently select the homes that a potential resident visits. While the resident makes the final decision in most instances, families are very important in the selection process and, thereby, families are also important to the reputation of the facility; a dissatisfied family can have a deleterious effect.

Clients/Residents

The most important constituency are the residents. In small and mid-sized nursing homes and especially in assisted living facilities, the administrator will make a point of becoming acquainted with the residents. For a resident, being able to talk with the administrator is very important. In most assisted living arrangements, the administrator or manager does a great deal of listening and problem solving outside the office. The relationship between resident and administrator tends to be very personal.

In larger and multi-facility organizations, the administrator is further removed from residents and must rely on direct care staff to know and care for the residents. However, even in larger institutions the administrator needs to find ways to be visible on occasions such as holiday celebrations, resident meetings, or by taking a meal in the resident dining room.

THE IMPORTANCE OF EXECUTIVE LEADERSHIP

There is a body of literature which says that the importance of executive leadership has been vastly overestimated in most management literature. Salancik and Pfeffer, for example, did a detailed study of the consequences of changes in mayoral leadership in 30 American cities. They analyzed 18 years of annual budgets for each of these cities sorting out the budgetary effects attributable to the city itself, the budgetary year, and the mayor. Changes in budgets were taken as changes in amount and quality of services provided by the city.

They found that the mayor had far less effect on budgets than did the city itself. In terms of budgetary influence attributable to the mayors, the median value was 9.9 percent of the variance in actual dollar allocations; the median value attributable to the cities themselves was 79.2 percent of the variance. The researchers further note that the mayors' greatest influence (approximately 14% of the variance) was in funding for libraries, health services, and parks and recreation. The mayors' smallest influence (approximately 7%) was in funding for police, fire, and highways departments. Salancik and Pfeffer suggest that these last three budget categories represent essential services. They are areas in which there are well organized and politically active special interest groups. They are also areas in which historic and continuing long-term commitments place constraints on how much budgetary change can be made in any given year.

The Salancik and Pfeffer study suggests that the organization has a momentum of its own and that changes in leadership have a relatively small effect in terms of influencing that momentum. On the basis of studies such as this one, Salancik and Pfeffer have also been instrumental in developing what is known as the resource dependence theory. This theory holds that the organization's dependence on resources in the external environment and the relative availability of those resources are the dominant factors affecting organizational performance. In this theoretical framework, the leadership of the organization is a factor of relatively smaller consequence–in fact, contributing perhaps a seven percent difference in essential aspects.

When youthful administrators are introduced to the Salancik and Pfeffer research, they are typically sobered by the findings. Why should they aspire to a career in long-term care administration when there is so little impact? What is to be gained by preparing themselves with graduate education and ongoing continuing education if it makes so little difference–perhaps no more than a seven percent difference regardless of their level of education?

It may seem to some that it is bad educational strategy to introduce the Salancik and Pfeffer research with youthful long-term care administrators. Indeed, we have a strong tradition in the United States of emphasizing the positives. It seems unnecessarily self-defeating to introduce negatives which undermine the enthusiasm and optimism which are so important for the long-term care field. Why project the politics of city government onto long-term care?

However, the Salancik and Pfeffer research is of high quality and makes an important contribution to our understanding of the role of executive leadership in organizational performance. For one thing, the data presented in this research is sobering. It promotes humility with respect to the real-world constraints on administrator influence as well as a sense of respect for the organization and how power is distributed both within the organization as well as in the external environment. A lack of appropriate humility and respect may lead to misguided expectations, frustration, a frittering away of organizational resources, and the risk of unnecessary degradation of programs or worse.

Salancik and Pfeffer are also very clear in stating that an understanding of how much influence the executive can or should have, and under what circumstances, is absolutely necessary to a realistic perspective on organizational action. Without this critical component, the perspective is distorted.

Finally, the Salancik and Pfeffer research did not include any qualitative evaluation of the effects of the budgetary changes associated with changes in mayoral leadership. This raises the question of the effects of those changes. It raises the idea that the seven percent difference is a vital difference and that the way an executive uses that seven percent difference makes the difference between excellence and mediocrity. What if the squandering of the seven percent difference in ill-conceived and misguided action is the hallmark of mediocrity while the mark of excellence lies in the stewardship and vision with which the seven percent difference is applied? Moreover, let your imagination grapple with the impact and significance of that seven percent difference when its effects are accumulated over several years. This makes the seven percent difference worth striving for and effective use of the seven percent difference is the contribution that competent executive leadership can make to the long-term care organization.

CONCLUSION

Someone has said, "We were trained to be managers, but we are called upon to be leaders." This remarkable statement sums up in capsule form what it means to take on the top senior management role, the executive role, in any organization. It is especially germane to the long-term care field as we face what promises to be an extended period of constricted resources and increasing competition for access to those resources. We may, indeed, be facing decline in terms of the constant dollar value of available resources. It has been suggested that in times of growth and prosperity, organizations can get along well with good managers. In times of scarce resources or decline, they need leaders. In this chapter, we have highlighted some of the themes in the literature of executive leadership. The intent has been to illuminate what is required to make the transition from good management to effective organizational leadership.

RECOMMENDED READINGS

Barnard, C. (1938). *The functions of the executive.* Cambridge: Harvard University Press.

Bennis, W.G., & Naus, B. (1985). *Leaders: The strategy for taking charge.* New York: Harper and Row.

Burns, J.M. (1978). *Leadership.* New York: Harper and Row.

Drucker, P.F. (1990). *Managing the non-profit organization.* New York: Harper Collins.

Gardner, J.W. (1986). The tasks of leadership, Part one: Getting things moving. *Personnel,* November.

Gardner, J.W. (1986). The tasks of leadership, Part two: Setting an example. *Personnel,* December.

Kotter, J.P. (1996). *Leading change.* Boston: Harvard Business School.

Mason, J.C. (1992). Leading the way into the 21st century. *Management Review,* October.

Olson, D.M. (2000). *How do leadership practices affect employee satisfaction?* Doctoral Dissertation, University of Minnesota.

Pfeffer, J., & Salancik, G.R. (1978). *The external control of organizations.* New York: Harper and Row.

Salancik, G.R. (1976–77). Constraints on administrator discretion: The limited influence of mayors on city budgets. *Urban Affairs Quarterly, 12:* 475–498.

Shortell, S.M., & Kaluzny, A.D. (1983). *Health care management: A text in organizational theory and behavior.* New York: John Wiley.

Chapter 5

DEVELOPING THE MANAGEMENT TEAM

RUTH STRYKER

"Administration: The Critical Long-Term Care Variable" is the title of an article written in 1977 (Smith et al.). Its message is even truer today. The external pressures in the field of long-term care do not allow a manager to be traditional, passive or merely reactive; administrators must learn to manipulate organizational variables in order to provide efficient and effective care.

Every facility is subject to internal pressures brought about by owners or boards, staff, residents and family expectations. In addition, every organization must respond to external forces such as the ever-changing political climate, new regulations, changing clientele, changing reimbursement mechanisms and community interests. As a result, the administrator is forced to spend more and more time dealing with the outside political world. It is therefore necessary to leave the day-to-day operational management of the nursing home in the hands of a qualified staff. The long-term care administrator must be competent in both internal and external affairs, but much internal management is accomplished through development of department heads and supervisory staff.

The success of supervisory (or department head) development is contingent first upon the administrator either having or seeking appropriate management knowledge and skill for her- or himself. Personnel cannot function unless the administrator knows how to keep the house in order. However, the administrator cannot do it alone. He or she must have supervisors who know how to supervise. They are the connecting links between employees and management. They represent management to workers, and workers to management. Their organizational position makes it possible for them to block both management and employee goals without being conscious of doing so.

On the other hand, this same position can increase the viability of the organization *if* supervisors understand their role and are given appropriate training.

Likert's Linking Pin Theory helps us to understand the delicate problems encountered in having a department head or supervisor position which links management and workers. Envision 100 chain links (100 workers) in five groups of 20 links with each group attached to one link (five supervisors or department heads) which are in turn attached to one link (the administrator). This visualization makes the dual role of the supervisor very clear. He or she must be both boss (supervisor) *and* subordinate (worker). This somewhat tenuous position requires clear lines of authority, clear areas of responsibility and special training for the job. When an administrator places new employees in the hands of an ineffective and/or untrained supervisor, conflict and turnover might well be expected.

Management skill at any level does have two aspects, personality and knowledge. An inept, insensitive, devisive or untrustworthy person probably can never become an effective manager regardless of knowledge and skill. On the other hand, a person who is competent in a job, sensitive and trustworthy cannot become an effective manager without learning management skills.

In reality, when a person enters any level of management, that person virtually makes a career change. Knowing how to do a job does not qualify, someone to manage others to do it. In fact, a supervisor may remain focused on the performance of the former job, because he or she does not know how to coach and supervise others to do it. A supervisor must become a doer of different things.

This position affects another area of employee-employer relationships: namely, union organizing. Frequently when a union initiates an effort to organize employees, the administrator is surprised. This usually results from a lack of knowledge about employee problems or a resistance to finding satisfactory resolutions. Administrators must realize that such employee efforts (including strikes) are often caused by supervisors as much as they are by the organization itself. Grievances that never surface or go unresolved at the supervisory level deprive the administrator of crucial facts. If this is accompanied by poor personnel practices, the stage is set for unrest and union organizing in order for employees to accomplish what they could not accomplish without union assistance.

In other instances, especially in small organizations, supervisors are labeled "inept" when in reality, their authority is usurped by a higher level of management. On the other hand, a supervisor may be willing to take the authority of the position but be reluctant to accept the responsibilities and accountability of the position. Because problems vary by individual and by organization, administrative assessment is necessary.

There is also a ripple effect among departments. Each department influences the work, attitudes and efficiency of others. For instance, unreliable and low performing housekeeping personnel influence the work and work-flow of nursing, dietary and activities. Poor food and erratic food service may influence food intake and behavior of residents which in turn affects their physical and psychological well-being which then makes nursing care more difficult. Poor nursing care influences resident behavior, which may affect attitudes toward food, activities, etc. Understanding, cooperation, efficient systems, and trained personnel in all departments are interdependent. As one administrator said, "whenever I improve one department, it always helps other departments. The entire organization is better off, not just that department."

The importance of the supervisor seems almost indisputable in terms of impact on employees, the administrator and overall organizational success. This chapter will examine organizational structure, supervisory responsibilities and what must be learned to perform in these capacities The terms, supervisor and department head, will be used interchangeably throughout.

ORGANIZING YOUR STAFF

Organizational Structure

Who are the key leaders in your staff? Each facility will have its own unique way of delineating leadership and responsibility but, almost without fail, it will be shown in an organizational chart.

The average nursing home will have an organizational chart that looks similar to the one in Figure 5-1. As a general rule, it shows the board of directors or corporation at the head of an organization, followed by an administrator who alone is responsible to that body. Then, responsible to the administrator, are the heads of all the different departments within the facility, all on a very long horizontal line depicting equal responsibility. Under the department head line may be figures delineating second and third line managers and other support staff.

The number of boxes on the long horizontal line could, be much greater, depending on the number of departments within an individual facility. The problem with this traditional organizational chart, of course, is that the various department heads or supervisors are responsible for unequal numbers of people and widely varying complexities. The director of nurses, for example, may be responsible for a department of sixty people, while the maintenance supervisor has responsibility for only two. This unbalanced delineation of

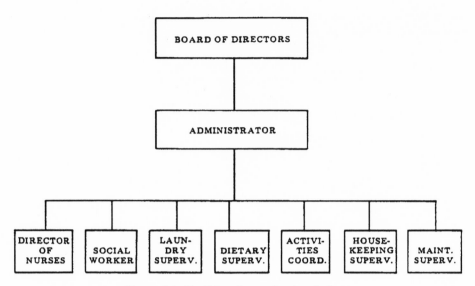

Figure 5-1. Traditional organizational chart.

responsibility may be a cause of conflict and certainly may lead to inefficiency if too many department heads report to the administrator.

An alternate organizational chart similar to Figure 5-2 may be better because it uses two lead assistants: a director of supportive services and a director of therapeutic services. Using this delineation, the personnel in the nursing, occupational and physical therapy, social service and activities departments would all be responsible to one person (who may or may not be the director of nurses). The remainder of the staff and their department heads would be responsible to the supportive services director. These two people would report directly to the administrator. The important thing is to arrive at a scheme that works well and then develop an organizational chart so that employees can easily see their niche in the system.

In assisted living and other residential settings, Figure 5-1 might be used but there are fewer workers in each department. In fact, there may be only one person as in the case of social service.

Responsibility

Once you have a chart to use as a visual aid, it is necessary to make very clear to first level managers what responsibilities you are delegating to them and what expectations you have of them. It is unfair to expect members of a management team to perform efficiently unless they know what decisions

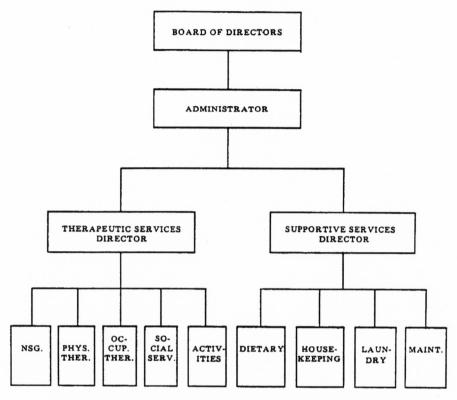

Figure 5-2. Alternative organizational chart.

and actions they can make on their own and which decisions you will reserve for yourself. It is also unfair to expect more than they are able to produce, so you should always keep in mind their educational level and experience.

Job Descriptions

Every administrator has worked with job descriptions until they are weary of the very term. However, they are an essential part of a well-managed facility. Here is an opportunity to sit down with a department head and very carefully discuss his/her responsibilities. Does the particular person have the opportunity to use his/her talents to the greatest extent? Has he/she been assigned responsibilities that are not appropriate? Do you expect your department heads to do their own purchasing and stay within a specified budget? Does the job description say so?

Job descriptions should include as complete a list of the employee's duties as possible. Not only will this help the employee to know what you expect, but it will provide a basis for job evaluations and training programs.

Delegation

We have spoken briefly about the importance of letting your first line managers know what responsibility you are giving them. It is equally important that you allow them to assume those responsibilities. Nothing is more discouraging to an employee than to be given a responsibility and then have the administrator refuse to support a decision. As an administrator, you take a risk when you delegate authority; but unless you allow your employees to make decisions and subsequently support those decisions, your department heads will stop making decisions, thus shifting their accountability to the administrator.

In the same manner, by delegating authority to your department heads, you are teaching them to delegate authority to their subordinates. When department heads see that they can successfully assume and carry out responsibility themselves, they are more likely to grant responsibility to their secondary managers.

Building up this spirit of trust and reliance can benefit the entire facility. When employees feel comfortable that they know what is expected of them and that their supervisors have confidence in them, they are more willing to assume responsibility. Thus, decision making is not limited to the administrator.

THE SUPERVISOR/WORKER RELATIONSHIP

Organizational charts usually diagram a hierarchy of centralized authority for decision making. However, what actually goes on in an organization is far more complex. The effect of the psychological environment, job design, and the function of work groups upon quality of care is hard to diagram. None of these factors shows on an organizational chart, yet they are critical to organizational success. All management levels need to attend to them if the goal of high quality care is to be achieved.

The relationship between supervisor and worker affects the interaction between staff and client. Disgruntled, frustrated, uninformed, and unappreciated workers do not give good care. They become preoccupied with themselves rather than their work. In addition to the usual worker frustrations, the diversity of today's work force compounds potential problems. Attention to misunderstandings of workers who speak English as a second language requires the supervisor to stay away from slang and idioms The supervisor needs to show respect for the many cultures and value systems that are held by workers from many countries. Diversity is but another example of complex educational needs of frontline staff, those nearest the client.

The organizations in the Wellspring Model are examples of management personnel who attend to many of these critical factors. In 1994, 11 Wisconsin nursing homes initiated a quality-improvement model. The stated philosophy is that "top management sets policies for quality and the workers who know the residents best decide how to implement those policies." To accomplish this, all management staff must learn a coaching/mentoring style of behavior which encourages empowerment of frontline staff.

Staff empowerment is accomplished with initial training sessions, the availability of care resource teams, and regular follow-up sessions. The training is led by a Geriatric Nurse Practitioner (G.N.P.) who is shared by the 11 organizations. Nursing assistants learn to make care decisions and are then expected to do so. They become aware of the value of their decisions and thus have greater respect for their work and for themselves.

This is exemplified by the use of the data the facilities collected on falls. Management discovered that one home had a greater number of falls than the other ten facilities. When this information was shared with the staff of the home, a nursing assistant noted that most of the falls occurred in one side of the building and in late afternoon. Was the glare of the sun causing the falls? The intervention was to lower the blind at sunset. This simple solution reduced the number of falls. Decentralized decision-making and staff involvement in monitoring quality of care not only improves quality but it provides staff with an opportunity to see how they can impact that quality.

Some of W. Edward Deming's management tips are at work here. First, employ a vigorous program of education and self-improvement. Second, supervisors should do less supervising and more problem solving. Third, drive out a fearful environment. The effect of implementing these and the above strategies is to change the organizational culture. The environment then becomes more rewarding for workers and it results in improved care of residents.

AN OVERVIEW OF MANAGEMENT LEVELS

Managers were not always managers. They have come up through the ranks of one or more organizations and held a variety of positions in those organizations. Success in previous jobs has culminated in their present managerial position. The question of what caused them to be hired as a manager must, of course, be asked. Was the manager a good cook, good accountant, good nurse, etc.? Did he or she show an ability to lead, to plan, to forecast, etc.?

Some managers will have been promoted for sound reasons: some for irrelevant reasons. Whatever the reasons for advancement, a new manager, regardless of the level, must look at his or her new position in relation to previous responsibilities and those of others. One way to do this is to examine three classic levels of management. Each differs in terms of job concentration, proximity of a manager to the environment where work is performed, the number of persons supervised, areas of planning and the kinds of problems for which one is responsible. A supervisor is physically close to the work situation in order to regularly assess workers, their performance, job outputs and the work environment. This requires short-range planning and problem solving for impediments to quality of outputs or services.

On the other extreme, top level management is responsible for all parts of the organization, which by definition makes it impossible to be at multiple job sites, and it is inappropriate because it would usurp supervisory responsibilities. This person's role with subordinate managers is more consultative, planning is long-range and problem areas relate to the future requiring conceptual and analytic skills. New earnings by persons moving into management for the first time or changing from one level to a new level are critical.

From Worker to Supervisor

When an employee with expertise in a specific work area is promoted to a supervisory level position, the major change relates to a reorientation from doing work to seeing that work is done. It also alters relationships to former peers. Learning can be obtained formally or informally, but requires the following:

1. Ability to withdraw from the doing of work except for teaching and role modeling purposes.
2. Ability to look for ways to improve efficiency, productivity, and effectiveness of all work done in an area.
3. Ability to coach and assist new and long-term employees.
4. Ability to rally a group of workers to cooperate with one another in order to maintain group identity and pride.
5. Ability to evaluate individuals on the basis of quality of job outcomes rather than personal characteristics unless the latter interfere with group performance and/or job outcomes.

From Supervisor to Middle Manager

When an employee assumes a middle manager position, the major change relates to a reorientation from technical mastery (how to) in one work area to knowledge of work requirements and goals of two or more areas in the organization. Formal learning will be useful in (1) the behavioral sciences to understand peer, supervisor and subordinate relations, (2) the management process and (3) budgeting. The position requires the following:

1. Ability to work with the informal system.
2. Ability to delegate tasks, authority, and secondary responsibility to others.
3. Ability to conceptualize problems related to function of departments and overall organizational function.
4. Ability to assist supervisors to perform, analyze problems, and seek solutions for improved performance at the unit/function level.

From Middle Management to Top-Level Management

When a person enters top-level management, the major change relates to a reorientation to the overall organizational performance and the relationships of the organization to the external environment. Demonstrated success in moving human and other resources toward organizational goals is essential. Broad formal and informal education is helpful to the development of both the person and the organization. In addition to the requirements of middle management, this position requires:

1. Leadership skills
2. Negotiating skills
3. Knowledge of long-term fiscal management
4. Knowledge of new and upcoming public policy affecting the function and direction of the organization specifically and the field generally.

These conceptual distinctions between management levels should certainly not be viewed rigidly. Indeed, there may be fewer or more than three levels. However, the framework does provide a basis for analyzing the various levels of management in one's own organization. It identifies the needs of newly promoted persons and provides guidelines for a facility-wide management structure.

The supervisory level of management is likely to be fairly similar in all organizations and is crucial to consistent quality of day-to-day organizational performance. The middle management and top level management levels are frequently blurred in small organizations because there are so few management levels. This may result in ill-defined levels especially when the informal organization dominates. Larger organizations frequently mislabel the supervisory level as a middle management level. For example, if the middle management group includes a food service supervisor, the social worker (a single person with a service function, not a department) and the director of nursing (responsible for 60 to 70 percent of the organization's personnel, with several levels of management within the department, and work performed in multiple sites), there may be many interdepartmental problems. In such an event, the administrator must reexamine the organization, not in terms of the importance of each (they are all important and interdependent) but in terms of management responsibility in the organization. If the administrator does not distinguish between management responsibility and a particular service or cluster of services, organizational success will be impeded by the structure itself.

Finally, multi-institution organizations have still a different problem because institutional administrators usually function at a middle management level in terms of the corporation. Multi-institution corporate leaders need to think through these issues as they relate to delegation of authority, responsibility, and accountability at both the corporate and institutional levels.

One other potential problem needs to be avoided. If one level of management usurps or impedes the authority and responsibility of another level, organizational performance is diminished. This can occur at any level. For example, an administrator may usurp the supervisory or middle management level in a job that he or she once held. This diminishes performance of the person currently holding the position, creates mixed expectations for workers, and detracts from the performance of the job at hand. If a person cannot be assisted to develop new skills, that person needs to be replaced.

This can occur in reverse. A supervisor can impede the function of the middle manager by demeaning and/or resisting that person's goals and authority. Such situations may be caused by interpersonal problems or management incompetence at any level. In any case, this is why persons at all levels need to have a general understanding of the responsibilities of each level of management and specific knowledge of his/her level in particular.

PROMOTING A WORKER TO SUPERVISOR

According to Section 2(11) of the National Labor Relations Act, "The term 'supervisor' means any individual having authority in the interests of the employer to hire, transfer, suspend, lay off, recall, promote, discharge, assign, reward, or discipline other employees, or responsibility to direct them or to adjust their grievances or effectively to recommend such action if in connection with the foregoing, the exercise of such authority is not of a merely routine or clerical nature, but requires the use of independent judgment."

In addition to the above, most supervisors need to participate in budgetary planning if they are to be truly accountable for their departments. The skills required for such a role are not learned in schools of nursing, physical therapy or other professional occupations, nor are they learned from being a cook, a housekeeper or a maintenance man.

While it is nice to receive a promotion, some people do not want to supervise others. Others may accept the promotion because they are complimented but not realize what the job entails. Therefore, it is crucial that job responsibilities be clearly described before a supervisor accepts such a position. While appropriate work experience and education about the work to be done may be necessary, willingness to expand into broader areas of responsibility is essential. Is the individual willing to accept responsibility for the work of others, to direct them, teach them and correct them? Is the person willing to participate in both budgetary planning and accountability? Does he or she wish to participate with a team of supervisors who help to establish organizational policies and procedures? Does the person have independent ideas for departmental changes? If the person is willing to do these things, then the administrator needs to assess the individual's potential for the job and be willing to arrange for training in the areas where previous experience is lacking.

The areas that trouble most new supervisors relate to mentoring, interviewing, evaluating performance, discipline, appropriate use of authority and communicating to staff. These concerns should be dealt with as soon as possible. When a worker is promoted from within the department where he or she has worked, there is a major disruption of social and group relations. Supervising friends and peers causes discomfort for all concerned. Especially in small communities, someone may have to supervise friends, neighbors and occasionally even relatives. How does one handle a good neighbor who is a poor worker? How does one become the boss of a former peer? Such problems need to be faced and discussed *before* a promotion. In addition, if there is any reluctance on the part of either the employee or employer (but they both wish to give it a try), the employee should be designated "acting" or "temporary" supervisor. Thus, if it does not go well, both parties will be spared embarrassment.

Time-framed goals need to be set and arrangements for supervisory training should be made immediately. Whenever possible, it should be completed or at least started prior to assuming the position. Community colleges, vocational schools, trade associations and some large hospitals offer regular supervisory development programs. Administrators who have teaching skills may do some of the training themselves. Readings can be suggested for independent learning, but there must be more to it than that. The administrator must be a good role model and coach the new supervisor, especially during the first few months. Regular conferences during the first few months will provide support and guidance when problems first arise with the new role. This also helps the new supervisor during the period when loss of the accustomed group identity is being replaced by a new more individual identity. In addition, it helps the individual to become acquainted with his or her new boss. Administrator assistance cannot be over-stressed. Good supervisors can help to protect the organization from a "them" vs. "us" posture between managers and workers, but both the administrator and the supervisor must work together to make this happen.

This chapter is not intended to be a supervisor's training text. Its purpose is to stimulate both administrators and supervisors to examine their own knowledge, to identify their own needs and to upgrade the skills that need strengthening. However, knowledge and skill in most of the following areas will be required.

1. The importance of the supervisor
2. The supervisor's impact on an organization—employees, clients and finance
3. Interviewing skills for:
   Screening applicants
   Evaluating employees
   Disciplining employees
   Emotion-laden problems
4. The art of listening
5. Appraisals
   Objectives
   Work-related vs. trait- or person-related criteria
   Goal-setting for weak performance areas
6. Discipline
   Legal aspects
   Disciplinary measures
   Effective methods
7. Handling grievances
   Getting the facts from all parties.
   Writing up the facts
   Following the steps of the grievance procedure
   Staying objective even if you are involved
8. Do's and Don'ts of a Union Organizing Campaign

9. Communications—English as both a first and second language
   Upward—employee problems, employee suggestions, unattended employee needs
   Downward—administrative changes (be ahead of the grapevine), organizational and personnel changes.
10. Basic problem-solving
11. Mentoring
12. Supervisory records
13. How to evaluate oneself

There are obvious other topics, but as supervisory development becomes an ongoing part of an inservice program, participants will generate their own topics. A basic teaching plan is required for all new supervisors and for each level of management. A one-event program is just a beginning, not enough to maintain supervisory skills. Episodic teaching is no guarantee of applied learning. Regular and diverse inputs are required to improve and sustain skills. Follow-up and appraisal will reinforce supervisory staff to apply their knowledge to supervisory behaviors. When an organization demonstrates a continuing commitment to employee development, employees will find their jobs more stimulating and satisfying as performance expectations rise. The organization will be rewarded by improved efficiency and more effective client care provided by a more stable, competent, and satisfied work force.

SUMMARY

Department heads are the primary managers of the long-term care facility. They should be carefully selected, they should have a good understanding of their role as a part of the management team, and they should be given every opportunity for self-improvement.

A creative administrator can do a good deal of the guiding, teaching and coaching of the management team including use of materials and knowledge from his or her own continuing education, both formal and informal. Administrators need to know their department heads well, analyze their needs and capabilities thoughtfully, and spend some time carefully planning their educational experiences.

The benefits to be reaped from building a strong management team include increased efficiency, more confident leadership at all levels, and freedom for the administrator to pursue external and long-range obligations.

REFERENCES

Bolman, L.G., & Deal, T.E. (1992). What makes a team work? *Organizational Dynamics, 21*(2), 34, Autumn.

Deming, W.E. (1997). Deming's management tips. *National Association of Working People 11,* 6, December.

Frawley-O'Dea, M. (2001). *The supervisory relationship: A contemporary psychodynamic approach.* Guilford Press.

Likert, R. (1961). *New patterns of management.* New York: McGraw-Hill, p. 14.

Reinhard, S., & Stone, R. (2001). *Promoting quality in nursing homes: The Wellspring Model.* Field Report, Commonwealth Fund, January.

Senge, P.M. (1990). *The fifth dimension.* New York: Doubleday, p. 424.

Smith, H.L. (1977). Administration: The critical long-term care variable. *HCM Review,* Fall, pp. 67–72.

Umiker, W. (1998). *Management skills for the new health care supervisor.* Germantown, MD: Aspen Corporation.

Wrzesniewski, A., & Dutton, J. (2001). Crafting a job: Revisioning employees as active crafters of their work. *Academy of Management Review, 26*(2), 179, April.

Zinn, J.S. et al. (1995). Organizing for nursing home quality. *Quality Management in Health Care. 3*(4), 37.

Chapter 6

FISCAL LEADERSHIP

BARBARA PORTNOY BARRON

Who makes financial decisions? The answer to this question reveals more about a long-term care facility than any other single question. The answer reveals the philosophy of the organization, how the organization is structured, how authority is distributed, the degree of centralization or decentralization, and the management style that is actually practiced, not just professed, by the organization.

The administrator in most long-term care facilities has primary responsibility for establishing a financial decision-making process. This responsibility may be in conjunction with a Board of Directors, or in the case of a multifacility organization, with the assistance of corporate personnel. However, the administrator usually retains operational responsibility for the financial management of a facility. Some basic principles for an administrator to consider in designing and implementing a financial process and a model for a financial decision-making process will be discussed in this chapter.

What is meant by a financial decision-making process and why should a long-term care facility have such a process? There is nothing mysterious about a financial decision-making process. It is merely a method for an organization to utilize in making financial decisions and solving problems or addressing concerns of a financial nature. Why should a long-term care facility adopt a financial decision-making process? A facility needs a financial system for the same reasons that systems are required or desirable in other areas of management. First, it is more effective and efficient for a facility to have an organized method, a logical progression for thinking through financial decisions, analyzing financial problems, and handling financial activities or tasks. Second, a facility needs a financial system to insure that appropriate, relevant information is considered whether the administrator is making a financial decision in the midst of a crisis or in a situation with a more flexible timeline.

DESIGNING A FINANCIAL DECISION-MAKING PROCESS

An administrator needs to review and consider a number of principles in designing a financial decision-making process. This review should always take place within the framework of the administrator's own facility.

1. A financial decision-making system should be designed to facilitate the achievement of the mission and goals of the facility (in the existing reimbursement system). This means that a financial decision-making process is not an end in and of itself. A financial process is a plan expressed in dollars or numbers and is only useful if it is designed to insure that goals are accomplished.

2. A financial system should encourage wise allocation of dollars through a program approach to budgeting. This must include establishment and justification of priorities and expenditures. A program approach in budgeting means that the dollars allocated for the various programs or services should be separately identified. For example, the budget for a therapeutic recreation (activities) department should clearly distinguish between the expenditures necessary for arts and crafts, daily living skill exercises, community activities, etc., rather than combine the dollars for supplies for all programs and services in the same line item. The budget should also distinguish between the expenditures related to the maintenance of existing programs versus the costs associated with expansion of new programs and services.

    This approach to budgeting is important because it facilitates making financial decisions, including, if necessary, reducing expenditures, based on the degree a particular program or service meets department and/or organization goals. In addition, since resources are limited, it is critical that the budget process include the development of systems for determining usage rates and standards for supplies and equipment, and performance and productivity standards for staff providing services.

3. A financial decision-making process should promote financial decisions being made at the **lowest** level possible in the organization. As in other areas of management, the parties that are most familiar with the area or closest to the provision of a particular program or service are usually best equipped to provide financial input and/or make the financial decision for administration.

4. A financial process should be designed to facilitate monitoring, evaluation, and the implementation of corrective action on a timely basis. A facility's financial process is not complete after the budget is developed and approved or a reimbursement rate report is submitted. Too often, management staff at all levels in an organization will believe that their

major financial responsibility is satisfied after the budgeting process is completed. A long-term care facility's financial situation is constantly changing and fluctuating. In order to insure that an organization is healthy and sound financially, the financial status must be continually monitored, assessed, and, if necessary, corrective action must be selected and instituted.

5. A financial process should recognize and be responsive to limitations and idiosyncrasies that exist in most long-term care (Medicaid and Medicare) reimbursement systems. For example, in many states there are delays and problems with the length of the rate determination process. Therefore, long-term care providers often find themselves paying current expenses with the reimbursement rate from the previous year or an interim or temporary rate. Again, the system needs to address and respond to resulting problems such as cash flow difficulties.

6. A financial decision-making process needs to be designed so that the participants can clearly understand and define their own role, responsibilities, the financial time-line, and the relationship between financial activities and financial decisions.

   Participants should receive financial technical training and computer assistance as needed, and receive guidance regarding budget guidelines and standards. In addition, modifications to prior year plans need to be fully explained to insure accurate incorporation of the changes. Participants in the financial process should also receive education regarding how decisions made at one level in the organization, or by a particular party, impact on the entire financial picture; that financial decisions are not made, nor are financial activities undertaken, in a vacuum. For example, it is important that department heads understand the relationship between how staff is utilized, including staffing patterns and schedules, performance standards, methods of delegation, and the facility's budget and financial requirements.

7. There needs to be a clear distinction between the roles and responsibilities of administration, controllers or accountants, and financial advisors. The role of a controller, accountant, or financial advisor should be to provide financial guidance and information for management, not to make management decisions for the administrator. In many situations, accountants/controllers are allowed either directly or indirectly through financial recommendations to establish priorities, actions, or decisions for administration. The contribution of a financial advisor is critical in the financial decision-making process; however, the process will be more successful and credible when there is a clear definition of

roles. The administrator must neither delegate his or her leadership role to advisors nor allow them to usurp that role.

8. A financial process should assure that department heads, as the primary managers in a long-term care facility, assume a major role in financial decision-making. This includes being held responsible and accountable for their role in meeting program, service and financial goals of the organization. In many long-term care facilities, department heads are held accountable for achieving program or service goals but similar expectations are not required when financial assignments are given. For example, the director of a social service department is likely to receive a goal of increasing family involvement in patient/resident care planning conferences. This is certainly an appropriate goal; however, the director should also receive goals regarding budget adherence, census maintenance, revenue generation, and per diem achievement.

9. A financial decision-making process should be designed so that general parameters are established in the operating budget arena, allowing department heads to retain the authority to reallocate or restructure expenditures within the guidelines. Assuming a department head is meeting organization and department standards and goals and is adhering to overall budget limitations for the department, the department head would retain considerable latitude in determining, appropriating, and adjusting expenditures. For example, if the original approved housekeeping supply budget contained $1,000 for plastic liners and $600 for light bulbs, the director of housekeeping would have authority to reverse the expenditures, i.e., spend $1,000 for bulbs and $600 for liners or spend the dollars for any items in the same or a similarly classified chart of account.

10. The financial decision-making process should be designed so that establishing service and program priorities for the organization as a whole within the existing reimbursement system is the joint responsibility of the department heads and the administrator. In other words, the problem(s) of reducing or adjusting budgets to meet reimbursement rates, limitations, or restrictions should be a shared obligation, rather than the sole responsibility of the administrator.

11. A financial process should include a formal, structured system for monitoring ongoing compliance with financial goals and targets. Monitoring and tracking systems and regular financial statements are essential to insure that there is an ongoing compliance with and achievement of the budget. If a budget is established and there are no monitoring and tracking systems or regular financial reports, the likelihood of the long-term care facility or individual departments achieving the budget is

minimal. There is a clear need for monitoring and tracking in addition to financial statements. Such statements are typically generated on a monthly basis and issued some weeks after month-end closing activities. Monitoring and tracking systems provide ongoing opportunities to intervene, correct a problem, and permit a department head or team of managers to respond in a quicker, more timely fashion.

The system may include daily, weekly, bi-weekly, or monthly tracking systems for labor hours and dollars, supply and minor equipment expense, capital expenditure purchases, and occupancy and revenue achievement. Department heads may find supply and minor equipment expense easier to manage by creating a checkbook-type tracking system. Many time clock and payroll systems generate reports, which can prove quite useful in monitoring labor hours and dollars. The system may track labor or expense on a per resident day basis and revenue on a per diem basis.

Participation in the tracking and monitoring systems should include all department heads. The accountability for such systems and making appropriate adjustments to get back into compliance with the budget is a shared responsibility and does not solely reside with the administrator. This shared responsibility includes, but is not limited to, the team of department managers reviewing and analyzing the monthly financial statements and weekly monitoring and tracking systems as a group. The synergy of the group process produces enhanced intervention strategies and reinforces shared accountability for the financial performance of the facility.

ESTABLISHING A FINANCIAL DECISION-MAKING PROCESS

Initially, the administrator must select the overall structure of the process. A basic structure, though the terminology may certainly vary, should identify the major financial components of the process, the specific activities and tasks which will be included in each component, the format or methodology which should be utilized, the responsible party, and time-line, including initiation and completion dates for each task or activity. A model for a financial decision-making process will be discussed.

First, the administrator should determine which components should be included in the system. There are five major components which summarize the type of financial decisions generally made in long-term care facilities: budget-operating expenditures; budget-revenue; budget-capital expenditure; rate setting; monitoring, evaluation, corrective action; and the purchasing component. Second, the administrator should determine the appropriate tasks for each financial component.

In the operating expenditure component, budgeting decisions regarding capital expenditures, salaries and wages, staffing patterns and ratios, benefits, lease/rental agreements, insurance, utilities, interest expense, property taxes, supplies, equipment, purchased services, consulting services, and raw food need to be made. Table 6-1 shows a way to organize financial decisions for the budget-operating expenditures component.

In the revenue component, projections regarding the number and distribution of patient/resident days and the utilization of other revenue-producing services such as physical therapy, occupational therapy, speech therapy, medical transportation, and other ancillary services such as salon services need to be generated. Table 6-2 shows a method for making financial decisions in the budget-revenue component.

The rate setting component includes financial tasks such as preparation of the reimbursement rate determination report for the Medicaid Program (including a determination of a daily rate for Medical Assistance residents) and determination of a rate for private pay patients/residents. Table 6-3 shows a format for making financial decisions in the rate (charge) setting component.

The component of monitoring, evaluation, and corrective action should encompass tasks such as projecting cash flow; tracking occupancy; monitoring expenditures, revenue, and census fluctuation, including comparing actual results to the budget; identifying deviations and unanticipated or unexpected financial events; evaluating the event or change and its effect on the financial picture; and determining and instituting corrective action when appropriate. Table 6-4 shows a system for making financial decisions in the monitoring, evaluation, and corrective action component.

The component of purchasing should include financial activities, such as determining appropriate product, service, contract standards; selecting vendors; and authorizing and processing purchases. Table 6-5 shows a way to approach financial decisions in the purchasing component.

Next, the administrator must determine what is the appropriate format and/or methodology for each financial activity or task. Particularly in a financial process, it makes sense to develop standardized ways to submit, display, and evaluate financial information. This need for standardization becomes extremely apparent if an administrator visualizes interpreting and attempting to consolidate ten department budgets, each prepared and submitted in a different format. The administrator's task would be, at the very best, frustrating and more likely would become an administrative nightmare.

In developing a format and/or methodology for each financial activity, there are a number of items to consider. There is no "correct" answer for the long-term care industry. Selection of an appropriate format or methodology

TABLE 6-1
FINANCIAL DECISION-MAKING PROCESS
Budget-Operating Expenditures
Fiscal Year–Calendar Year

Tasks	Format/Methodology	Completion Date
A. Capital Expenditures/ Depreciation	A. Label and describe capital expenditures as mandatory, necessary, or desirable. Propose alternative to purchase, e.g., repair and maintain, lease, rental.	A. 10/7
B. Salaries/Wages 1. Wage Schedules 2. Staffing Patterns, Full-Time Equivalents	B. Submit staffing pattern by job classification, shift, floor/station/assignment. Submit wage schedules designed on basis of performance and tenure. Provide research data regarding salaries/wages offered in competitor communities and other nonhealth care industries recruiting from the same labor pool. Calculate full-time equivalents required for each position.	B. 10/1
C. Benefits	C. Forecast costs associated with maintenance of current benefit level (including premium or eligibility changes). Proposals for new benefits must include description of service and explanation of associated costs.	C. 9/15
D. Leases/Rental Agreements	D.–H. Project maintenance of current status and	D. 9/15
E. Insurance	costs associated with additions/changes,	E. 10/7
F. Utilities	and submit documentations of rate	F. 10/7
G. Interest	changes.	G. 10/7
H. Property Taxes		H. 10/7
I. Supplies and Equipment	I. Establish system for determining standards and usage of supplies and minor equipment.	I. 10/7
J. Purchased Services	J. Describe the scope and frequency of utilization of consultants and contract personnel.	
K. Raw Food	K. Determining the cost of raw food–distinguish between meals, nourishments and other nutritional supplements, and costs associated with special events, activities, and sales/marketing functions.	K. 10/7

RESPONSIBLE PARTY(IES)

Department Heads: As individuals, develop and propose budget for own department in all operating expenditure areas. As group, with administrative guidance, propose capital expenditures for facility.

(Continued on next page)

TABLE 6-1. (continued)

RESPONSIBLE PARTY(IES) (continued)

Administrator:	Develop budget forms and methodology. Review and revise department budget proposals. Ensure continuity between budgets and goals. Do research necessary for budget development. Develop general facility and administrative budget.
Accountant/ Controller:	Calculate impact of budget proposals and financial alternatives.
Board:	Approve final budget and general financial strategies through adoption of resolutions.

TABLE 6-2
FINANCIAL DECISION-MAKING PROCESS
Budget–Revenue
Fiscal Year–Calendar Year

Tasks	Format/Methodology	Completion Date
A. Projection–Number of Patient/Resident Days	A. Project admissions and discharges and profiles of new residents by reviewing/discussing historical information and outlining future trends. Project information on monthly basis for fiscal year. Consider average length of stay.	A. 10/15
B. Projection–Utilization of Revenue Producing Services	B. Project utilization of services by reviewing/discussing historical information and outlining future trends. Project information on monthly basis.	B. 10/15

RESPONSIBLE PARTY(IES)

Department Heads:	Sales/Marketing Staff, Directors of Nursing Service, and Social Service research and prepare census projections. Directors of revenue producing centers (such as physical therapists, occupational therapists) project utilization of services.
Business Office Manager and Accountant/ Controller:	Project revenues.
Administrator:	Provide assistance. Review and approve final projections.

must fit the requirements of the administrator's facility and staff and the reimbursement structure. It is usually dictated by how the financial information will ultimately be utilized, both internally and externally, and the type of financial decisions which will be generated from the information. In other

TABLE 6-3
FINANCIAL DECISION-MAKING PROCESS
Rate (Charge) Setting
Fiscal Year–Calendar Year

Tasks	Format/Methodology	Completion Date
A. 1. Projection–Number Medical Assistance Rate	A. Project current year-end costs and cost changes for new year. Predict allowable maximum reimbursement rates and	A. 1. 11/1
2. Medical Assistance Reimbursement Report Preparation	increases for new year. Generate Medical Assistance reimbursement rate for new year.	2. 2/1
B. Determination of Private Pay Rate	B. Determine private pay rate based on budget projections. Medical Assistance rate determination, and market research.	B. 11/1

RESPONSIBLE PARTY(IES)

Administrator and Controller (or Financial Advisor): Prepare rate reimbursement report and determine Medical Assistance rate and private pay rates.

words, by looking at the desired outcome, the administrator should be able to determine format. The administrator will also want to consider who will be utilizing the information, both internally and externally, and the frequency of the utilization. For example, will the information be utilized in negotiations with financial institutions? Will the information be utilized in the rate determination process with the Medicaid (Medical Assistance) Agency? Will department heads use the information on a monthly basis for budget adherence purposes? Designing a format or methodology which is simple, clear, and easily understood and interpreted by the parties involved in the financial decision-making process is certainly a critical consideration. Finally, in making format or methodology decisions the administrator needs to determine the type of financial information to be generated by each financial activity and how the information should be devised and developed. For example, in regard to specific financial activity, is year-to-date information relevant and/or significant?

The administrator is responsible for the delegation of financial decisions and activities by determining who is best equipped or prepared to handle the authority and responsibility. The administrator will need to determine what role, if any, the following parties will play: department heads, other supervisory personnel, an accountant/controller, the board of directors, in the case of a multifacility organization the corporate staff, bookkeeping staff, line staff, and consultants. An administrator may want to consider expanding the roles

TABLE 6-4
FINANCIAL DECISION-MAKING PROCESS
Monitoring, Evaluation, and Corrective Action
Fiscal Year–Calendar Year

Tasks	Format/Methodology	Completion Date
A. Project Cash Flow	A. Develop monthly/annual cash flow projections. Identify areas of cash flow concern and establish solutions.	A. 11/30
B. Monitor Budget–Expenditures,	B. Develop monitoring system including review of invoices, payroll summaries, labor and time clock reports, census sheets, financial statements. Explain discrepancies between actual experience versus budget on monitoring summary sheet, at manager meetings, and through financial variance reports.	B. Daily, Weekly, Monthly
C. Attain Budget Projections	C. Propose and initiate actions to correct discrepancies and attain budget projections.	C. Weekly, Monthly

RESPONSIBLE PARTY(IES)

Administrator and Controller: Prepare cash flow projections.
Department Heads: Monitor department budgets and implement corrective action to assure adherence to budget.
Administrator: Ensure adherence in the general and administrative areas and to overall organization budget.

and responsibilities of the participants over time in the financial process, if he/she is working with a staff with limited financial expertise, education, and experience. In other words, just as in instituting any major organization change, an administrator may need to gradually design and implement a financial decision-making process.

As the final segment of the financial decision-making process, the administrator must determine when financial decisions and activities should occur and be completed. There are a number of considerations, some imposed by external agencies and factors, others attributable to the operation of the administrator's particular facility. Probably the major factor in establishing or determining a time-line is the facility's fiscal year, as certain parameters are almost naturally established by the fiscal year. Certain time guidelines are dictated by such things as when staff of a facility are prepared to work and meet with outside auditors and the length of the audit process. If a facility's

TABLE 6-5
FINANCIAL DECISION-MAKING PROCESS
Purchasing
Fiscal Year–Calendar Year

Tasks	Format/Methodology	Completion Date
A. Determine Product/ Service Standards	A. Design studies/tests of supplies and equipment to determine standards.	A. 10/7
B. Select Vendors	B. Establish an initial vendor selection system and a semiannual evaluation process. Include assessment of delivery process and schedules, technical abilities of salespersons, willingness of salespersons to provide assistance.	B. 10/7
C. Authorize Purchases	C. Establish a purchase requisition system including mechanisms for placing and processing orders, checking goods received against orders, approving invoices, authorizing preparation of payment.	

RESPONSIBLE PARTY(IES)

Department Heads:	Develop studies/tests for supplies and equipment used in own department. Complete evaluation forms during initial selection of vendors and semiannually thereafter.
Administrator:	Assist in designing and analyzing studies/tests and the results. Develop vendor selection and evaluation criteria. Design and implement a purchase requisition system.
Controller:	Assist Administrator in designing a purchase requisition system with emphasis on the internal bookkeeping process.

reimbursement rate report is prepared or reviewed by an outside financial advisor, the administrator must consider the time required by the process and when the reimbursement rate determination report must be submitted. The administrator also needs to consider how and when private pay residents must be notified of changes in rates. The degree of experience and exposure to a financial decision-making process by key participants will certainly dictate the time-line that the administrator establishes. In fact, an administrator may wish to revise the time-line as the staff becomes more familiar and experienced with the financial decision-making process. Finally, the administrator will want to develop a time-line that allows the necessary time for the administrator to review and revise financial information and activities.

SUMMARY

The administrator must assume fiscal leadership for the organization. This requires clearly defined responsibilities for all persons who need to be involved in advising and decision making. Second, the decision-making process must be established with identifiable needs and goals, realistic time-lines, congruency with state and federal agencies, and a monitoring system.

Part III

HUMAN RESOURCE MANAGEMENT

Chapter 7

HUMAN RESOURCE MANAGEMENT OVERVIEW

RUTH STRYKER

Human Resource Management (HRM) is defined by Hall and Goodale as the "process through which an optimal fit is achieved among the employee, job, organization, and environment so that employees reach their desired level of satisfaction and performance and the organization meets its goals." Human Resource Management deals with the ways an **organization** treats individuals. An organization is obviously a collection of individuals, but employees perceive vacation time, compensation, and training as **company** systems as opposed to an individual CEO's way of handling staff. At the personal level, employees also expect to be treated fairly and honestly by their immediate supervisor.

Human resource management is guided by the philosophy that there are methods of organizing and treating people at all levels so that they will give their best to the organization and achieve personal satisfaction while they are performing their work. HRM is an ongoing responsibility of all levels of management. Immediate supervisors are responsible for performance appraisal, interpreting and implementing personnel policies, hiring, and orienting new employees, etc. Higher levels of management are responsible for compensation planning, record systems, personnel policies, hiring systems, and monitoring and evaluating all components of the overall HR system.

THE CLIMATE OF LONG-TERM CARE AS A WORK ENVIRONMENT

Every employer must be cognizant of inherent factors that influence employees in a particular work environment. First, one must acknowledge the negative factors. For example, nursing home work is not easy work emotionally or physically, yet it is both challenging and satisfying to many workers.

Pressure by external agencies often forces nursing homes to fill vacancies quickly and thus encourages the hiring of inappropriate or younger workers who are known to turn over rapidly in any organization.

Nursing homes have gone through rapid change during the past decade. They are heavily regulated yet some regulations have not changed much in spite of the fact that resident populations are sicker, more debilitated and continue to grow older. Nursing homes have been encouraged to provide higher quality care but with a preponderance of unskilled workers.

All of this seems to suggest that long-term care administrators have some very special tasks. They obviously need to develop competitive pay scales, fringe benefits, equitable distribution of less popular work times etc. However, the need to control public spending conflicts with some of these goals as well as some of the standards set by law.

Public image also influences nursing homes and nursing home employees. The poor practices of some have been widely described in the media. In turn, this has had an impact on the self-esteem of all persons who work in nursing homes and certainly makes new clients afraid of what they might find.

The knowledge of staff in many homes is limited. Even when nonprofessional employees are trained, it may have been done without adequate training criteria and there are still many professionals who lack geriatric expertise.

The high proportion of nonprofessional workers to professional workers in nursing homes results in the fact that most direct care is given by nonprofessional workers. This creates a circularity of nursing home problems. A small number of supervisors must do more supervision, especially in the nursing department, and opportunities to learn better supervisory skills are usually limited.

Finally, patient outcomes are not likely to be dramatic, and death can be anticipated for many. However, the goal of rehabilitation, to maintain and improve function, must be coupled with helping to provide meaning to the lives of residents, maintaining comfort, and enhancing self esteem and dignity whether death seems imminent or not.

The factors that make the climate of geriatric work unique must be continually addressed by the administrator and department heads. Remember, these obstacles are shared by all homes. Quality homes with good personnel relations and low turnover experience the same external problems as poor nursing homes with high turnover. Therefore, it is the immediate work environment that must be scrutinized by the administrator.

The work environment in geriatric organizations not only affects employees but it directly influences the welfare of residents. Therefore, governing boards, administrators, owners and department heads must be willing to analyze their own organizations, monitor their own practices and take appropriate actions in order to develop new organizational strengths. Those who are willing to do this will find cost benefits, improved quality of resident care and a richer work environment for their employees and for themselves:

HRM practices were studied in Texas and Florida nursing homes by Sheridan, White, and Fairchild. Their findings suggest that HRM practices, policies and procedures are the underlying factors contributing to poor nursing home care. They found that ineffective HRM fosters cold and impersonal feelings and interactions between staff and residents. In other words, staff discontent and poor care feed on each other. Tellis-Nayak and Tellis-Nayak describe this problem in the context of two parties who are powerless and little respected.

> In too many nursing homes the institutional culture prevails. Within it aides are only hired hands; no one provides for their affective needs nor cares if it alienates them. And being in constant company of dependent elderly residents, the aides, too, begin to individualize their problems. They make their wards the ready target of their discontent and resentment. And that completes the vicious cycle.

With so much evidence that sound management of human resources can impact an organization positively, why do so few companies take advantage of it? Is it inertia or complacency? John Donnelly, former president of Harmon International, believes that managers are afraid of losing authority. The typical organizational pyramid limits the capacity for growth of managers and it artificially reinforces the notion of unquestioned authority and wisdom of the person at the top.

This is also seen in long-term care facilities. Thomas notes that the style of management in nursing homes is similar to an "army regiment." He goes on to say that it is very difficult to produce warm and nurturing care surrounded by this kind of command structure.

Sheridan notes that the criteria for the Malcolm Baldridge National Quality Award places 30 percent weight on leadership and human resource management actions needed to build a strong organizational climate. He goes on to say that Deming's Total Quality Management (TQM) requires a foundation of effective HRM policies, practices, and procedures. In fact, many researchers believe that ultimately this will prove as important as any regulatory strategy for improving the quality of care in nursing homes.

THE HIGH COST OF EMPLOYEE TURNOVER

In 1975, when the author first reviewed the literature on personnel turnover in nursing homes, five articles were found, compared to hundreds for hospitals and business organizations. When the literature was again searched from 1980 to 1993, only 18 more articles were found, but only five described data-based studies. The others consisted of opinions, essays, or described only one organization. Six more data-based studies were found from 1994–2002. With almost 70 percent of a nursing home budget going to personnel, and national data indicating that the turnover rate for nursing assistants averages 100 percent (varying from 40% to 500%), it is astonishing that more information is not available.

Employee turnover has been studied in almost all types of organizations from baseball teams to assembly line workers. While there are many commonalities among organizations which can provide practical help to long-term care administrators, long-term care organizations have special qualities that need identification. Therefore, the studies cited will speak to long-term care organizational issues as they relate to employee turnover and retention.

First of all, why reduce personnel turnover? What are the issues? Turnover almost always has a negative influence on the effectiveness of an organization in three major respects: (1) financial costs, (2) lower quality of care, and (3) disrupted personnel relations. Because turnover can be used as a measure of HRM effectiveness, it is important for the administrator to know as much about it as possible.

Financial Costs

Financial cost to the organization includes the time required for terminating, recruitment, selection, interviewing, checking references, placement, training, and greater supervision time for the new employee.

Overtime of other employees may be required during the learning period. Salary costs of new less productive workers and lowered productivity of the helping workers must also be added. Of particular interest to nursing home administrators is a report by two hospitals that it costs more to replace nursing assistants than it does to replace either the LPN or RN because of the training needs and longer period of low productivity.

Health care is a labor intensive industry, accounting for 60 to 70 percent of its budget. Therefore, unnecessary labor costs cannot be treated lightly. While the replacement cost of different positions vary, the formula of four times the monthly salary is a useful estimate of the cost of turnover of short-term employees. The estimated cost of replacing an RN is $7,000 to $10,000 and the estimated cost to replace a nursing assistant is $4,000.

Every department head and administrator needs to think about costs. How many persons and how much time are required for paper and records that must be closed and opened for new and terminating employees? How much overtime is paid because of loss of one or more employees? What is the cost of using temporaries from employment pools? What is the loss of supervision time to employees when the supervisor spends hours interviewing job applicants? How much breakage and waste of supplies, linen, and equipment is caused by new employees? How much down time is required of other employees who assist new personnel? How many back injuries occur with newer employees? What is the cost of want ads, posters and bonuses for finding new employees? What is the cost of regulatory fines? Is occupancy affected? Every organization needs to flush out their actual costs. Unnecessary acquisition, training, and separation costs are unacceptable to a competent administrator.

Unfortunately, some administrators claim that turnover is cheaper because of the high number of base salaries and fewer employ benefits. Research on the subject does not support this short-sighted view nor does an accurate account of turnover costs. Turnover may be the greatest cause of fiscal loss in personnel management. The real costs result in failure of the organization to develop, the inability to attract good workers because of its poor reputation as an employer, and reduced work output and inefficiency resulting in low productivity during the never ending learning periods of new personnel.

Reduced Quality of Care

Another effect of employee turnover relates to quality of care of residents. This has been known for 40 years. Kahne relates the acquisition of new personnel to an increased number of patient suicides in a mental hospital. Burling reported a downward effect on nursing care standards when there was rapid turnover in hospitals.

There are only a few studies on the effect of high turnover on patient outcomes in nursing homes. However, one must speculate about such influences on frail elderly residents who have suffered innumerable losses of close persons such as spouse, friends, siblings and children. It is entirely possible that depression might increase, the desire to disengage from others might increase, disorientation might increase and so might a sense of isolation, hopelessness, and disappointment. Because personnel in long-term care institutions serve not only as caretakers but also as friends of residents, negative treatment outcomes are entirely possible. Certainly new employees are more likely to function at a custodial level than at a therapeutic level and there are frequently a greater number of incident reports with new employees.

Studies looking at the relationship between quality of care and personnel turnover cannot be compared because quality is difficult to measure and its definition varies among studies. Do discharge rates indicate quality? Do death rates indicate lack of quality? Does patient satisfaction indicate quality? How many and what kind of state and federal citations reflect poor care? What about rates of falls, urinary tract infections and decubitus ulcers? The administrator needs to identify what people are talking about when they talk about quality of care.

For example, a vice president of an Ohio nursing home chain reports that their quality of care criteria (citations, resident and family complaints) are consistently lower in their low turnover homes. Halbur and Fear studied personnel turnover and resident outcomes in North Carolina. They found a higher rate of discharges in homes with a *higher* RN turnover rate. They speculate that the introduction of new and more flexible RNs may explain this.

Munroe measured quality of care in California by the number of official survey citations. She also looked at the ratio of RN hours to LVN hours per resident day. She found that poor quality homes had a greater proportion of Medicaid days, higher employee turnover and a lower ratio of RNs to LVNs. Higher quality homes had just the opposite pattern for these dimensions.

In Sweden (Backstrom et al.), 214 nursing home residents who required feeding were studied for a month. In that time, each resident had 16 to 30 persons feeding them. The authors make a case for patient vs. task assignments of personnel so that the effects of turnover is not increased by the constant change of personnel because of an assignment system. In this instance quality of care was reduced because of inattentiveness to the impact of assignments.

In a study of Wisconsin nursing homes (Kruzich et al.), satisfaction with the nursing home was greater when the director of nursing, the director of social services, and nursing assistants had low turnover rates. Interestingly, the authors also found differences among units in each home, even good ones. This finding emphasizes the need to look at individual units even when a home's overall turnover rate is low.

Working at a more "professional" level also tends to increase employee tenure. A more professional level of course implies a higher level of care. Steven's Square, a Minneapolis nursing home, instituted a wellness program which used a holistic approach to care. Their employee average length of stay was 16.1 months prior to the program in 1980 and it went to 63.4 months in 1986 when the program was fully implemented.

More recent attempts to reduce turnover have had success. Self-Managed Work Teams (SMWT's) is a system that allows a group of caregivers (they could all be nursing assistants) to make their own assignments and to make care decisions (Yeatts and Seward). Like the Wellspring model, improved care comes when staff learn to make care decisions. Similar findings were found in dementia care (Beck).

Concern for residents is certainly an added incentive for administrators and department heads to become more attentive to a stable staff. While low turnover cannot guarantee quality of care, certainly high turnover makes it almost impossible.

Disrupted Personnel Relations

The third cost of high turnover is associated with the morale of personnel and their relationships with one another. Price reports that high turnover decreases staff integration. Work groups do not have time to form. The crucial socialization process of workers is disrupted by the constant coming and going of new members. Weakened agreement on standards of care causes dissension among staff and lack of uniformity of care. Loyal and dedicated staff who must routinely shift their time from residents (their reason for working) to assist constantly arriving new employees may also resign because of reduced work satisfaction. This is true whether the employee works in the kitchen, the laundry, housekeeping, nursing or activities.

"Stayers" may have a sense of being exploited by the extra load. In addition, morale deteriorates because of disrupted work routines, disrupted work schedules, and a sense of guilt that residents are receiving less than desirable quality of care.

On the other hand, very low turnover or none could result in a stagnant organization, devoid of fresh ideas and the stimulation of new personalities. Therefore, the goal of reducing turnover to near zero is unsound and probably impossible in any event. If one examines the "leavers" of an organization, turnover can sometimes have a positive influence on staff relationships and resident care. When low performers leave, morale of both personnel and residents is likely to rise. When the organization introduces innovative programming, new employee performance standards are expected. If employees block progress or are reluctant to change their performance level, they are not a loss to the organization when they leave.

The importance of supervision may be even more important for nursing assistants. Waxman concluded that when nursing assistants perceived the management environment to be highly controlled, turnover was high. He concluded that turnover is more influenced by a supervisor's management style than by wages and benefits. Even in quality homes, turnover was greater if there was a rigid management environment.

Administrator Intervention Study to Lower Turnover

What can administrators do to reduce turnover? Emphasizing unavoidable factors such as size, location, or unemployment rate leads administrators to feel helpless or excuse high turnover. This is untenable. Too many questions go begging. Why do some homes in large communities have low turnover? Why do some proprietary homes have low turnover? Why do some large homes have low turnover? To answer these questions, it seemed logical to study only high turnover homes. The goal was to determine which administrative interventions would be most successful in reducing turnover.

Thirty-two nursing homes with an employee turnover rate of 70 percent or higher agreed to enter the study. There was ongoing education with the administrators for the two-year study. Of the 32 facilities, 19 stayed in the study. The reasons given by the homes that dropped out were "too much work," "too many internal problems," "change of administrator," and "there is nothing you can do about turnover."

Two of the above homes are worth special note as they remained in the study for 18 of the 24 months. In one instance, the administrator had managed to reduce the turnover rate from 113 percent to 46 percent by the end of the first year. When the home was sold, the administrator resigned and the new administrator felt the problem had been solved.

In the second instance, the administrator worked very hard to reduce the turnover rate from 87 percent to 66 percent by the end of 15 months. The turnover jumped to 45 percent (180% annual if this had persisted) the following quarter. When I asked him what caused the sudden increase, he stated that the owner walked in one day and fired the director of nursing. Many personnel resigned in protest, as did the administrator.

Findings. Table 7-1 presents the prestudy turnover rate, the rate at the end of the second year of the study, the amount of change and the percent of change for each home. The percent of change was important. For example, compare home number six with number nine. They ended with virtually the same turnover rate (60 vs. 63 percent), However, home nine reduced its turnover by 40 percent while home 6 only reduced its turnover 10 percent.

For the final analysis, seven homes lowered their turnover 39 percent to 76 percent and were classified as successful homes and 7 homes with a change of 10 percent or less are classified as unsuccessful homes. It should be noted that three of these homes increased their turnover rates.

The five moderately successful homes considered themselves successful also. Indeed, they were better off. All of them reduced their turnover, in some instances quite substantially (see home seven ending with a 59 percent turnover rate) and all but one ended with a turnover rate of 66 percent or less.

Five administrative interventions distinguished the successful from the unsuccessful homes at a significant statistical level. They were (1) increased supervision of new employees, (2) revised personnel policies, (3) increased recruiting measures, (4) supervisory training, and (5) avoidance of use of personnel pools.

Table 7-1
CHANGE IN TURNOVER–
PRESTUDY RATE COMPARED TO RATE
DURING SECOND YEAR OF STUDY

Classification	Home No.	Owner	Prestudy Turnover	Turnover 2nd Study Year	Amount of Change	% of Change
7 homes	1	P	217%	53%	−164	−76%
classified	9	NP	100%	60%	− 40	−40%
successful	11	P	78%	39%	− 39	−50%
	8	NP	81%	45%	− 36	−44%
	10	P	83%	50%	− 33	−40%
	5	NP	81%	49%	− 32	−40%
	3	NP	70%	43%	− 27	−39%
5 homes	12	P	88%	64%	− 24	−27%
moderately	4	NP	84%	61%	− 23	−27%
successful	7	NP	79%	59%	− 20	−25%
	2	NP	81%	66%	− 15	−19%
	15	P	92%	80%	− 12	−14%
7 homes	6	P	70%	63%	−7	−10%
classified	13	NP	77%	70%	−7	− 9%
unsuccessful	17	P	84%	79%	−5	− 6%
	19	P	85%	80%	−5	− 6%
	16	P	80%	81%	+1	+1%
	18	P	73%	85%	+12	+16%
	14	NP	77%	94%	+17	+22%

Successful homes also mounted more effort as evidenced by the greater number and greater variety of interventions (71 vs. 34 interventions or 10.1 per home vs. 4.8 per home). For the significant variables, there is even a more striking difference, 35 interventions by the seven successful homes compared to nine of the same interventions by seven successful homes (4.7 per home vs. 1.2 per home).

This seems to confirm the need for multiple administrative actions because of the interrelated effects of these actions. In addition, it suggests a priority for certain ones. If high turnover begets high turnover, the same can be said for low turnover; low turnover promotes low turnover. The goal is to break into the cycle in as many ways as possible.

Training of supervisors and department heads apparently will not reduce turnover unless the content is appropriate and other factors are in place. New employees require a significant amount of supervision. A supervisor training program may not help unless it includes techniques for supporting employees.

The frequent use of pool personnel constantly introduces new employees who do not know the work routines, the residents or the standards of the organization, and the supervisor has little or no authority over a person employed by another organization. In addition, it disrupts the group relations of regular employees and produces many of the same problems that a new employee does. Hoped-for outcomes of supervisory training can also be hampered when inappropriate personnel are hired. The latter comes about when recruitment efforts do not provide enough available applicants to permit choices for employee selection. Finally, supervisory training cannot compensate for lack of direction when personnel policies are unclear, unwritten or unfair.

Departmental Differences. The nursing department should be examined in terms of numbers and proportional contribution to the organization's turnover. If 70 percent of the total staff is in the nursing department, but it only, contributes to 50 percent of the organization's turnover, then other departments (30% of the total staff) are contributing 50 percent also. In eight of the 18 homes, nursing departments were not the major contributors to the problem. In order of frequency, the dietary department reported the highest turnover most frequently, the housekeeping department the second most frequently and nursing was the third most frequently reported.

When And Why They Left. The 4,482 persons who left the 19 organizations during the two-year study period, left for the following reasons:

24%–personal reasons
28%–job competition
11%–returned to school
17%–job caused
20%–discharged or did not show up

While the reason for leaving and the reason given for leaving may not always be the same, it at least is information that administrators can study.

Study Summary

In summary, five administrative interventions distinguished the successful from the unsuccessful homes at the statistically significant level. They were:

1. Revised personnel policies.
2. Increased recruitment efforts.
3. Supervisor training program.
4. Avoidance of use of personnel pools.
5. Increased supervision of new employees.

Some of the other interventions included use of primary nursing, increased staff, increased in-service education, use of Buddy system for new employees, increased employee recognition, and replacement of a nursing assistant by an LPN. While probably supportive to the above five, they were not statistically significant. There was no indication that either organizational characteristics or external forces influenced the reduction of turnover in the successful homes. The conclusions of this study should provide optimism for resolving many personnel problems. It indicates that even if turnover is in part influenced by external factors, controlling internal management problems can negate those influences and result in remarkable changes.

IMPLEMENTING A SOUND HRM PROGRAM

Many important and expensive decisions are made by administrators on the basis of unexamined opinions and assumptions about the behavior of employees. Administrators can benefit greatly from research-based conclusions and recommendations, especially when recommendations to the field of practice are found to be beneficial in a variety of settings. When an administrator applies such findings to his or her particular organization, success is far more likely to be achieved. It is important to underscore that the studies cited in this chapter have examined internal organizational factors that can be changed by administrative action.

An effective Human Resource Management program is critical to the main organizational goal, high quality care of clients. An HRM program can be organized in a variety of ways. Because it is not economically feasible for small organizations to employ HRM specialists, many administrators must personally attend to the HR function. In this case, an administrator might use a personnel consultant to assist in setting up personnel policies, developing job descriptions, preparing a system of personnel records, setting wage and salary scales, and recommending appraisal systems. An alternative method is for several small organizations to employ a personnel manager. In this way, recruitment, selection, retention, and personnel records can be monitored by an expert at a proportionately lower cost. In other words, the human resource function may be managed by the administrator with the help of a consultant, by shared HR services, or by a full-time HR manager.

The next chapter will explore worker motivation, attitudes and perceptions in order to lay the foundation for recruitment, screening, selection, and staff development. Monitoring and evaluating HRM policies and practices will provide direction in merging personnel expectations with organizational expectations.

REFERENCES

American Health Care Association. (1999). *Facts and Trends: The Nursing Facility Sourcebook*. Washington, DC: AHCA.

Backstrom, Ake, Norberg, A., & Norberg, B. (1987). Feeding difficulties in long-stay patients in nursing hones: Caregiver turnover and caregiver's assessments of duration and difficulty of assisted feeding and amount of food received by the patient. *International Journal of Nursing Studies, 24*(1), 69.

Beck, C. (1999). Enabling and empowering certified nursing assistants for quality dementia care. *International Journal of Geriatric Psychiatry, 14,* 197.

Bowers, B. & Becker, M. (1992). The nurse's aides in nursing homes: The relationship between organization and quality. *The Gerontologist, 32*(3), 36.

Burling, T. et al. (1956). *The Give and Take in Hospitals*. New York: Putnam.

Cohen-Mansfield, J. (1997). Turnover among nursing home staff. *Nursing Management, 28*(5), 59, May.

Eaton, S. (2000). Beyond unloving care: Linking human resource management and patient care quality in nursing homes. *International Journal of Human Resource Management, 11*(3), 591.

Halbur, B., & Fear, N. (1986). Nursing personnel turnover rates turned over: Potential positive effects on resident outcomes in nursing homes. *The Gerontologist, 26*(1), 70.

Hall, D.T., & Goodale, J.G. (1986). *Human Resource Management*. Reading, MA: Addison-Wesley Educational Publishers.

Kahne, M.J. (1968). Suicides in mental hospitals: A study of the effects of personnel and patient turnovers. *Journal of Health and Social Behavior, 9*.

Kruzich, J.M. et al. (1992). Personal and environmental influences on nursing home satisfaction. *The Gerontologist, 32*(3), 342.

Leon, J., & Marcotte, J. (2001). *Pennsylvania's frontline worker's in long-term care: The provider organization perspective*. Jenkintown, PA: Pennsylvania Intra-Governmental Council on Long-Term Care.

Munroe, D.J. (1990). The influence of registered nurse staffing on the quality of nursing home care. *Research in Nursing and Health, 13*(4), 263.

Price, J.L. (1997). *The study of turnover*. Ames, IA: Iowa University Press.

Remsburg, R.E. et al. (1999). Improving nursing assistant turnover and stability rates in a long-term care facility. *Geriatric Nursing, 20*(4), 203k, July–August.

Sheridan, J.E. et al. (1992). Ineffective staff, ineffective supervision, or ineffective administration? Why some nursing homes fail to provide adequate care. *The Gerontologist, 32*(3), 334.

Singly, D.A., & Schwab, R.C. (2000). Predicting turnover and retention in nursing home administrators: Management and policy implications. *The Gerontologist, 40*(3), 310, June.

Smyer, M. et al. (1992). Improving nursing home care through training and job redesign. *The Gerontologist, 32*(3), 327.

Stryker, R. (1981). *How to reduce turnover in nursing homes*. Springfield, IL: Charles C Thomas.

Tellis-Nayak, V., & Tellis-Nayak, M. (1989). Quality of care and the burden of two cultures: When the world of the nurse's aide enters the world of the nursing home. *The Gerontologist, 29,* 307.

Thomas, W.H. (1994). *The Eden Alternative: Nature, hope, and nursing homes.* Sherburne, NY: Eden Alternative Foundation.

Waxman, H.M. et al. (1994). Job turnover and job satisfaction among nursing home aides. *The Gerontologist, 24*(5), 503.

Yeatts, D.E., & Seward, R. (2000). Reducing turnover and improving health care in nursing homes: The potential effect of self-managed work teams. *The Gerontologist, 40*(3), 58.

Chapter 8

WORKER MOTIVATION, ATTITUDES, AND PERCEPTIONS

GEORGE KENNETH GORDON

A nursing home does not function in a vacuum. It is, in sociological terms, a social institution; the way the nursing home works on a day-to-day basis as a reflection of the beliefs of the local community as well as the larger society in which the home exists. These beliefs are especially expressed in the interchange among the staff, the residents, and residents' families. How this interplay of beliefs is meshed or mismatched has important implications for the outcomes of the care provided. This is a difficult area of inquiry. Nevertheless, the consequences of the way these beliefs interface and are expressed in the daily round of activity in the nursing home are so important that prudent managers cannot afford to ignore them.

The term "beliefs" has been introduced above as a very general term. What follows is an attempt to examine three specific areas in which beliefs are involved—work motivation, staff attitudes, and ageism. These are all areas which not only can be scrutinized and monitored by managers but they also can be influenced by managers. The last part of this chapter will explore how managers can develop a work environment which can exert positive influence on these beliefs.

A FRAME OF REFERENCE

During the 1960s and 1970s, there was widespread interest in Japanese management practices among American managers and management researchers. One of the things that some of the American managers and researchers discovered was that when they immersed themselves in the study of Japanese management, they unexpectedly found themselves occupying a new vantage point from which to observe and study management practices in America. Some of those researchers said that, in fact, they learned more about American managers than they learned about the Japanese.

Richard Pascale and Anthony Athos were among those who gained a new perspective on American management. From that new perspective, they characterized American managers as appearing to be preoccupied with strategy, structure, and system. They go on to contend that this preoccupation can produce organizations which are arid wastelands, which reduce the people who do the work of the organizations to cogs which are required to respond mechanically to changes in strategy, structure, and system. They present an unpleasant picture of the organization as an inhumane machine in which the demands of strategy, structure, and system wear away at each other and grind each other down.

These authors do not in any way denigrate the importance of strategy, structure, and systems as primary management responsibilities. Indeed, they are quite explicit in expressing their admiration for the excellence with which certain organizations fine-tune these three management functions.

They contend, however, that there are other elements of managerial function that must be tended to in order to convert strategy, structure, and system into outcomes and accomplishments. There can be no outcomes, in fact, apart from people to enact them. Strategies, structures, and systems are nothing more than pure abstractions until real flesh-and-blood people accept them, or claim ownership of them, and enact them into performance and accomplishment.

Pascale and Athos thus present a challenging question: what does it take to develop and cultivate a lively organization which can attain a high level of effectiveness across time? They present the suggestion that it is entirely possible to design an elegant, parsimonious, and thoroughly rational organization, which simply will not work.

What Pascale and Athos say is perhaps illustrated by the Hamm's beer advertising campaign of a few years back which featured a woodsman and a grizzly bear. For years, the Hamm's beer commercials had featured an animated cartoon presentation of a bear who encountered "the Perils of Pauline" in segment after segment on behalf of Hamm's beer sales. The woodsman and the bear, however, were not animated cartoon presentations. They presented a real man and a real bear doing very ordinary things together.

Viewers were enthralled. The woodsman and his bear gained the status of celebrity and had a nationwide following of admirers.

In their swing on the celebrity circuit, the woodsman (really, the bear's trainer) was frequently asked how he got the bear to do the things the bear did in the commercials. His stock answer to this question was, "I never ask the bear to do anything that will embarrass him."

In essence, the trainer was saying that if you want to work with a bear (a wild animal that has never adapted to domestication), you had better start by understanding the nature of the bear. And you never ask the bear to do something which contradicts or violates the bear's fundamental nature. If you do, you run the risk of reducing the bear to a caricature of itself, on the one hand, or of provoking the bear's active resistance and hostility on the other hand.

Probably the charm of the Hamm's beer commercials was that the bear conveyed a sense of great dignity in performing his part in the commercials. The bear was not degraded or reduced to a caricature of what a bear should be nor was he provoked into expressions of rage and resistance under coercion.

There is an important point here with respect to organizational management. Simply put, it is entirely possible for managers to design elegant and rational systems, structures, and strategies for organizational performance which are not acceptable to the people who must implement them. If it is organizational performance that you are concerned about, you had better take time to consider the requirements of the people who must accomplish the performance—and "never ask the bear to do anything that will embarrass him."

This point is not to be taken lightly. There are, in fact, specific cases to illustrate the point, and perhaps none is more pointed than the mechanization of coal mining in Great Britain.

There can be no doubt that the mechanization of coal mining was a great boone to the miners. It relieved them of the tedious and backbreaking labor of cutting the coal by hand and then loading the cut coal, again by hand, into a hutch. Mechanization obviously made the work much easier.

Surprisingly, however, grievances and work disruptions increased with the introduction of mechanization and productivity suffered. It simply, did not make sense.

It did not make sense, that is, until management discovered that a persistent fear in the back of every miner's mind was the fear of being caught, alone, isolated in an underground disaster.

Under the manual labor procedures through which mining had been carried on for 200 years, it was not likely that an individual miner would be caught as an isolated individual in event of a cave-in or explosion. Miners always worked close together in cooperating groups.

Mechanization had the unwitting effect of dispersing and isolating the miners from each other, each man efficiently operating a particular machine. Mechanization thus presented a thoroughly rational system of mining which was elegant and efficient. Moreover, it freed the miners of much of the grinding hand labor they had known. But the mechanized system also contradict-ed a very fundamental human value that was critically important to the min-ers as people.

The thoroughly elegant and efficient technical system of mechanized min-ing had to be adjusted and accommodated to the distinctly human needs of the people who implemented (and were among the major beneficiaries of) mechanized mining procedures. The potential excellence of the technical sys-tem had to accommodate to the psychosocial system of the miners.

This is akin to what Pascale and Athos are driving at when they say that good management involves more than a preoccupation with strategies, struc-tures, and systems. Management thinking must also account for the needs and motivations of the people who must do the day-to-day work of the organ-ization.

WORK MOTIVATION

When we turn our thoughts to work motivations, there are two basic con-cepts that managers need to keep in mind:

1. The workers need to know that you care about them.
2. The workers need to be their own unique selves.

On first reading, these two propositions sound like they come directly from the humanistic psychology which was popular among many organizational consultants during the 1960s and 1970s. One observer has suggested that those human relations consultants played the role of court jesters to American corporations in those decades.

No such "straw-man," satirical, sarcastic, or cynical context should be attached to these propositions currently. Frederick Herzberg laid down these two propositions, quite simply, as guiding principles for what managers must do to develop organizations through which well-conceived strategies, systems, and structures, can be implemented.

Before proceeding any further, it is probably useful to review briefly the origins of Herzberg's two-factor theory of work motivation. Herzberg's for-mulation is appealing because of its empirical derivation. Basically what Herzberg did was to ask workers to write descriptions of things that happened at work that made them feel good about their jobs and, on the other hand, things that made them feel bad. When these descriptions were sorted out, it was found that most of the work situations that made them feel bad had to do with the environment in which workers do their jobs while most of the situations that made them feel good had to do with the nature and content of the jobs themselves.

It is out of this context that Herzberg developed his two propositions regarding what managers must do to develop effective organizations. In very homely fashion, these two propositions define the difference between excellent and ordinary organizations. It is commitment and attention to these two propositions in excellent organizations that provide the lubricant that keeps strategies, structures, and systems from grinding each other away.

The innovative manager who aspires to excellence in organizational performance grasps these two fundamental propositions and translates them into action principles for the organization. This is the point at which formal theories become useful guides to action.

Caring

How, for example, does a nursing home organization express to its rank-and-file employees that the organization cares about them? Herzberg's two-factor theory of work motivation suggests that you express that you care about them by treating them well, that you treat them as best you possibly can by providing them a decent place to work.

According to Herzberg, that means that you provide the best possible work environment that you are capable of providing. Herzberg goes on to list the components or categories of consideration through which the management conveys to employees that the organization cares about them:

Wages
Benefits
Policies and Administration
Supervision
Human Relations
Security
Status

It is useful to note that these elements are listed in descending rank order of the frequency with which workers mentioned them as being sources of dissatisfaction in the workplace. Herzberg contends that it is through the above that management expresses to nursing home employees that the organization cares about them. He is unrelenting on this point. Any toleration of less than the best possible conveys shabby treatment to rank and file employees; it says that the management does not really care about them.

Some managers may conceive "caring about the employees" in terms of being able to address each employee by name or maintaining a "tickler file" of birthdays and employment anniversaries which are to be acknowledged.

Herzberg's list goes far beyond such techniques. A careful elaboration of what constitutes excellence in terms of each item in the above list will quickly reveal that the nursing home organization and its management must be both up-front and out-front in committing the resources of the organization and accepting responsibility for the pursuit of excellence. That is how the organization expresses caring for the rank and file employee.

Employees are not dumb. They may lack technical competence and precision in defining the constraints within which the nursing home must perform, but they are not dumb. Generally, they are forgiving with respect to external constraints on organizational operations but they have a fine sensitivity to the authenticity of a manager's commitment to excellence in providing a decent place to work. They know when management cares about them.

Performance

The manager who is a student of formal work motivation theories will recognize, at this point, that Herzberg's itemization of how an organization expresses caring about employees only has to do with providing a decent place to work. It does not guarantee employee performance.

When we focus on performance, we get back to the analogy of the bear in the TV commercials. The trainer said that he never asked the bear to do anything that would embarrass the bear. He studied the nature of the bear and never asked the bear to do anything that contradicted or violated the nature of the bear. The result was that the bear performed with apparent dignity and ease.

Human beings are far more diverse, complex, and adaptable than bears. In this sense, it is better to forget about the bear. Human performance in the provision of nursing home care takes us to an entirely different plane of sophistication and values.

Nevertheless, the point is well taken. If it is performance in the delivery of nursing home services that you are concerned about, and you must manage the organization and delivery of those services, you must take account of the nature of the people who deliver those services. The design and organization of the work must include opportunity for the people providing the services to be their own unique selves. This should not be read to mean that people can do as they please. It means, rather, that the work is organized and conducted so as to allow the workers to use their talents, skills, and knowledge in ways that respect and provide appropriate expression for their personhood. This is a management ideal which is perhaps best expressed by W. Edwards Deming when he wrote: "It is the responsibility of management to remove the barriers that rob people of the pride of workmanship—which is the hourly worker's birthright" (*Out of the Crisis,* p. 77). In other words, the provision of services must fit the people providing the services in order for them to perform with the sense of dignity and ease which derives from pride of workmanship.

With respect to designing work so that people can be their own unique selves, Herzberg is helpful again. What he says is that you must design work so that you **use** people well. That means that the work must fit the capabilities of the people doing the work and provide appropriate opportunities to advance and refine those capabilities.

Earlier, Herzberg was quoted as saying that you express the fact that you care about employees by **treating** them well and that is a matter of providing a decent work environment. With respect to motivating employees for quality work performance he says that you must **use** them well and that means designing jobs which provide opportunity for:

1. Achievement
2. Recognition for accomplishment
3. Challenging work
4. Increased responsibility
5. Growth and development

Herein lies a challenge to the creativity, problem solving, and moral commitment of nursing home administrators. A great deal of the day-to-day work of nursing home employees is repetitive and routinized. There is a challenge, therefore, in recruiting and selecting employees who will find challenge and opportunity for achievement in the provision of nursing home care. More important, there is the challenge of developing effective, multiple ways of providing recognition, of expanding work responsibilities for employees as they mature in their work capabilities, and of redesigning jobs and training programs so as to maintain appropriate growth and development for individual employees. The administrator needs to understand the employees and cultivate the options for growth and development in the work itself.

It should be noted, again, that the five elements displayed above are listed in rank order of the frequency of their mention as sources of satisfaction in the workplace. Of course, there can be distinctive variations associated with individual organizations or groups within organizations. As a matter of fact, one research report (Rantz et al.) concludes that "interpersonal relations" now ranks first ahead of "achievement" and all others as a work motivation factor.

All of the foregoing brings us to a key question: what are the characteristics of nursing home employees that must be taken into account in the design and management of the work itself? What are the needs and requirements of the workers which the work must satisfy?

Generalizations are always risky because as soon as they are stated they are likely to generate thoughts and recollections of specific exceptions. With that limitation in mind, the following generalizations are presented for your consideration:

1. **They tend to be service-oriented.** They are likely to be consciously committed to the belief that service to fellow human beings is a self-validating good which needs no further explanation or justification. Furthermore, they tend to believe that providing such service is legitimate work. They like to work with people and they get personal satisfaction out of helping others.

2. **They tend to be relations-motivated.** Such people believe that people are the most important things in the world, that organizations exist for people and not the other way around, and they place high value on being able to develop and maintain congenial and mutually supportive human relationships. They expect their work to provide an arena in which their relationships-motivation can be expressed and satisfied.

3. **They have a need for recognition.** It is a secondary characteristic of relations-motivated people. When good human relationships have been established, then the need for recognition of quality performance emerges and may become a dominant influence on behavior and performance.

    This is especially true of nursing home personnel. Most of their work consists of providing personal care and services which are transient events in time leaving no concrete residual or artifact demonstrating the quality of the caring act or service. They need recognition from others, especially from co-workers and management, in order to sustain high quality work performance over time.

4. **They tend to be group-centered.** They are not loners but prefer to work in stable, interdependent teams with predictable and dependable co-workers.

5. **They increasingly see themselves as professionals.** The body of knowledge about nursing home residents and their care has mushroomed during the past decade. Consequently, many nursing home employees are aware that there are special skills and know-how in providing quality nursing home care. Not just anyone can do it. Therefore, nursing home personnel increasingly see themselves as having "careers" in long-term care, and career people are not simply job-holders. They have valuable competencies to be nurtured and developed. How do organizational practices accommodate such employee perceptions and expectations?

6. **They are conflicted about their work.** Nursing homes are a fairly recent social innovation; there is widespread misunderstanding, confusion and controversy over the role and function of nursing homes in

our society. For some people, nursing homes are a source of guilt and shame. There are, therefore, ample opportunities for nursing home personnel to encounter a sense of personal contradiction or conflict over their employment in the nursing home.

Organizational practices which stimulate or aggravate the sense of conflict or contradiction are debilitating to personnel performance. This is especially true with respect to how organizational policies and practices influence control versus independence of the residents.

These six characteristics of nursing home employees present a global description and they suggest the areas of concern that managers need to take into account in order to develop and maintain a motivating work environment. Managers who do not tend to these employee needs or who develop work systems and practices which subtly subvert the work requirements of personnel thereby undermine the potential for commitment and quality performance in the provision of care. The resultant discontent of employees (though they may not be able to define precisely the cause of discontent) will be expressed in poor work performance, high levels of tardiness, unplanned absences, use of sick leave, high turnover, and a general sense of mediocrity communicated to residents, families, and the community at large.

THE EXTERNAL ENVIRONMENT

The matter of conflict, contradiction, and controversy over the public image and opinion of nursing homes is an area that deserves clarification. As indicated earlier, public controversy over nursing homes is a fact of life for the nursing home field. Moreover, nursing home personnel frequently express their dismay and sense of personal hurt because of across-the-board condemnations of nursing homes which are sometimes made by nursing home critics. This cannot but influence the way personnel feel about their employment in a nursing home—and the most committed personnel are likely to feel most disturbed.

FEAR

It is important, therefore, for everyone connected with nursing homes to clarify the nature of the controversies wherever possible. The literature of the field includes multiple suggestions and explanations for the sources of the controversy and quite possibly all of them have some credibility and are worthy of scrutiny. One of the most provocative suggestions is that the controversy stems from deep-seated fear. An advocate of the "fear hypothesis" writes as follows:*

Antipathy toward nursing homes by the general public, potential employees, and potential clientele, as well as policymakers, stems from eight distinct sources. Several of these are more related to *the job nursing homes are asked to do* rather than the institutions themselves. They include:

1. Fear of one's own possible physical and/or mental deterioration which might cause loss of control of body and behavioral functions resulting in intolerable dependence or strain upon family members, strangers, or public dollars.
2. Fear that a family member will become so dependent and/or disruptive to other family members that outside services or institutional care will be required. This is a two-edged sword—the patient feels rejected by the family and the family feels guilty for being unable or unwilling to care for the person.
3. Fear that all nursing homes are like the worst portrayed in the media. While the purpose of such exposés is to close incompetent and unscrupulous homes, it creates a generalized suspicion of incompetence, lack of humanity, and lack of ethics in all nursing homes.
4. Fear that a prolonged period of physical or mental dependence will deplete one's own financial resources.
5. Fear that anger and guilt from present and/or past family relationships may result in inappropriate decisions for care.
6. Fear that knowledge needed for distinguishing between appropriate and inappropriate nursing homes is inadequate if one must be selected.
7. Fear of the unknown associated with any move to a new community, new job, or new role experienced by persons of all ages.
8. The sense of permanency associated with nursing home placement has a potential for drastically reducing an individual's sense of control and independence.

This "fear hypothesis," as elaborated by Stryker, is very persuasive both in scope, explanatory power, and intuitive appeal for people who are well acquainted with nursing homes.

Several years ago, Charles Salewski, Jr., a graduate student in the School of Business at the University of Minnesota, conducted a small marketing study which quite unintentionally produced a set of data which lends credence to the fear hypothesis. He surveyed a group of older adults living in a high-rise in Michigan. They responded very positively in their assessments of various aspects of the nursing homes they were acquainted with: cleanliness, quality of care, food services, staff attitudes, activities programs, etc. Nevertheless,

---

* Ruth Stryker, personal communication.

when asked how they would feel if they were informed that they needed to be admitted to a nursing home the next day, the overwhelming response was the expression of depression, sadness, and despair. When asked to comment on the reasons for this response, the explanations had to do almost entirely with the loss of personal freedom. Summing up, the respondents had very few complaints about the way nursing homes perform their functions, but the prospect of personally requiring nursing home care was depressing and, perhaps, hateful. The study supports Stryker's statement that some of the fear of nursing homes seems to relate to *"the job nursing homes are asked to* **DO** *rather than the institutions themselves."*

The Michigan study described above was a limited, small scope, preliminary inquiry. Nevertheless, it is worthy of note because there is all but a total lack of systematic study of the public perceptions of nursing homes. This is most unfortunate because it leaves every citizen with the difficult task of making sense out of the tangle of rhetorical arguments about nursing homes encountered in the media and legislatures of our nation.

AGEISM

Not only nursing home employees, but the elderly themselves meet a host of contradictory behaviors wherever they go. Ageism, a prejudicial attitude toward the elderly, is an all too common social phenomenon manifested by discriminatory practices and bolstered by unsubstantiated stereotyping. Kastenbaum states that health professionals hold these same societal attitudes, resulting in a reluctance to work with the elderly. Indeed, even elderly persons sometimes have a gnawing sense of self-reproach that seems to stem from actually becoming what they once were prejudiced against. This is both insidious and elusive because the causes go unidentified and many false beliefs go unchallenged.

Studies of the attitudes of health care professionals toward the elderly, while sometimes contradictory, indicate generally negative attitudes across the professions. Physicians, nurses, social workers, and dentists are of particular interest because they have so many elderly clients.

Much of the research with these groups has employed Palmore's *Facts on Aging Quiz*–a standard instrument used both in research as well as program development. The *Facts on Aging Quiz* yields two kinds of scores: (a) factual knowledge about aging and (b) bias or prejudice toward or against aging and the aged. The *Facts on Aging Quiz* has been administered to thousands of health care professionals during the last 40 years. Following are some of the salient findings for health care personnel.

West and Levy surveyed 170 physicians across 28 medical specialties in Texas. All age cohorts, except those aged 60-and-up, tended to be negatively biased toward the aged. Most of the physicians' knowledge scores were no better than university undergraduates' scores. In addition, physicians in practice areas most likely to treat the elderly did no better than did pediatricians. On a more positive note, Green found that third year medical students were quite positive about their feelings toward, and contacts with, elderly patients.

Michael Strayer's study found that over 45 percent of Ohio dentists chose the elderly as their least preferred patients. The dentist's scores on the *Facts on Aging Quiz* were similar to those of the general population. However, dentists with the largest percentage of elderly patients and those who worked in nursing homes had the most negative attitudes toward the elderly.

Wolk and Wolk's study of 220 social workers found that only 25 percent chose to work with the elderly. Among 4,000 student nurses, the aged were identified as the least popular age group to work with (Feldbaum and Feldbaum).

Education, but not experience, is a critical variable related to positive attitudes in many studies. The more educated social workers, nurses, supervisors in nursing homes, and home health care personnel had more positive attitudes than less educated persons in similar positions (Kosberg, Cohen, and Mendlovitz). Similar results were found in a study of home care aides in South Carolina (Timms and Fallat). On the other hand, Brower's study of Florida nurses found that the greater the contact with elderly persons, the greater the amount of negative stereotyping. Nurses' stereotypic expectations of the aged (Bernard 1998; Carr, 1982; Olsen, 1982) included slow recovery times, general deterioration, and extra time requirements for performance of ordinary tasks. Those with positive grandparent relationships tended to have more positive attitudes (Robb).

On a more optimistic note, Grant says that misconceptions of the aged have decreased somewhat among health care providers although there is still a great need to reduce and eliminate prejudice and age discrimination. And there is an encouraging report from Germany (Brendebach and Piontkowski) that did not find the negative stereotypes of the aged that would be predicted on the basis of professional ageism.

In summing up 40 years of research on attitudes toward aging, Palmore (1999) said that health care professionals tend to have the same (or worse) attitudes toward aging as are found in the rest of our society. He went on to say that it is apparent that extensive professional training is not enough to correct the ageism that is embedded in our American culture. Moreover, health care professionals typically know very little about normal aging and the well elderly. Their beliefs about the elderly, he suggested, may be based largely on the pathologies they observe among their own elderly patients rather than on acquaintance with patterns of aging among the well elderly (Palmore 1998).

Administrator sensitivity to these issues and awareness of these findings should guide the selection, training, and evaluation of employees in any type of geriatric service or program. It is certainly critical to realize that mere exposure to the elderly is as likely to generate negative attitudes as positive ones.

THE MOTIVATIONAL WORK ENVIRONMENT

The preceding exploration of characteristics of the external environment leads clearly to the expectation that long-term care employees bring to their jobs a very mixed array of attitudes, expectations, and prejudices toward the elderly as well as fundamental ignorance about aging. Consequently, the long-term care organization faces the continuing task of developing and melding a diverse aggregation of people into a staff that is able to work together consistently and effectively. This requires development of a work environment which is clear with respect to expectations of staff attitudes and desirable work behavior. There is also a need for the operating environment to be rewarding for personnel who cultivate and demonstrate the desired attitudes and behaviors. The rest of this chapter will deal with the development of such a work environment.

Of course, what is under scrutiny here is worker motivation and how to build an environment that will reward motivated behavior. Therefore, it is well to begin with the question of how to go about motivating another person. The simple answer to that question is that no one can motivate another person. Rather, people have motives and these motives are the sources of energy to drive behavior if a person finds linkage between her or his motives and a source of satisfaction, a "payoff," in the environment. The development of the motivating environment, therefore, begins by taking the employees seriously. It means identifying the motives that are available to drive their behavior and building an environment which, on the one hand, clearly identifies and rewards desirable behaviors and which, on the other hand, **equally clearly** provides no reward for undesirable or unacceptable behavior.

Educational Component

A cornerstone for building such an environment is education and training. In the first place, the orientation of all new employees needs to be consistent in developing and explicating the ideals of the organization, the body of knowledge on which the provision of care is based, and the standards of desirable behavior in carrying out one's work. Secondly, inservice and continuing education must enable individuals to continue to grow and achieve in their jobs.

The Motivational Environment

Beyond this educational cornerstone, the management and supervisory systems need to develop a day-to-day working environment which clearly and consistently rewards desirable employee behavior as it occurs. Charles McConnell says that there are certain principles which can be used to build such a work environment:

- Reinforcement of behavior encourages its repetition.
- The faster the response to behavior, the stronger the effect on future behavior.
- Positives are better incentives than negatives.

These principles, McConnell contends, seem to prevail regardless of whether one uses Herzberg's framework, Abraham Maslow's, or some other.

Reinforcement Encourages Repetition

Reinforcement, very simply, is a positive response to an act or behavior. Reinforcement is thus a rewarding response and it may be as simple as complimenting good performance with the statement, "Well done."

One of the difficulties with reinforcement is making sure that the person performing the behavior sees the clear connection between the act and the reinforcement. Typically, there are a lot of things going on in the work environment and an individual may perform several behaviors in fairly short order. When a compliment is given, therefore, it may be important to make explicit for which behavior the compliment is given.

This may be especially important when there is a string of behaviors not all of which are desirable. The fundamental dynamic of reinforcement is that it encourages repetition. There should be no misunderstanding in the employee's mind about which behavior is being reinforced.

A corollary to the behavior-strengthening effect of reinforcement is that behavior which goes unreinforced is likely to dwindle and fade away. With the passage of time, the unreinforced behavior is likely to be extinguished.

There is quite another set of issues with respect to punishment for undesirable behavior. As a matter of clarification, any negative response to a behavior is classified as "punishment" just the same as any positive response is classified as "reinforcement." There is contradictory evidence with respect to the effects of negative response—that is, punishment—on the persistence or elimination of undesirable behavior. Indeed, there is some possibility of punishment producing an unintended perverse kind of reinforcement of the undesirable behavior.

It is also important that reinforcement of behavior be consistent across time and instances. If one individual is rewarded for desired behavior while another is not, this presents a confusing environment. Again, if one individual presents a mixed bag of behavior which draws undifferentiated reinforcement this can be viewed by the individual as well as co-workers as approval of the whole bundle of behaviors–and the basic principle is that behavior that is reinforced is likely to be repeated and it may be copied as well.

Effects of Quick Reinforcement

In general, the faster a reinforcing response is made, the stronger the effect of the reinforcement. This is one reason why it is important to encourage staff to reinforce each other for good performance. While it is true that the supervisor is typically a very powerful person with respect to reinforcement, it is also true that the supervisor can't be everywhere at once. By comparison, co-workers–especially teamed co-workers–may be a rather constant presence in the work environment.

The time lapse between performance of an act and recognition for the excellence of the act also becomes a problem with organizational feedback systems such as annual performance review and merit raises. Simply put, they lack immediacy in terms of providing reinforcement. There may, in fact, be weeks or months separating the performance of tasks and reward for that performance. Moreover, there may have been significant changes in behavior by the time a formal review is scheduled. Supervisors need to be attentive and creative in developing fast-response reinforcement for desirable behavior, especially when the behavior is in a formative stage of development and mastery.

Positives Versus Negatives

There is a proclivity among some supervisors to want to "stamp out" undesirable behavior. That is, the resort to negative, punishing responses may be nearly automatic and couched in compelling supporting arguments. However, there are compelling countering arguments. Consider the following:

- Positive reinforcement for performance of desired behavior is likely to issue in repeated performance of that desired behavior in the future.

- Accomplishment of the intended effects of reinforcement is more likely than the possibility that punishment of undesirable behavior will eliminate repetition of undesirable behavior.
- It is unlikely that punishment of undesirable behavior will issue in performance of the desired behavior.

Building the Motivational Work Environment

One of the enduring truths of organizational life is that the behavior of senior managers is likely to become the "gold standard" for the behavior of subordinates. That is to say, department heads tend to treat their subordinates in ways that echo or reflect the way the senior manager treats the department heads. Moreover, the credibility of the way department heads and supervisors behave toward their subordinates is enhanced if they are, in fact, replicating the behavior of the senior manager. And the behavior of the senior manager has much more durable impact if the manager can say "Do as I do" rather than "Do as I say."

Managers and supervisors need to be trained and helped to become adept in the rationale and behaviors appropriate to enacting a motivating work environment. They also, themselves, need reinforcement as they experiment and attempt the behaviors. While it is true that they can reinforce each other with support and recognition and that this is very important, nevertheless it is also true that the demonstrated commitment of the senior manager is irreplaceable.

SUMMARY

Creating a motivational environment for employees is a management function in nursing homes just as it is in any organization. The execution of this management function needs to be grounded in a clear understanding of work motivation and this understanding must be based on the best research available. Frederick Herzberg's pioneering development of his two-factor theory of work motivation provides a highly regarded research and theory framework. A systematic exploration using the Herzberg framework can be invaluable for identifying points for management initiatives in a specific nursing home environment.

From time to time, there have been instances in which the workers in a specific organization present a configuration of work motives that contradicts what would be expected according to the Herzberg formulation. It is very important for managers to be able to identify such variations and set motivational strategies accordingly.

Some of the variability in work motivation may be caused by the attitudes and personal expectations of the kind of people who self-select to work in nursing homes. Additional variability may be traceable to the confused public image of nursing homes, aging, and care of the elderly which are current in our American culture.

A major challenge for management is to shape and develop what may, in fact, be a disparate set of employees into a functional and effective work force. This requires a major commitment on the part of management to design, model, and enact a reinforcing work environment.

REFERENCES

Bernard, M. (1998). Back to the future? Reflections on women, ageing, and nursing. *Journal of Advanced Nursing, 27,* 633–640.

Bowker, L. (1981). *Humanizing institutions for the aged.* Lexington, MA: Lexington Books.

Brendebach, C., & Piontkowski, U. (1997). Old female patients at the family doctors: A contribution to gerontological attitude research. *Zeitschrift fur Gerontologie und Geriatri, 30,* 368–374.

Brower, T. (1981). Social organizations and nurses' attitudes toward older persons. *Journal of Gerontological Nursing, 11*(1), 17.

Carr, C. (1987). Giving the hospitalized elderly the best care possible. *Health Services Manager, 15,* 6.

Cass, E.L., & Zinner, F.G. (Eds.). (1980). *Man and work in society.* New York: Van Nostrand Reinhold.

Deming, W.E. (2000). *Out of the crisis.* Cambridge, MA: Massachusetts Institute of Technology, Center for Advanced Engineering.

Feldbaum, E., & Feldbaum, M. (1981). Caring for the elderly: Who dislikes it least? *Journal of Health Politics, Policy and Law, 5,* 62–71.

Grant, L. (1995). Effects of ageism on individual and health care providers' responses to healthy aging. *Health and Social Work, 21,* 9–15.

Green, S. et al. (1983). Medical student attitudes towards the elderly. *Journal of American Geriatrics, 31*(5), 305, May.

Hersey, P., & Blanchard, H. (2000). *Management of organizational behavior* (8th ed.). Englewood Cliffs, NJ: Prentice Hall.

Herzberg, F. (1968). One more time: How do you motivate employees? *Harvard Business Review, 28*(1), 58–61, January–February.

Herzberg, F. et al. (1993). *The motivation to work.* New Brunswick, NJ: Transaction Publishers.

Kastenbaum, R. (1963). The reluctant therapist. *Geriatrics, 18,* 296–301.

Kosberg, J., & Harris, A. (1978). Attitudes toward elderly clients. *Health and Social Work, 3*(3), 69–90, August.

Kosberg, R. et al. (1972). Comparison of supervisors' attitudes in a home for the aged. *The Gerontologist, 12*, 241–245, Autumn.

Olsen, I. (1982). Attitudes of nursing students toward aging and the aged. *Gerontology and Geriatric Education, 2*, 233.

Palmore, E. (1998). *The facts on aging quiz* (2nd ed.). New York: Springer.

Palmore, E. (1999). *Ageism: Negative and positive.* New York: Springer.

Palmore, E. (1999). Ageism in gerontological language. *The Gerontologist, 40*(6), 645.

Palmore, E. (2001). The ageism survey. *The Gerontologist, 41*(5), 572–574.

Pascale, R., & Athos, A.B. (1972). *The art of Japanese management.* New York: Warner Books.

Rantz, M. et al. (1996). Employee motivation: New perspectives of the age-old challenge of work motivation. *Nursing Forum, 31*(3), 29–36, July–September.

Robb, S. (1979). Attitudes and intentions of baccalaureate nursing students toward the elderly. *Nursing Research, 28*(1), 43–50, January–February.

Salewsky, C.S. Jr. (1982). Perceptual image of the elderly toward nursing homes. Unpublished research report, University of Minnesota.

Strayer, M. (1885). Dentists' stereotyped knowledge of the elderly in relationship to personal problems in patient management. Unpublished Master's thesis, University of Minnesota.

Timms, J., & Fallat, E.H. (1996). Assessing homecare aides with Palmore's facts on aging quizzes. *Gerontology and Geriatrics Education, 17*(1), 83–94.

West, H., & Levy, W. (1984). Knowledge of aging in the medical profession. *Gerontology and Geriatrics Education, 4*, 23–31.

Wolk, R., & Wolk, R. (1977). Professional workers' attitudes toward the aged. *Journal of American Geriatrics Society, 25*, 624–639.

Chapter 9

RECRUITMENT, SCREENING, AND SELECTION OF PERSONNEL

RUTH STRYKER

Recruitment, screening, and selection efforts are the major steps to attracting and obtaining the right persons for your positions. To be successful, these initial efforts involve putting to use many of the ideas and suggestions which originate from research and well-established personnel practices.

Every organization must abide by more than a dozen federal labor laws when recruiting, interviewing, hiring, promoting, and transferring employees. The Federal Equal Employment Opportunity (EEO) law is actually a group of labor laws which prohibit discrimination based on race, color, religion, sex, national origin, disability, and age over 40 years. Other laws require equal pay for men and women who do substantially equal work and family and medical leave for birth, adoption, an ill family member or illness of the employee. All of the following functions must be carried out in ways that do not give an employee cause to file a charge of discrimination.

RECRUITMENT

Recruitment is the attraction of multiple applicants for each position opening in order to give you choices in filling your positions. In other words, it gives you an opportunity to select the best person(s) from a pool of applicants. Recruitment is only a first step to lowering turnover. Unless an organization provides a support system, recruitment will be a never-ending cost with no payoffs. It can be compared to running water into a bathtub with an open drain. You can never fill the tub unless you have some mechanism to hold the water. An organization must be able to both attract and retain desirable employees. Recruitment, however, is the first step. It is particularly difficult in a tight labor market.

The number of recruitment methods is endless. Newspaper ads, bonuses, radio, the Internet, public service teas, church contacts, community signs, former employees, present employees, announcements, families, local schools and employment agencies are commonly used. A brief comment on a few of these methods seems warranted.

First of all, a satisfied employee, former employees, and affiliating students are your best available recruiters. One gains a reputation as a good employer from these persons. Disgruntled and unhappy persons who have left the organization can seriously harm your recruitment efforts. Employees and former employees are not neutral. They either enhance the image of your organization as a good employer or discourage every potential employee (and client also) they meet.

This consideration suggests an often forgotten recruitment method; namely, transfer and promotion. Does a nursing assistant want to be a dietary aide or vice versa? Would the maid on 2 East be a good housekeeping director? Posting all job openings in the organization is frequently fruitful, as lateral moves may be desired by some employees.

Newspaper ads, unless you are the only home in a community, must highlight some special or worthwhile aspect of the job or the organization. For instance, what does, "Wanted: Nursing Assistants, all shifts," convey to a reader? It tells me that this organization has a lot of openings and I wonder why. Second, it does not state any personal or education requirements, so I wonder what if any, there are. It also looks like a lot of other ads. The more thoughtful applicant, the one you want, is going to search for an ad that mentions some interest in its employees and/or some standards of care. Ad 1 invites applicants who do not care about such things.

Administrators should read the Want Ads in order to compare themselves with their competitors and learn how to capitalize on the assets of their own organization. Here are two examples taken from a Sunday newspaper.

AD 1–RN'S LPN'S
Part time, full time, 7–3, 3–11 shifts.
Contact Jane Jones, Mon–Fri 8–4. EOE*
Lake Hill Nursing Home 438-1218.

AD 2–NURSES WHO WANT TO GET INVOLVED
Tired of constant patient turnover?
Why not become a geriatric nurse?
The Community Nursing Home takes pride in its personalized care and its geriatric rehabilitation education program. We offer competitive salaries, flex-

---

* Equal Opportunity Employer

ible scheduling and a new opportunity to practice your profession more independently. Call Mary Johnson, 436-8121, for an appointment at your convenience. EOE*

The author happened to know the administrators of both homes and called to inquire about the response to the ads. Lake Hill received only one call from an L.P.N. The Community home received calls from six R.N.'s and 17 L.P.N.'s! While their ad was more expensive, it paid off. They understood their "specialness," tried to locate disenchanted hospital nurses, and offered training, flexible scheduling, and competitive salaries. They had a target, and it did not invite just anyone.

Knowing what long-term care nurses like about their jobs can assist in identifying nurses for long-term care. According to Kaye White, job satisfaction comes from: (1) greater autonomy in decisions regarding delivery of care, (2) closer relationships with residents and families, (3) more opportunities to use professional and administrative skills, (4) time to talk to and understand patients, (5) seeing the results of well-planned team care plans, (6) use of a greater variety of skills including teaching, and (7) less organizational bureaucracy than hospitals. Some of the stresses of the job relate to (1) death and dying, (2) communication problems with residents, (3) emotional commitment as a family surrogate, and (4) difficulty in separating work concerns from one's personal life. Seeking nurses who like the autonomy and responsibilities of a nursing home position and helping them to deal with the emotional and regulatory stresses that go along with the position will certainly encourage them to stay and continue to feel challenged.

Too frequent advertising, inappropriate timing and other factors may actually do an organization more harm than good. Timing may be important. September and January are considered good recruiting months by some health care providers. Such differences may vary among communities and should be observed on an individual basis.

If you know your turnover cycles (one reason for monitoring turnover quarterly), you can plan ahead for recruiting new staff. Waiting for a predictable resignation to occur pressures an employer to accept questionable applicants. Recruiting for predictable vacancies in advance is no more costly and gives you a chance to choose from a greater number of applicants.

Bonuses to employees for locating a new employee may backfire. First, a bonus tells the world that you are desperate. This could be due to a 2 percent unemployment rate in your area or because your home has a bad reputation. In either instance, a bonus game among employees may develop, leaving you where you were, but after considerable expense.

---

* Equal Opportunity Employer

Other good recruiting methods include neighborhood teas for potential applicants, using the home as a site for a geriatric nurse refresher course and inviting nurses from the community to your inservice programs. Your reputation as an employer and the way your adjacent community perceives your organization is particularly important in rural areas and blue collar neighborhoods in metropolitan areas.

Families can be another ally in recruitment. One nursing home formally called in families to explain the problem of short staffing. Within a month, they had three new R.N.'s, two L.P.N.'s and seven nursing assistants. Again, this assumes that you are giving good care to residents. This obviously will not work if families have their relatives on the waiting list of another home.

Some homes find that they benefit over a period of time when they serve as a training site for nursing schools, vocational schools, training dietary workers and others. This can have a positive impact if the training is made challenging *and* the students like the organization. If a nursing home allows itself to be a training site for routinized custodial care, it is unlikely to gain employees in the end. On the other hand, these persons will look to you for employment if they found some challenges, learned to care for the elderly and found personnel working well together.

Another source of labor is the so-called "New American." Immigrants come to the United States for a variety of reasons. They may come for family reunification or a better life. They are very likely to be strongly motivated to get a *job* and to have a positive attitude toward work. Many also have a great reverence for the elderly. Some women even view the job of nursing assistant as a career rather than a job. Finding immigrants requires dissemination of information where they are, such as cafes, social or informal organizations and social service agencies serving them. This varies from community to community.

There are challenges when employing immigrants. Language and cultural barriers need to be addressed. Outside community resources, such as available English as a second language classes will be needed. In addition, residents, families, and employees will need to share and understand one another's cultures and values. This is a critical internal management issue if "diversity in the workplace" can become a positive thing.

The demography of potential employees is changing just as it is for the elderly. School closings due to smaller numbers of school children translates to fewer part time students in the labor pool. It will be incumbent upon nursing homes to look to other age-groups such as the middle-aged woman whose children are in college, some of the young old (65 to 75 years of age) and allow more flexible working hours for women with children still at home. Over half of the older age group want to work and 40 percent do work. Older workers tend to have better attendance, a higher productivity rate, a lower accident rate, and they like to learn.

Finally, more and more people want to work part-time. It gives them more flexibility and more time for family and friends. Having a cadre of available part-time employees who know your facility and residents is invaluable and is far better than calling in pool workers who are unfamiliar with the facility, its residents, and its routines.

In summary, recruitment efforts should indicate both an interest in the potential employee and a concern for residents. The ideal goal is of course to recruit more applicants than you need so that you have choices. Even when you do not have this luxury, screening the recruit or drop-in applicant is necessary to prevent the acquisition of persons who may do more harm than going short-handed.

SCREENING

Employers either distort or disregard the employment process when they talk about "recruiting employees." One recruits *applicants*. Within a group of applicants, you may or may not find an employee you want. If you recruit employees (employ anyone who comes to your door), it is almost predictable that you will not only have high turnover, but absenteeism, low morale among employees and poor quality of patient, care as well.

Let us examine this concept a little further. Two of the high turnover homes in one of our studies reported at least eight to ten "no show" or "no call" terminations every quarter. Both homes also had a very high absentee rate. Physical and emotional exhaustion from carrying extra work loads or working extra shifts, resulted in more absenteeism, more sick time, and more resignations. Desperation then caused quick employment of high-risk persons and the cycle was never broken.

The full screening process prevents unnecessary absenteeism and turnover by screening out undesirable persons with a history of job hopping and unsatisfactory work. Screening recruits may also be thought of as a first step to a quality assurance program.

Some administrators screen unskilled workers but will, immediately hire any R.N., L.P.N., R.P.T., or other professional, assuming that their education and/or license makes them suitable job candidates. This fallacy leads to still different problems. Because such persons must assume supervisory positions and program direction, it is imperative that they do not have a personality disorder and that they either have geriatric knowledge or are willing to learn. In other words, the first step in having a stable workforce is to try to recruit applicants, not employees. You then screen the applicants, a process of filtering out undesirable candidates and then looking more closely at seemingly questionable and desirable ones. This helps to prevent employing the wrong person, which merely results in a temporary body count anyway.

Some administrators will argue that they cannot do this as they will receive a deficiency and/or fine from the health department because they may go below the required hours of care per patient. An administrator must address this or turnover problems will be hopelessly locked into the organization. First of all, an organization can hire above the minimum requirements in order to catch up on training and increase the confidence of employees and residents. This will begin to break the turnover cycle. Secondly, the organization can document its recruiting and screening efforts. Some health department surveyors currently accept this as evidence of effort to increase staff and realize that a short staff may be preferable to a staff of inappropriate short stay or no show workers. Nursing home organizations should work with local officials to help them to understand this dynamic.

So much for the importance of screening applicants. What does screening entail?

The Application Blank. Traditionally, the application form has been viewed as a screening device, rightly or wrongly. The application form will probably not predict tenure, but it will give you some basic information on which to build. It is imperative that your application form does not violate fair employment practice standards.

Barbara Portnoy studied the applications of 311 nursing, dietary, and housekeeping assistants, employed by the three long-term care organizations where she was the executive administrator. The purpose of the study was to determine if certain items on the application form could predict whether an employee would have short or long tenure. This exhaustive piece of research concluded that it did not. However, reflection upon her lack of findings led to some startling conclusions and recommendations for managers. Some of Portnoy's findings and suggestions are as follows:

1. Supervisors and administrators employ persons on the basis of characteristics they *believe* to be associated with tenure, such as previous health care experience, personal references, tenure on previous jobs, graduation from high school, distance from job, etc. Since none of these were statistically associated with tenure, new criteria for selection must replace these false assumptions. Indeed, previous health care experience and distance from employment were inversely related to tenure at one of her organizations!

2. Employee exit interview information should be studied in depth.

3. At the time of interview, all management staff should review selected organizational and job information to be given to applicants so that actual work is portrayed accurately. Both monetary and nonfinancial rewards

should be included. This will lessen misunderstandings before, rather than after, employment.

4. Application forms should be clear and understandable to the least educated applicants.

5. Interviewers should be more diligent in pursuing omitted questions, gaps in employment history, and incomplete or ambiguous responses on the application blank. In fact, one nursing home discovered that most of their short stay employees gave incomplete work histories and vague answers when questioned about these items.

Checking References. Obtaining an honest work reference is often difficult. However, it necessitates reasonable efforts. Obtaining an At-Will Agreement or a written release of information from an employee is recommended. Certainly a telephone call to verify if employment and the dates did in fact occur is in order. Sometimes a question such as "Would you rehire?" will be answered. Other desirable questions include: Was this person's work above or below average in terms of amount and quality? What were his or her strengths and weaknesses? Was there a problem with attendance, interpersonal relations or work performance? Why did he or she leave? You may not obtain all you want, but some information is better than none. At the minimum, you will have verified a previous job. For nursing assistants, the State Nurse Aide Registry can be checked for reports of abuse, neglect, or theft.

Because interpretive guidelines for federal regulations say that "facilities must be thorough in their investigations of the past histories of individuals they are considering hiring," many organizations request criminal background checks (CBC's). First, the application form asks if the applicant has a felony conviction. Second, the applicant signs a *release* stating, if they are offered employment, it is conditional until a background check is completed. Information usually comes from the State Bureau of Criminal Apprehension for a small fee, and any findings are usually discussed with the administrator and ultimately with the applicant. While every case is considered individually, theft, assault, and chemical abuse are thought to be reasons for denying employment in a long-term care setting.

Checking personal references is usually nonproductive unless you are also acquainted with someone listed. Success or failure in a previous job may predict the same result in your organization. However, there are exceptions, and talking to the potential employee about an unsuccessful job experience may elicit information about factors that would not be relevant in your situation.

Interviewing. Entire books have been written on interviewing. Administrators and department heads must learn interviewing skills. This should include learning the distinction between direct and nondirect methods, subjective and objective information, reading and sending non-verbal and verbal messages, dealing with one's own prejudices, generalizing from one characteristic, legal implications of some questions, preparing for, conducting and terminating the interview, improved listening skills, etc. In addition to obtaining information about the applicant, the applicant will need to know about the job–the hours, the pay, the non-monetary satisfactions, etc. The applicant should also see the job description.

Basically, a screening interview should be well planned and provide information about the applicant's past work experiences, intelligence/education and motivation/career aspirations. Questions related to the likes and dislikes, performance and accomplishments in previous jobs may provide some insight into the candidate's fit for the position. For jobs requiring problem-solving skills, questions about how he or she analyzes problems, and the educational content of a major may help you to assess if knowledge is applied to performance. Lastly, it is helpful to know the special interests and career aspirations of applicants to assess both the fit and possible tenure.

It is important to adhere to EEO interview rules. First, ask questions that directly relate to job performance only. You want to know if the person has the ability to perform the job. Job performance is the only issue and that must be the focus of the interview. Second, do not ask any questions about the individual's personal life. If there are any personal problems that might affect attendance, for instance, it is up to the employee to solve the problem, not the interviewer. Personal questions are not only irrelevant but they are illegal.

There are a few special areas of concern for long-term care organizations. They should be dealt with in openness initially. Why does the individual want to work with the elderly? How did or do they feel about their parents and grandparents? It is important that they realize that older people are just like any other age-group. Some are more likable than others and some are more difficult to get along with than others.

Interviews should try to explore certain attitudes and feelings that relate to the clientele. If the clientele is aged, one might want to explore some of the following questions:

- Do you have an interest in a client relationship that will last for a prolonged period?
- How uncomfortable do you feel in the presence of mentally and physically disabled persons? Note: You do not want employees who are uncomfortable with their own aging, who wish to have people depend on them, or have patronizing or infantalizing attitudes.
- Do you believe that most elderly have a rehabilitation potential, at least to some degree?
- Tell me about the older relatives or friends you have known. This might elicit feelings of affection, hostility and/or realism. Usually, it is only

when someone is unconscious of anger or fear of parental authority that there is a potential danger of acting out such feelings with residents.

- Do you feel you know yourself well enough not to act blindly if a resident reminded you of someone you disliked?
- Have you ever experienced the death of a close relative or friend?
- What did you like best and least in your previous job?
- If the applicant is a professional, you might ask, "To what extent do you think that the typical professional role interferes with a resident's needs?"

Several organizations have developed small case examples of likely events in a nursing home. The applicant responds to the interviewer and discusses the cases. These responses are then used to assess applicants. Both applicants and interviewers report favorable responses to this approach. The Penn State Mental Health Caregiving Questionnaire provides excellent ideas for development of case situations (Spore et al.).

Some research has shown that turnover is high when the employee and the employer differ in job expectations. Therefore, it is important to mention some of the special features of long-term care. Then, if it is not what the applicant expected, he or she can reject the job *prior* to employment. Factors that fall into this area include such things as the following:

Long-term involvement with residents can sometimes become emotionally draining when a favorite resident becomes ill and dies. The role of an employee is often that of a friend, especially for a resident with friends or family living at a distance.

The role of an employee is to help the resident stay as independent as possible. The long-term care organization does not need or want employees who obtain their satisfactions by feeling superior to the infirm, by fostering dependence or by infantalizing the confused.

The interview is not considered a very accurate way of assessing a potential employee. Because of this, it is often wise to have two persons interview (separately) an applicant. Each person is likely to see different strengths and weaknesses so the applicant is assessed with greater accuracy. Certainly, one of the interviewers should be the department head.

An interview can also assess inservice and training needs for an individual. For instance, a nice young college freshman would like to work three evenings a week for at least two years. She likes older people and has been close to a widowed grandmother. She is also going to become a social worker. She has never experienced the death of a close friend or relative and has never read anything about bereavement or care of a dying person. If you hire this young woman, you would want the inservice director to give her some readings in this area and make sure that she attended any inservice classes on this subject. She would then be less uncomfortable about her skills when such a situation occurs.

Every interview should include a tour of the work area under consideration, an introduction to any coworkers on duty and an introduction to one or more residents. A potential employee cannot envision his or her work from the interviewer's office. The sights and sounds of the nursing home must be viewed first hand before an applicant is in a position to decide to work there.

The DeKalb-County Nursing Home reports that residents participate in this process (Bahr). Volunteer residents have some briefing on interviewing and take applicants on a tour of the home. They observe the person's reaction to the disabled, the helpless and the disoriented. They watch for non-verbal communications such as acceptance, boredom, interest, etc. Besides the positive benefit of having another opinion and observation of an applicant, it provides a perspective that supervisory personnel could not judge from their conversation. While an applicant may say he/she likes older people, this method provides a sort of pre-test for behavioral responses. This home reports that new employees express appreciation for meeting residents prior to employment and residents of course feel very positively about being a part of the employment process.

In summary, the interview should include a discussion of the job itself, the various tasks involved, the salary, and the many personal ramifications of the job. This will help to make the interview as predictive as possible. Discussing these things prior to employment sets the tone and expectations of the job initially. If the applicant is later employed, there will be better congruence or agreement about job expectations. Those who did not agree with the stated expectations will most likely not agree to work for you. Thus, many poor matches can be prevented.

SELECTION

The final decision to hire should be made by the immediate department head. This person knows best the job requirements, the personalities of present employees, and the dynamics of the work environment. Therefore, the department head has the most insight into the total work situation. In addition, this helps to develop a sense of responsibility and accountability for his or her department.

Every organization is affected by the quality of its selection decisions, but labor intensive service industries such as nursing homes suffer the greatest consequence of hiring someone who will be a poor employee (Kettlitz et al.).

As mentioned before, a poor decision is costly financially, detrimental to other employees, and impacts care of residents.

Casio reports that a thorough examination of the personal history data on the application blank is often overlooked. He goes on to say that personal history data predicts performance twice as accurately as interviews and is as accurate as peer assessment and personality inventories.

Kettlitz et al. studied this aspect of selection for nursing assistants. First, they found that those who stayed in a new job had stayed in their previous job up to 65 weeks compared to only 38.4 weeks for those who were short-tenured in a new job. Similar findings appeared in the second most recent job. Short-tenured employees also had had more previous jobs, were more likely to be unemployed at the time of their interview, were more likely to omit information about educational courses they had had, but they filled in more information about their previous work, possibly to look good. Short-tenured employees were more likely to be referred by an employee in the organization which implies that referral rewards may not always be useful. On the other hand, a long-tenured employee was more likely to be a walk-in, employed at the time of the interview, had had fewer previous jobs, were more likely to complete educational information, and had stayed longer at both the last and the second last job.

A thorough selection process includes the assembling of all available information about an applicant, the assessment of this information and the decision to employ or not to employ one individual among several applicants. It is crucial that all steps be followed if management is serious about its mission. This of course does not mean that you will have no doubts about the person you hire. Selection is always an act of faith. However, you will know what those doubts are and you will be prepared to deal with them if they present themselves. In addition, you will know ahead of time what inservice areas of assistance that may be warranted.

You are ready to select an employee for employment if:

- All federal and state guidelines are met.
- The application form is complete and checked for completion and accuracy.
- The interviewer(s) has been trained.
- The trained interviewer feels that the applicant should be assigned to a particular job (not any job).
- The interviewee has seen the job description, knows what hours s/he will be assigned, wages to expect, visited the work area and met some peers as well as residents.
- License of professional persons verified.

- Reference checks have been attempted and preferably received by letter or telephone.
- The applicant has a "stayer" profile (older, longer tenure in other jobs, racial minority, does not job hop).

Employers in health care often overlook one very important concept in the selection process. People are more likely to stay challenged and interested in a position if they can work at their *higher* level of ability. Working at one's lowest capability soon results in boredom and lack of interest. Therefore, the selection process should attempt to match the person's ability as well as interest on the job. If a job requires repetitive tasks and dependability rather than analysis and judgment about changing situations, a borderline retarded person might be the ideal employee. Professional persons would, on the other hand, be allowed to use the widest, not the narrowest, range of judgment for which he or she is educated. In other words, employing a person who has education and ambition beyond which the job can offer, incurs risk of early turnover.

If you tend to hire persons who have more than one dubious recommendation, a reminder not to hire someone else's rejects is in order. However, if such a situation arises, it is wise to pursue the matter with the applicant to see if there is a plausible reason for a poor recommendation in the past. After all, there are bad employers, just as there are bad employees, and most of us have experienced both sides of such a situation. If you are satisfied with the explanation about a particular job, it is not out of order to employ the person.

There is one other important consideration when administrators and department heads are selecting persons who will give direct care to residents. It relates to attitudes. An untrained person with positive attitudes toward a particular clientele, especially the disabled and the elderly, often has a more therapeutic effect than a trained person with a negative attitude. The latter may actually cause increased fear or psychological withdrawal by patients. It is far easier to teach technical skills than to change attitudes. At this juncture, it is important to point out the license to practice a particular profession does not guarantee positive motivations for dealing with a particular clientele. In other words, knowledge and skill is important, but attitudes can either dilute or strengthen those skills.

The final point in selection is to prepare an initial plan of orientation for the individual. This is best done with the individual and can be explored during the interview, discussed in a letter or telephone call when the position is offered, or it can be developed in greater depth on the first day on the job. It of course may need revision during the first few weeks of employment.

SUMMARY

Recruiting, screening and selection efforts will have many benefits. Not only will they reduce turnover, but they will improve organizational function. First, the number of gross misfits entering your organization will be reduced. This in turn will reduce the number of persons needing to be discharged. Second, by giving the employee a chance to learn about the job, applicants will have greater information on which to base their decision to accept or reject the position. Those who are unsuited for the job are more likely to withdraw before going on the payroll. This is far preferable to having someone come to work and then not show up or quit during the first days or weeks of employment. Thus, the facility will be spared some of the financial cost of non-productive work and wasted teaching time. Third, other personnel will be spared a great deal of unexpected and erratic work requirements caused by having such persons on staff. Fourth, residents and patients will not be subjected to inept, uncaring or fearful employees. Lastly, it sets standards and expectations upon which you can build new employees. This will give present employees a sense of confidence in management and will give residents a sense of confidence that the organization does not wish to subject them to inappropriate care givers.

In other words, a new employee will not attach much importance to the job unless the organization does. Present employees will not respect the organization unless the organization demonstrates respect for their working conditions. Residents will be better able to maintain their self-respect if they are not forced to deal with preventable changes and disruptions in their environment.

REFERENCES

Bahr, J. (1980). Residents participate in selection of new employees. *Journal of Gerontological Nursing, 6*(1), 43, January.

Casio, W. (1992). *Managing human resources.* New York: McGraw Hill.

Kettlitz, G. et al. (1998). Validity of background data as a predictor of employee tenure among nursing aides in long-term care facilities. *The Health Care Supervisor, 16*(3), 26, March.

Portnoy, B. (1979). A study of usefulness of employee application items in predicting tenure. Unpublished Master's thesis, University of Minnesota.

Spore, D. et al. (1991). Assessing nursing assistant knowledge of behavioral approaches in mental health problems. *The. Gerontologist, 31*(3), 315, June.

Stolte, K., & Meyers, S. (1995). Reflections of recruitment and retention at the unit level. *Health Care Supervisor, 13*(3), 36.

Straker, J., & Atchley, R. (1999). *Recruiting and retaining frontline workers in long-term care: Usual organizational practices in Ohio.* Scripps Gerontology Center, Miami, University.

Tai, T. et al. (1998). Review of nursing turnover research, 1977–1996. *Social Science and Medicine, 12*(12), 1905.

Wething, L. et al. (1993). Applicant background checks. *The Informer, 13*(3), 29, May/June.

Chapter 10

PERSONNEL POLICIES WITH SPECIAL IMPACT ON EMPLOYEES

RUTH STRYKER

GENERAL COMMENTS

Personnel policies and procedures reflect the concern of management for its workers and influence the success of many organizational goals. Certain policies are especially helpful in producing a positive corporate culture.

Perhaps the best way to view the importance of the content of this chapter is through Herzberg's two-factor theory. He calls these Motivation and Hygiene factors. He describes adequate and appropriate wage and personnel policies as positive "hygiene factors." They are important to the work climate, but they do not motivate. He goes on to say, however, that if wages and policies are inadequate and unfair, they cause job dissatisfaction. The removal of such dissatisfiers, however, does not create job satisfaction. The removal of these dissatisfiers merely makes a more "hygienic" work environment.

Once an organization has fair and adequate wage and personnel policies, it can go on with the business of job satisfaction. Job satisfaction involves motivation which in turn encompasses the nature of the tasks performed and opportunities for achievement. This chapter concerns improving the general hygiene of the work environment by removing dissatisfiers. It will include (1) definitions to differentiate policies, procedures and rules, (2) guidelines for writing policies and procedures, and (3) suggestions for content of personnel policies that have been selected because of their special impact on personnel.

The existence or nonexistence of certain policy content and its wording warrant the scrutiny of the administrator. Some policies should be removed from an organization's policy book because they pertain to either a bygone social era or outdated circumstances. For example, one administrator found a policy on employee meal hours which stated that all employees had to eat at either 11:00 AM or 11:30 AM in order for kitchen help to serve patient meals by 12:15 PM. However, for five years they had been serving employee meals cafeteria style from their expanded kitchen between 11:00 AM and 1:00 PM. This kind of situation makes a joke of policy books and deters personnel from using them or being able to rely on them.

Outdated policies are one problem. Unwritten policies are still a different problem. Sometimes things are done, but no one knows just why, nor can they be found in writing. Unwritten policies especially confuse new employees because situations are handled differently and inconsistently by supervisors. Lack of uniform standards and expectations of course make employees anxious. This was evident at one nursing home where nursing assistants complained that evening charge nurses expected different things of them. One evening charge nurse required that fresh water be given to residents at meal time. Another insisted that it be given after meals and at bedtime, and a third did not allow residents to have any water at the bedside after 8:00 PM because there were fewer calls for assistance to the bathroom at night. The nursing assistants complained about these different expectations and expressed their disappointment that only one of the charge nurses seemed to be more concerned about fluid intake than work for the night nurses. This situation required a written policy—in this case, one that benefited resident care.

In some instances, a written policy may be perfectly adequate, but implemented only on whim or by certain individuals. All of the above situations reduce the effectiveness of policies, decrease respect for management personnel and cause conflict between personnel.

The actual content of a policy or procedure may cause problems and frequently explains inconsistent implementation. If a policy interferes with day to day supervision or causes frequent frustration for, either employees or supervisors, it needs to be analyzed and reviewed with the staff whom it affects and then changed accordingly.

Finally, the wording of policies is crucial. They must be clear and concise in order for the reader to understand the intent. Wordiness and imprecise words can easily result in unclear meanings and a variety of interpretations. It helps to have an outsider read your policies in order to prevent wording like this: "Emergency Exit, do not use under any circumstances" (a sign at an automotive factory). The way a policy is stated is also important. Because health care organizations have historical roots from both the church and the military, there is a frequent tendency to make dogmatic statements that sound very much like military orders. Administrators and supervisors should select their language carefully in order to guard against this pitfall because it can produce both resistance and resentment on the part of personnel.

While all personnel policies and procedures have a collective influence on personnel, certain ones are particularly important and may even provide grist for union organizing in some cases. In fact, one segment of the literature suggests that poor institutional personnel policies and practices, is the single most important factor in attracting unions. The same discontent that makes some employees seek unionization of course makes other employees leave an organization. The following policies have been selected for discussion because of the strong influence of these issues: paid time away from work (holidays, vacation and sick leave), disciplinary measures, handling grievances, and compensation.

DEFINITIONS

Before we discuss specific policies, it is important to define our terms. All too frequently, a policy is confused with a rule, a procedure or a regulation. The following definitions will help the reader to think through the differences:

DIRECTIVE. A directive describes a specific course of action for a one-time event. For instance when a patient unit closes for some reason, a directive is required to establish a system for moving patients and supplies.

Directives are misused when they describe new rules, policies or procedures for repeated use. They are then lost and rarely incorporated into the general policy manual.

RULE. A rule describes a required course of action in a given situation. Rules do not allow for individual judgment. "No smoking" in certain areas or in the presence of oxygen are examples. Because of the rigidity of rules, it is best to use them only when necessary and to have as few as possible.

REGULATION. A regulation describes a course of action required by law.

PROCEDURE. A procedure describes the steps in performing a task. Filling out organizational forms and performing passive range of motion exercises are examples.

POLICY. A policy describes a recommended course of action for carrying out an organizational goal.

"Recommended" is the key word in this definition. A policy allows for individual judgment in determining the appropriateness and method of an action in different situations. In general, the purposes of policies are to (1) convey the thinking of management in order to assist middle management and other employees in their daily activities, (2) express and guide the implementation of organizational goals and (3) provide information and reference material for employees.

In practice, however, most policies have both guidelines for action and some rules. As you read the following policies try to identify the rules imbedded in each policy, so that you understand which statements allow for flexibility and those that do not.

FORMAT FOR WRITING POLICIES

When policies are written, they need to have a consistent and easily readable format. Generous use of headings and subheadings are important for easy reference, especially for someone who merely wants to look up one part of a policy or just the procedure for carrying it out.

Title

The title should describe the subject of the policy as clearly as possible. For example, a policy entitled Passing Water could mean passing drinking water to patients, or it could mean helping paraplegics to pass urine while on a bladder training program. In one organization, the policy entitled Passing Water meant the latter. This kind of surprise content is found more frequently than one would like to think.

Purpose

Every policy should begin with a purpose. This has several functions. First, it forces the management of an organization to think through why a policy exists. Is it needed at all? If things are done "just because it says so," there may be less enthusiasm for carrying it out. It also helps administration to evaluate each policy to see if it actually carries out its purpose.

Secondly, it provides a mind set for the reader before he or she starts to read the policy. It provides some understanding of the thinking behind it and will seem a more reasonable thing to do. The stated purpose should reflect administration's beliefs and position on a particular subject.

Third, policies should rarely result from a one-time incident or situation. An outside reader can identify these because they are so obviously developed in lieu of counseling an individual staff member in a particular situation. Policies should guide behavior for all employees. If it is developed because one employee or one supervisor did not do something properly, it can insult other employees.

Policy

There are usually multiple facets to a policy. In other words, there are sub-policies to an overall policy and they usually cluster around several aspects of the policy. This is handled by the use of headings. Organizing ideas under headings is illustrated in some of the sample policies on the following pages.

Procedure

Many policies stand alone and have no accompanying procedure. For example, there may be a policy that all employees use the parking lot in the rear of the building. There is no need for a procedure. However, if a policy requires all employees to use a time clock, a procedure may be needed to tell employees what to do if they make a mistake, forget to punch in and out or become ill at work. This author recommends that if a procedure relates directly to a policy, it should accompany that policy rather than be placed in a separate Procedure Book.

SOME SAMPLE POLICIES

Grievances

Most personnel directors agree that an ideal grievance policy probably does not exist. There are two principal reasons for this. First, no grievance policy can possibly anticipate the great variety of gripes, conflicts, complaints and offended feelings that are usually lumped under the rubric, grievances. In addition to the policy itself and the nature of a grievance, the attitude of those implementing the policy strongly influences the outcome. In spite of these problems, it is essential to have some mechanism for both surfacing and resolving employee problems.

Not having a grievance policy can merely provide another reason for someone to join the ranks of terminating employees. It is also known that when organizational discontent is exhibited by turnover, and there is no way of airing conflicts, union organizing is a distinct possibility.

The purpose of a grievance policy is to provide a formalized method of upward communication of a problem. If a lower level of management blocks or does not resolve a problem, it allows review of the matter by persons who are further removed from the immediate situation. The following policy and procedure is one way of accomplishing this.

Grievance Policy

I. Purpose: To provide a mechanism for resolving problems and misunderstandings between management and employees or pool personnel in a fair and equitable manner.

II. Policy: Each employee shall be afforded the opportunity to express grievances without fear of retribution or termination. If the employee does not feel that the problem has been resolved to his/her satisfaction, he/she shall have the opportunity to request that it be presented to a higher level of management.

III. Procedure:

   A. Grievances should first be discussed with the immediate supervisor.

   *B. If the immediate supervisor does not resolve the grievance to the employee's satisfaction within five days, the employee may direct the grievance in writing to the administrator.

   C. After receiving the written grievance, the administrator shall meet in person with the employee and the supervisor together or individually, and present a written decision to the employee and the supervisor within five days.

   D. If the employee is still not satisfied, he/she may present the issue to the Grievance Committee, which will be composed of:
one board member
one employee representative selected by employees
one person selected by the person presenting the grievance
one department head selected by the department head involved.

   E. The Grievance Committee's decision shall be final.

Discipline

Disciplinary action can be a source of much friction between employees and supervisors if it is not dealt with consistently for all employees. In addition, employees need to know what constitutes unacceptable behavior. Therefore, a disciplinary action policy needs to be well thought out and clearly written. It is recommended that such a policy be checked by an attorney so that it is consistent with the many labor laws that govern employment practices.

---

* In larger institutions, there may be other levels of redress, such as the department head or personnel director, before it is taken to the administrator.

Disciplinary Action

PURPOSE. To protect the welfare of and property owned by patients/ residents, families, visitors, personnel, and the organization.

POLICY.

1. The disciplinary procedure will be initiated for the following reasons:
    a. Performance—the inability or failure to perform assigned tasks or to follow departmental rules.
    b. Absenteeism
    Irregular or excessive absenteeism
    Being absent for one or more days without notifying the immediate supervisor
    Giving false excuse for absenteeism when sick time is paid.
    c. Misuse, damage, or theft of property owned by the facility, patients, visitors, or other employees.
    d. Falsifying facility records such as time cards, resident records, application forms, health records, etc.
    e. Verbal or physical abuse of patient/residents, other personnel, or visitors.
    f. Unbecoming behavior such as use of alcohol or other chemicals on the job, possession of illegal narcotics on facility property or reporting to work under the influence of alcohol or illegal narcotics, or fighting on the premises.
2. Levels of Disciplinary action:
    a. Disciplinary probation or extended probation period may be instituted to enable an employee another opportunity to demonstrate fitness for his/her position. This action will depend upon the circumstances in the individual situation, the employee's previous record and any special factors that may be pertinent.
    b. Suspension without accrual of benefits will be instituted when (1) no improvement or minimal improvement results from disciplinary probation, (2) during an investigative period or when discharge is under consideration, and (3) immediately in the case of intoxication, drug induced behavior, or alcoholic odor.
    c. Discharge may be immediate and with forfeiture of accrued time in the following instances:
    Unauthorized possession of deadly weapons.
    Unauthorized possession, use, or sale of narcotics, barbiturates, or any habit-forming or controlled substance.
    Fighting.
    Physical or verbal abuse of patients/residents or other staff.

Theft.

Conduct or actions which might endanger patients, visitors or hospital personnel.

Willful damage or destruction of hospital property.

Insubordination.

Falsifying patient records.

Falsifying personal records.

Sleeping while on duty.

Two (2) occurrences of "No Call–No Show."

PROCEDURE (except in the case of immediate discharge)

Note: May be initiated at any point in the procedure depending upon the nature of the infraction.

1. Counseling by supervisor who places a report of the incident and conference in the employee's personnel file.
2. Counseling and written warning of suspension or discharge notice to employee and copy for employee's personnel file.
3. Suspension for three to five days without pay for review of incident(s) for consideration of immediate discharge or permission to return to work.
4. Discharge in the event of repeated events, multiple infractions or unsatisfactory outcome of the above steps.

CONSIDERATIONS FOR OTHER POLICIES

Wages and Salary

While it has been clearly demonstrated that people do not rate money as their primary incentive for work, especially in health care occupations, salary and/or wages can obviously deter or encourage workers. High pay rarely holds someone in an unsatisfactory work situation or job, just as low pay rarely causes someone to quit who is well satisfied. Again, this is just one of many factors to be considered in trying to maintain a stable staff.

Compensation management should be studied in detail elsewhere. However, it would be remiss not to discuss a few guidelines that relate pay to attracting qualified personnel.

First of all, administrators must carefully review their wage and salary schedules and benefit packages. The following questions are basic to beginning such a review:

1. How many positions in my organization begin at the minimum rate required by law? Since this is also required of all competitors, it should be examined in terms of any position that is difficult to fill. Entry wages may be an obstacle.

2. How many positions are currently open? Is this fairly usual? Are the same positions usually open? If the number and kind of job openings are fairly constant, the wage and salary structure should be examined.

3. How does this organization compare to similar organizations in the community? Do wages contribute to the reasons for resignations? Every health care organization must stay informed of how its pay scales compare with comparable jobs and similar organizations in the community. The Employment Office in most states provides regional data that describes salary ranges for major occupational groups. Many organizations do their own surveys, either formally or informally, and some professional associations have such information available.

One large nursing home regularly had about 90 openings among 400 positions. This situation obviously mitigated against a stable work force, locating competent staff and the ability to provide quality of care. After considerable study, the organization discovered its starting salaries were in the lowest quartile in that community for similar positions.

In another instance, an administrator attempted to justify noncompetitive wage scales by saying, "If they just work for money, then we don't want them." His lack of understanding of employee motivation and competitive job opportunities perpetuates a chronic staff shortage. First of all, health care organizations are indeed lucky. If most of their employees "just worked for money," they would have to close down. Second, research in this area clearly reveals that health care workers place money about sixth or seventh among their reasons for staying in a job. In large metropolitan areas, applicants can usually choose between several very fine organizations. One could hardly expect a potential employee to select the lowest paying organization for an employer. If an organization becomes complacent because of its philosophy and goals, it will lose good employees and thus strengthen one's competitors.

4. Is the wage structure designed to encourage tenure? If an employee likes a job, he or she is more likely to leave if the top of the pay scale is reached in two or three years. A minimum and maximum wage level for each job level is essential. The range between the two must be wide enough to provide some incentive for an employee to stay. Some organizations have as much as a 30 percent range between minimum and maximum salaries.

The timing of wage increases must be spread over a period of years. Some organizations give rather substantial raises during the first year, then taper off rather drastically and sometimes even stop after three or four years. Some organizations take into account ten to fifteen years of employment. In addition, most experts recommend that the increases become greater toward the end of the time frame rather than early in the schedule. In addition, experienced new employees may enter somewhere midway in the scale.

Finally, do **all** employees receive regular raises or are they tied to performance standards? Good employees deserve financial recognition.

5. Do jobs with similar requirements for education, experience, hours to be worked and job stress have the same pay scales? For instance, should the dietary aid, the housekeeping aid and the nursing assistant all have the same pay schedules? Should the Director of Nursing receive more pay than the Social Worker because the size of the staff and budget is greater? In other words, on what basis have wage differentials been determined? While there are probably no precise answers to these questions, it is imperative that administrators think through these issues in order to provide a defensible rationale for decisions in these matters.

6. What benefit package is provided employees? Does it compare to competitive organizations? Overall, benefits range from 20 percent to 40 percent of the annual salary depending on the size of the organization. Benefit packages may include paid holiday and vacation time, hospital, medical and dental insurance, retirement plans, group life insurance, educational stipends, as well as the availability of savings plans and profit sharing.

In summary, adequate wages and benefits are critical to (1) attracting competent employees to an organization, (2) keeping competent employees and (3) reducing competition from other organizations. While adequate pay scales will not substitute for other organization deficiencies, they will contribute to the hygiene of the work environment and not be a source of dissatisfaction.

Paid Time Away From Work

Time away from work is paid by an organization when employees take vacation, holiday and sick time. Vacation and holiday time can be scheduled, but sick time usually comes up unexpectedly and is rarely scheduled. In addition, most organizations find, or at least suspect, that sick time is frequently abused by one or two day absences which are taken to fulfill personal or psychological needs. While this may arise from legitimate needs, personnel policies often leave employees no other option but to call in sick when fatigue, the need for personal time or family pressures accumulate. For this reason, some organizations do not pay for one, two or three day absences in order to discourage their frequency. However, this penalizes someone who gets a migraine headache or twenty-four hour flu and tends to encourage employees to come to work when they might spread colds or flu. In addition, it penalizes conscientious workers who do not use sick days indiscriminately.

Several systems have been initiated to encourage employees to use sick leave more discriminately and to reduce one and two day absences. Before starting such a program, it is critical to calculate the cost of absenteeism and sick leave (the cost paid to sick employees plus the cost of replacing the sick employee, added overtime or the use of an employment agency). Then a new system can be evaluated accurately when it is initiated. One hospital did just that. Its absentee rate went from 3.9 percent to 2.1 percent in one year when employees received a bonus every six months if one day illnesses were reduced to one in that period. They estimate that this saved about $34,000. The cost of their innovative policy was $30,000 compared to an estimated cost of $64,000, had their former sick leave policy remained in effect.

Another system is to bundle holiday time, accrued vacation time, and a certain amount of eligible sick leave into one unit of paid leave. This is some-times referred to as "employee incentive time." Each employee accumulates a bank of paid leave days and hours which he or she can then use when the individual chooses. That way, paid time off is never classified as vacation, sick time, or holiday time. It is simply paid leave time.

Whether an organization decides to have a separate sick, holiday, and vacation policy or one that bundles one or all of these, clear definitions are necessary. Whatever system an organization adopts, definitions of full-time and part-time are necessary. Beyond that, the employee needs answers to many questions. How do I handle my time card when I am sick or on vaca-tion? How is my vacation and sick time calculated? What are the limits on accumulating sick and vacation tine? When do I need a doctor's permit to leave and/or return to work in case of a prolonged illness? Fair treatment of all employees results from clear policy statements.

Harassment and Discrimination in the Workplace

There are two main kinds of harassment, sexual and ethnic or religious. Unfortunately, harassment occurs in our society but when it occurs in the workplace, there are laws prohibiting it. Therefore, clear policies must be in place to help prevent occurrences and all management levels must be aware of possible problems and be sensitive to the hesitancy of victims to come for-ward. Parenthetically, an internal grievance policy is not adequate to address harassment.

Sexual harassment is exemplified by unwelcome sexual propositions, offensive touching, and explicit jokes and pictures. Sexual harassment may occur with same sex and opposite sex encounters. Ethnic and religious harass-ment is exemplified by ethnic slurs, demeaning remarks, overt gestures, and threatening physical conduct.

Not only managers, but all personnel need to be alert to potential problems. Beyond that, a harassed individual needs to know where to go in such an eventuality. The person's supervisor may be the obvious one to report to, but that may not be appropriate or comfortable in many cases. As a result, one or two designated investigators in the organization need to be known and available.

Any incident should be investigated immediately when it is reported. The possible victim needs to be assured confidentiality and guaranteed there will be no retaliation for reporting an episode. It is sometimes wise to suspend the accused employee while the investigation is going on. During the investigation, the administrator may want to consult with the facility's own attorney and/or the local E.E.O.C. office. If an incident is found to be harassment, the offending employee may receive a written reprimand, a warning that a second incident will mean termination, or immediate termination of employment may be warranted.

As a last resort, a person subjected to harassment may file a charge at the nearest E.E.O.C. office. This outcome may be avoided if an employer has an effective and clearly communicated policy and procedure addressing harassment and if the complaint was dealt with in a timely fashion and done thoroughly and fairly. Harassment is prohibited by law and employees must understand the consequences of not respecting the right of coworkers.

SUMMARY

This chapter has been concerned with selected human resource management policies and procedures. Both research and experience have shown that these policies are especially important to healthy employee relations.

REFERENCES

Herzberg, F. (1976). *The managerial choice: To be efficient and to be human*. Homewood, IL: Dow Jones–Irwin.

Mathis, R.L., & Jackson, J.H. (1991). Personnel/human resource management (6th ed., ch. 13 and 14). St. Paul, MN: West Publishing.

U.S. O.E.O.C. (2001). www.eeoc.gov/facts/fs-relig_ethnic.html, October 16.

Chapter 11

STAFF DEVELOPMENT

RUTH STRYKER

A good staff development program has always been an important element of a quality organization. Today, however, it has become critical to staff performance on a daily basis. This does not mean that classes are held daily, but it does mean that informal teaching is going on daily. It also means that some lower level staff need to be prepared and brought into the teaching (becoming role models at the very least) of peers.

There are basically three levels of staff education. The first is that which takes place outside the facility, including the range of licenses, certifications, and degrees that people earn at vocational settings, colleges, and universities. The second is the indoctrination and introduction of a new employee to a specific setting at a particular facility. The third level is that of ongoing improvement of staff. The latter may mean presentation of new knowledge that comes to a field, development of staff a step further than his or her traditional role, or all that is required to bring workers from foreign countries together to form a working team.

Introduction to a job must be done in the facility. However, staff development is usually done both inside and outside the facility. This implies that the staff development director must be aware of the community resources available for his or her current needs.

The highest rate of turnover occurs during the first three months of employment. This is true of hospitals, nursing homes, and business organizations. Most evidence points toward two principal causes, (1) selection of the wrong person for the job and (2) the training and manner in which a new employee is introduced to the workplace. Turnover after the first three months is more likely to be caused by other factors such as how the employee is treated by the immediate supervisor, the need for extra assistance, the way a team functions, and other factors that affect the person's comfort level

152

at work. This chapter will deal with assisting the new employee to stay rather than leave the organization.

INTRODUCTION TO THE FACILITY

The literature gives us many clues about the reasons for breakdown in employee-employer relations during the early months of employment. The endeavor to match organizational goals and values with employee goals and values is not an easy task, nor is it achieved overnight. Some researchers refer to this element as congruence or agreement of goals by both parties. This is one aspect of the process of assimilating a new person into an organization. Perhaps a more important and often overlooked aspect of job introduction relates to the socialization process. Work is not performed in a social vacuum especially for minorities and foreign-born. Therefore, far greater attention needs to be given to this basic human need on the job.

Graen and Ginsburgh introduced another way of looking at this issue. They not only examined role orientation (the tasks and work itself), but leader acceptance of the new employee also. Both were related to the assimilation process and both affected turnover.

If the greatest amount of turnover occurs during the first three months of employment, then it behooves administrators to examine organizational dynamics during this period. In other words, what in the system produces this undesired outcome? The following discussion of the practical aspects of the assimilation process is based on some of the things that are known about (1) agreement on goals and values, (2) social aspects of work, (3) job and role orientation, and (4) acceptance of the new employee by the leader.

Orientation is the first step toward retention. It requires two basic aspects; one, that given to all employees and second, that part which is planned for a specific individual. For example, if you have just employed a new inexperienced nursing assistant, she will require a great deal of on-the-job training and assistance, especially during the first six weeks of employment. If at the same time, you have also employed a nursing assistant who has worked in the same capacity at another organization for five years, her training needs will obviously differ. In other words, an employee's orientation must be individually planned around the knowledge and experience he or she brings to the organization.

The quality of the initial job experience communicates a great deal about an organization. It sets the tone. It will promote displeasure with, indifference toward or regard for the organization. The outcome in terms of length of employment and job satisfaction is greatly influenced by this introduction.

If negative experiences continue to dominate, leaving is an almost predictable outcome. If positive experiences predominate, the individual is likely to stay.

Orientation is comprised of several aspects. First of all, it must include an introduction to the physical environment. This means a general tour of the building so that the individual knows the general layout. The tour should emphasize obvious personal needs, such as the location of lockers, bathrooms, dining rooms, time clock, etc. It should be followed by a more in depth acquaintance with the immediate work area and with any equipment that will be used.

In addition to the physical environment, every new employee must be introduced to the people in the work environment, both employees and residents. In one's own home, you would not think of bringing in a stranger without introducing that person to anyone who lived or worked there. It is the same in a health care organization.

Orientation must also include a description of the routines with which the employee will be working. What are the meal hours for both residents and employees? What about coffee breaks? If the individual is in the housekeeping department, when is it appropriate to clean a patient's room and when should it be postponed? If the new person is a dietary worker, when are food trays prepared, delivered, collected, etc.? The new employee needs to know what the rhythm of his or her day will be.

Employees must be introduced to procedures and equipment in a planned systematic manner. If the job description is accurate, it will identify the needed content. Teaching should be spaced over a period of time so that learning occurs gradually. Too much, too soon is not only overwhelming; it is ineffective. Two hour segments are recommended. Selected resources such as books from the library and procedure books from the station or office should be provided. Time to review them at the individual's own pace needs to be planned into the first few weeks of employment.

Every new employee should be immediately assigned to work with an experienced employee during the first week or so. This is sometimes called the buddy or hostess system. Whatever you choose to call it, it allows the new person to identify with one person as a helper. This arrangement could mean days, weeks, and sometimes months to work up to full speed or quality. The system provides someone nearby to answer questions until the job feels comfortable to the employee and until it is done well from the supervisor's viewpoint. This does not mean that two people are doing one job constantly; it means that a specific individual is designated to assist the new employee in addition to the supervisor.

The buddy system is also a way to recognize experienced employees with good work performance. Some organizations pay a slightly higher hourly rate for this recognition, while others merely use it to demonstrate confidence in the individual. The buddy must be carefully selected, as it is just as easy to learn the wrong things as the right things, and new employees will not know the difference until they are criticized for doing something wrong. Once in a while, you will find an experienced employee who finds this a burden. If so, such an assignment should not be forced, as you may lose the very employee you want to keep. In most instances, however, this responsibility is sought after when it is approached properly.

The buddy system does not absolve the supervisor or department head of responsibility to the new employee. It is simply a back up system which helps the employee to become assimilated into the work group (something that a supervisor cannot do) and to feel comfortable initially. It keeps new employees from eating alone, from feeling at loose ends, and it gives them someone to identify with until their own relationships become established.

Initial work loads should be lighter than those of experienced employees. New employees need to feel a sense of accomplishment and success. They will only have a sense of frustration and defeat if they are constantly disappointed by having to skip over things while they are learning their job and getting a feel for organizing their work.

A Negative Case in Point

This is the description of one nursing assistant's experience in a large metropolitan area nursing home of 150 beds.

> I came on duty on my first day of employment at 3:00 PM. When I arrived at the nursing station, a stranger told me that I was assigned to six residents. She pointed in the direction of their rooms and walked away. No one introduced me to the staff or the residents. I then went to each resident and introduced myself because I thought that seemed like the thing to do. Throughout the evening, I had to ask each resident how to take care of them–things like, which is the best side for me to stand on when you get up? where is the dining room where you eat? what time do you like to go to bed? etc. I thought it was terrible that I had to learn what to do from the residents themselves.

This nursing assistant's prior nursing home experiences had been positive, so that she was completely unprepared for this introduction to her new job. She resigned after six weeks because (1) the home did not seem to respect its residents (she never saw anyone visiting them unless they had some request or physical need), (2) the home placed the burden of orienting personnel to nursing care on the residents, (3) personnel did not help one another when there was a difficult situation, (4) there was no supervision of her work, and (5) there was constant bickering and tension among the staff.

I asked her what reason she gave for leaving. She told the home that her school load was heavier than anticipated, so she could not work that semester after all. If that home kept a record of leavers, they would have determined that this resignation was "employee caused," and that would have been the end of it. If that home had been aware of the need for organizational self-analysis, it would have learned something about itself. This was certainly a golden opportunity because this young woman had excellent references from her former employer and did not need theirs. Besides, as she put it, "I wouldn't even put that job down on my record because it would look like I had had trouble there. If another organization called them, they would have said that I had stayed only six weeks and that would not help me to locate another job." Fortunately, she had had a very positive experience at the home in which she worked in another state, so she simply found a home that was more like her prior employer.

This classic case demonstrates how recruiting, screening and selecting by itself has no relation to retention. This organization had found a good employee, but they did nothing to make the job or the organization attractive. They had ignored (1) the impact of anxiety-inducing job experiences and (2) the need for new employees to have time to assimilate knowledge and to integrate their personalities into a cohesive work group.

Parenthetically, the reader should know that the author was acquainted with the administrator of the organization involved in this story. This administrator explained in one of our classes that they did everything possible about their turnover problem. "We run ads regularly, pay bonuses, give teas and hire every ablebodied comer. Our hands are tied because all our leavers leave for personal reasons. Turnover is inevitable." As long as this tragic lack of administrative insight and refusal to analyze the internal causes of turnover persists, turnover will indeed be inevitable at this organization.

Supervision of the New Employee

The immediate supervisor or department head is responsible for a great deal of training, whether the organization has an inservice education director or not. The most convincing literature and research concludes that the basic integrity of the organization lies with the quality and quantity of communication at the supervisory level. The supervisor is the human resource program representative as well as the responsible manager for his or her assigned area.

The supervisor must prepare a recommended outline for orientation and initial training for each position (in his or her department) in writing. It should be based on the job description and the supervisor's knowledge of what each position entails. The written plan for orientation and initial training content should be geared to the least trained and least experienced worker who might be expected to fill a particular position. It can always be shortened for the more educated and experienced new employee. This method provides each department in the organization with a written plan that details each aspect of training. Its purpose is to prevent superficial, hit or miss teaching of new employees.

The written plan should stipulate some minimum and maximum time limits. In other words, a laundry person who folds linen should not take months to learn the job, while a new administrator may need several months, not only to learn general duties but to become acquainted with the personnel, the systems, the problems and the strengths of the organization. In neither case does it mean that the worker is totally unproductive during the early weeks of employment. It merely indicates that it takes longer to learn some things than others. One can learn and do simultaneously in many instances. Nonetheless, some outside limits for teaching and learning should be specified. This will be equally helpful to the new employee.

Once the written plan for a position is developed, it can then be discussed with a new employee and specific goals can be planned for part of each day. This may range from a few minutes to a formal class. It should be most intensive during the first week or two and gradually taper off in intensity for a period of about three months. It should never just drop off, leaving the employee to dangle. Supervision is an ongoing process which maintains and develops the staff of a particular department.

The supervisor needs an inservice educator to assist in carrying out initial training. Such backup support is essential, even if the organization is small and can only afford it part time. This position should be viewed as a key resource for all supervisors and new employees. Even when such a person is available, there is nothing he or she can do about a disruptive work situation. Training cannot assist an individual to tolerate working in a department with unfair work schedules, inefficient work loads and an untrained supervisor. The training role of the supervisor is stressed because of its critical relationship to tenure as shown by the research. Because of this emphasis, the author wishes to underscore the necessity of having an inservice educator help supervisors to plan and conduct on-the-job training. This is definitely a shared responsibility.

The following is a general guide for the first four months of employment of a nursing assistant.

First Two Weeks of Employment. This period of time might be considered a work/study period in which a new employee:

1. Receives both formal and informal instruction about the job and any equipment or procedures that are required.

2. Is assigned an hour or so for several days to read appropriate policy, equipment and procedure manuals as well as selected articles or books related to the job.
3. Is assigned to work with another employee (the hostess employee or buddy).
4. Is assigned to independent regularly scheduled work but with a somewhat reduced work load. This can be increased gradually on the basis of a decision made jointly by the employee, the supervisor, the inservice person, and perhaps the buddy.
5. Meets with the supervisor at the end of each week to determine the needs and progress of the individual.

Weeks Three Through Six. Weekly conferences with the supervisor should continue. These conferences need not be lengthy, but they should not be done on the run or in passing. The purpose of continued conferences is to identify any further learning goals, feeling of confidence, any interpersonal problems encountered, and general adjustment. They should be discussed from the point of view of both the employee and the supervisor. The supervisor's role is to support the individual, not to undermine with judgmental observations or evaluations. This can be accomplished by conveying acceptance and a desire to coach and assist in any weak areas. It also provides an opportunity to give positive comments about the quality of work done.

Early problems can be approached as goals to be achieved in the upcoming week. When conferences are regularly scheduled, the impulse to call someone in only when there is a problem is averted. There is a long-run effect of early and planned conferences; they set in motion a supervisor/subordinate relationship based on mutual interest in the person, and an interest in good work as well as poor work. This lays the ground work for better communications in the future. If the supervisor is approachable early on, the employee will feel freer to discuss problems at a later date. If adequate help is given initially and a good relationship has been launched, the employee is more likely to bring up future problems rather than let them smolder.

Weeks Seven Through Twelve. Supervisor conferences begin to taper off to two, three and then four week intervals. The general tone and purpose are the same as in previous weeks.

Weeks Thirteen Through Sixteen. These are crucial weeks, as the employee is, for the most part, left on his own. During this time, the individual comes to terms with the work group. It is now that the employee chooses friends, decides to become an informal group leader or not, notices if the supervisor has favorites and integrates his or her personal life with work. During this period, the employee decides whether there is congruence or agreement about job expectations and what the job actually offers. This is true across all job levels. For instance, if a professional person expects to use higher levels of skill than the job allows, he or she may request greater responsibility.

It is also at this time that an individual can become bored. The challenge of learning is pretty much over and the overly qualified person becomes restless. Managers should realize that a poor match of an individual's intellectual ability and ambition with the job will show up at this time. If there was a good match, the person is likely to stay. If not, the person will be looking for a new challenge and will be interested in leaving or being promoted. If the job holds little or no opportunity for promotion, the less ambitious person is probably the best choice if turnover during the third to sixth months is high. This, of course, assumes that all of the factors discussed thus far have been considered.

INSERVICE EDUCATION

During the first months of employment, the role of the inservice educator includes helping to plan orientation schedules, conducting facility tours, teaching formal classes and locating resources for the various departments. Because so many inservice positions are filled by nurses, there is a tendency to neglect the needs of other departments. However, classes on body mechanics, safety, fire and disaster procedures, confidentiality, and many other topics are needed by all employees. The job description and budget for this position should not be limited to the nursing department in any health care organization.

The inservice educator must have had or obtained some teacher training. If not, he or she will have very limited vision and skill on the job. Courses in teaching adults and leading group discussions are not difficult to locate, nor are they expensive. Nearly all area vocational schools, community colleges and state colleges and universities offer such courses. Some professional associations and the Red Cross also offer courses in some localities.

Whether the inservice department has several staff, one person full time (or part time) or shares staff with a hospital or another nursing home, such a department is essential. Not only must the educator understand how adults learn and possess some teaching skills, this person must also have knowledge of the needs of the special clientele being served.

In the case of the nursing home, knowledge about the well elderly, the physically disabled elderly, the mentally impaired elderly, rehabilitative and environmental factors must be in hand. An educator cannot be expected to be all-knowing about everything. Therefore, a major task is to know resources. These can be in the form of books, journals, audiovisual materials, persons in the community or employees within the organization.

The actual role of the educator has many facets. Some of the primary responsibilities include:

1. Assisting with work related problem solving and educational needs assessment.
2. Improving on-the-job skill and performance.
3. Developing all staff to grow with organizational changes.
4. Helping staff to understand and handle their emotional reactions to feelings of inadequacy, hopelessness, anger and grief.
5. Helping staff to accept the attitudes and feelings of others by not inflicting their values on others and yet maintain their own values. (This problem becomes especially apparent when residents are sexually active.)
6. Gathering resources for the training needs of all staff, which of course includes the needs of department heads untrained in management.
7. Orienting and participating in the teaching of all new personnel on all shifts. This implies flexible hours for this person.
8. Assist in career development and promotion of individuals who need greater personal and professional goals.

SPECIAL CONSIDERATIONS FOR A DIVERSE WORK FORCE

In many parts of the United States, the nursing home workforce is almost entirely composed of immigrants or so-called "New Americans." This brings a host of new educational and psychological demands on workers, residents, and families. To meet these challenges, the organization will need to address them in a variety of ways.

The first and most obvious difficulty is language—reading, writing, speaking, and understanding. Many applicants and employees will have to attend an English class as a Second Language (ESL) program. The administrator may wish to have ESL classes held at the facility as well as encourage the inclusion of the specific vocabulary that will be needed to work in long-term care. Immigrants are very embarrassed and fearful of being seen as not understanding their new language so they may pretend to understand, hoping that it is not important or that they can get help later. For this reason, supervisors and staff must learn to help New Americans by speaking a little slower, avoiding slang and idioms, and asking for feedback to assure understanding of what is being said to them.

The second challenge relates to cultural differences, attitudes, and beliefs about the elderly and their health problems, especially dementia. For example, caregivers from India may view mental illness as embarrassing and something that should be hidden from the public. Because India's average age at death is much younger than that of the United States, dementia in the elderly is rarely seen there, but dementia is equated with mental illness in their minds. People from some cultures place high value on caring for their aged at home and therefore believe that U.S. families are abandoning their elderly when nursing homes are used for their care. Some religions have special taboos. For example, in some Muslim cultures women are not allowed to give physical care to a man who is not a blood relative.

One of the more difficult cultural differences relates to the position of women in many of the immigrant societies where men are dominant. Because nursing home and assisted living employees are nearly all women, some immigrant men have a very difficult time taking orders from women who are in a superior work position. This often takes time and individual guidance to work through.

These differences require new understandings. This is a two-way street. The New American will have to learn to adapt but so must the facility and those who work and live there. One way to promote such accommodations is to hold classes that explore differences through discussion of other beliefs and cultures. Along with employees, families and residents can be invited to such sessions. To help New American workers adapt to their work environment, it is helpful for coworkers to develop an understanding that will be respectful, nonjudgmental, and accepting. To foster these attitudes, some facilities have culture fairs, flag displays of all the home countries, food fairs, and special articles in the facility newsletter.

When New Americans are employed, they may need to have a slower paced introduction to the facility and the workplace. They may also need mentoring over a longer period of time. The extra time and effort required for these people is very likely to be time and money well invested because most of them have a strong desire to have a job, most have a deep sense of respect for the elderly, and some women hold the belief that a position in long-term care is a career, not merely a job.

EDUCATIONAL STRATEGIES TO INCREASE EMPLOYEE TENURE

Long-term care facilities are unique in the health care system because the least skilled and lowest paid workers are the ones who spend the most time with residents and their families. In addition, the highest turnover rate is among this same group of employees. This is contrary to common sense because on the one hand a facility avows that quality care is its major goal but, on the other hand, low level workers are minimally appreciated or valued.

Many organizations are attempting to improve care, lower employee turnover, and provide more recognition to the employees on whom they most depend. Many different strategies have been reported.

Pine Valley Care Center in Richfield, Ohio developed a nursing assistant career ladder. Initially, the administrator, director of nursing, staff education director, and a nursing assistant met to analyze problems and try to find answers. They developed a three-tier ladder. Each level has a curriculum that increases the nursing assistant's knowledge about nursing care. They set measurable nursing care goals which allow workers to see the positive results of their care. With their baseline turnover rate of 82 percent in 1996, turnover went to 73 percent in 1997, 33 percent in 1998 when there was a full complement of level three workers and to 16 percent in 1999. Their success was gradual, but it was also fundamental to the goal of improving care and reducing employee turnover.

Because a large number of residents of both nursing homes and assisted living facilities have dementia, increased training of nursing assistants in the area of dementia is reported in many studies. Certified nursing assistants (CNA's), those who have had the minimum number of hours of training required by federal regulations in addition to whatever number of additional hours required by a particular state, are still unprepared to cope with the more severely demented residents whom they will encounter. Those who received additional training in understanding dementia, learning how to redirect difficult behaviors, new strategies to perform ADL's, and better communication methods had reduced stress and lowered turnover (Grant et al.).

Grant et al. also found that a variety of training methods (films, videos, reading materials, role playing, use of outside and in-house experts) was particularly beneficial to the nursing assistant group. Greater knowledge leads to other ways of empowering and enhancing the self-esteem and role of the nursing assistant. Nursing assistants become part of the care team and have a say in the way residents are cared for. It is regrettable that nursing assistants, even those who have not had additional training, are not used more often to help determine care needs. Who knows better how to describe what an individual resident needs and wants than the person who is with the resident the most time? Chapter 5, Developing the Management Team, discusses this aspect of training further.

In addition, more radical restructuring of jobs has been attempted. There is the "single task employee" who is minimally trained to do only nonnursing and nonmedical tasks to assist other staff. This is a little like waiter assistants in restaurants who only fill water glasses and clear away dirty dishes.

At the other extreme is the "universal worker," one who is prepared to give total care to a resident. This concept is based on the Swedish Service House. Caregivers are generalists who give direct care, prepare meals, do laundry and housekeeping, and arrange social and leisure activities for one or two residents (see Chapter 18 for more details).

PERFORMANCE APPRAISAL

The purpose of performance appraisal is to improve the job performance of employees. It is a part of staff development, but is seldom thought of as such. However, personnel experts agree that many systems fall short of this goal, mainly because they so often place the supervisor in the untenable position of judging the worth of subordinates. This aspect of conventional appraisal programs produces widespread uneasiness on the part of both the employee to be evaluated and the person doing the evaluation.

The performance appraisal system in many organizations is detrimental to employee relations. At best, it usually does nothing to enhance supervisor subordinate relationships. Both parties usually dread the process, but many reasons for this are correctable. First, supervisors do not like to use trait-based evaluation forms because they criticize the person instead of setting clear performance goals. Second, supervisors are frequently untrained in the appraisal process. Third, the employee is not involved in the process. Perhaps using the term, performance analysis, would make the task less onerous.

A sounder approach places some responsibility on the subordinate for identifying new performance goals. These might include areas of new learning and growth that are desired by the worker. He or she might suggest ways of accomplishing and assessing progress of those goals. In addition, the employee might identify obstacles in the work environment that affect work performance negatively or positively. A supervisor should be looking for ways to assist workers and a performance appraisal meeting is a good opportunity to probe for ideas to improve the work climate.

There should be no surprises when the formal annual performance conference takes place. If a problem arises, it needs to be dealt with at the time, not months later. Throughout the year, expressions of appreciation for a job well done should be expressed spontaneously and with some frequency.

The attainment of optimum performance by an employee involves factors within that individual *and* those in the organization. While an individual's ability affects performance, there is little he or she can do about that; other factors are within the person's control, however. By the same token, the job structure and organizational relationships are within the control of the organization. Therefore, a manager who appraises an employee must appraise all of the factors, including his or her influence in relation to an individual employee's performance on the job.

In general, there is no known panacea for performance appraisal. However, most systems can be improved by addressing three of the most commonly found problems:

1. There should be frequent feedback, not just in the form of an annual evaluation. Any feedback that tends to discourage, alienate or patronize should be avoided. Praise motivates better than criticism.

2. Keep the approach to evaluation future-oriented rather than rehashing the past. Positive suggestions from both the supervisor and the subordinate for future goals and ways of accomplishing them should be emphasized. Remember, the vast majority of employees want to perform at their highest capacity and to take pride in their work.

3. The appraisal form itself should not contain trait-oriented items that require subjective judgments that tend to insult rather than instruct. The form should contain observable objective and measurable performance standards TAKEN FROM THE JOB DESCRIPTION.

A recommended approach to performance appraisal is that of the Work Plan & Review (WPR). There are variations on implementation, but the major thrust is to make it a joint planning session with the involvement of both the supervisor and subordinate. In order to accomplish this, five steps are recommended.

Step 1–Together, both should review the job description to make sure that there is agreement on the major areas of responsibility and accountability. Step 2–The employee sets performance targets for the next few months or year. Step 3–The employee again meets with the supervisor to discuss these targets and they select ways of measuring progress. Step 4–Checkpoints for measuring progress are established. Step 5–They meet at the end of the period to discuss the results of the targeted goals. The process can then be repeated.

Properly executed, performance appraisals can become a useful management tool. While the major purpose is employee development, they can also help to identify persons for promotion, demotion, transfer and executive development. They can be used by the training director to identify training needs, and finally, they can help to identify persons for merit raises, special bonuses and special recognition.

SUMMARY

Once the organization has recruited, screened, and selected the best, or perhaps the most appropriate person for a particular position, it is incumbent on the inservice educator and the supervisor to plan and provide the best possible work environment for learning. While this should involve the input of an inservice educator, the primary focus should be on the application of learning to the job. Close supervision during the early weeks and months of employment are crucial if the organization wishes to retain its employees during the highest turnover period, the first three months. These measures, along with ongoing inservice education, will reduce the amount of job stress and anxiety and tend to increase both tenure and organizational commitment of employees. Finally, a good performance appraisal system will help to develop individual employees to their fullest capacity. The ultimate goal of course is to engage the total organization in providing high quality care to residents.

REFERENCES

Beck, C. et al. (1999). Enabling and empowering certified nursing assistants for quality dementia care. *International Journal of Geriatric Psychiatry, 14,* 197.

Gipson, G. (1999). Building a network of stayers. *Contemporary Long Term Care,* May.

Graen, G., & Ginsburgh, S. (1977). Job resignation as a function of role orientation and leader acceptance: A longitudinal investigation of organizational acceptance. *Organizational Behavior and Human Performance, 19,* 1.

Grant, L. et al. (1996). Staff training and turnover in Alzheimer's special care units: Comparisons with non-special care units. *Geriatric Nursing, 17*(6), 278, November/December.

Hoban, S. (2001). Recruit, retain, reward. *Nursing Homes,* p. 20, April.

How we developed a nursing assistant career ladder. *Nursing Homes,* p. 53, March 2000.

Jung, F. (1991). Teaching registered nurses how to supervise nursing assistants. *Journal of Nursing Administration, 21*(4), 32, April.

McGillis-Hall, L., & O'Brien-Pallas, L. (2000). Redesigning nursing work in long-term care environments. *Nursing Economics, 18*(2), 79.

Mass, M. et al. (1994). Training, key to job satisfaction. *Journal of Long-Term Care Administration, 22,* 23.

Performance appraisal series. *Harvard Business Review,* 1972 and 1982.

Chapter 12

MONITORING AND EVALUATING
HRM PRACTICES

Ruth Stryker

It is essential that the administrator use data from all available sources in order to have adequate information for sound decision making. Many sources of information can provide the administrator with important organizational insights.

First of all, it is critical to assure the organization's compliance with the many Fair Labor standards, Equal Employment Opportunity legislation, Right to Know laws, the Disability Act and many others. Your state Department of Labor and professional association will supply up-to-date details of these laws.

To better understand employee perceptions about an organization, an employee satisfaction survey can be useful if the responses guarantee anonymity. Items about the organization, the job, supervision, pay, training, benefits, co-workers, etc. should be included. This assessment tool is sometimes painful, so it is easy to become defensive. If that is management's reaction, then the survey can do more harm than good. On the other hand, if the findings are taken seriously enough to create organizational changes, it can be of benefit.

The administrator will certainly want to know the costs of recruiting, selection, screening, training, sick time, overtime, and employee pools. The cost of Worker's Compensation insurance might be reduced by reviewing employee accident reports. What can be prevented by better training, better equipment, and an improved safety program? Does sick time reflect fatigue from small injuries that go unreported because they are barely noticed? For instance, repeated lifting may cause a small weakening of back muscles on a daily basis until a more acute strain occurs and is reported. To reduce back injuries, some nursing homes require all direct care personnel to wear a back support in addition to teaching proper body mechanics, using a gait or transfer belt and doing warm-up exercises before giving cares.

Many resident incidents and complaints uncover personnel needs. They may reveal a need for training, attention to safety, counseling of thoughtless employees or even demonstrate the need for a new resident program.

Both the number and content of employee complaints and grievances should be approached with the attitude that they will help to understand personnel feelings and perceptions about the organization. Complaints of favoritism, lack of consideration of employees, broken promises etc. should be taken very seriously. While these problems usually seem like opening a can of worms, dealing with them openly and fairly can often correct a long-standing issue that has exasperated personnel for months or even years. Allowing problems to fester is poor management.

THE IMPLICATIONS OF TURNOVER

The employee turnover rate is one of the best information tools for evaluating a human resource management program. Along with knowing the stability, wastage, and absentee rates of employees, the administrator can identify the strengths and weaknesses of human resource management in the organization.

First of all, it is important to know how much turnover is avoidable. If turnover is over 20 or 25 percent, there undoubtedly is avoidable turnover. Because nursing homes have a greater proportion of nonprofessional employees compared to hospitals, nursing homes will usually have a somewhat higher turnover rate than hospitals. That is because professional employees tend to have lower turnover rates in almost all occupations, and there are proportionately more of them in hospitals. Therefore, a 20 to 25 percent turnover rate would be considered high for a hospital but only borderline high for a nursing home.

High turnover is organizationally caused in spite of the reasons employees give for leaving. Therefore, rather than excusing it, administrators and department heads need to identify the causes and attend to those causes appropriately.

Many years ago, Asis concluded that 65 percent of all turnover is avoidable. When this author studied turnover a decade later. 75 percent was classified as avoidable (in 25 nursing homes) and 25 percent was thought to be unavoidable. Unavoidable turnover might include family relocation, change in marital status, or a serious personal or family illness. More recent studies have remarkably similar findings; namely, at least two-thirds of nursing home turnover is avoidable. This should be encouraging because it means that there is something managers can do about over 65 percent of their turnover.

In your home, why do personnel leave? It is imperative to find out. Whether you inquire through exit interviews by someone removed from the immediate work situation or by an anonymous followup letter, it is crucial information that can help to select some administrative interventions. Remember, many employees will be reluctant to give their real reasons for leaving if they fear a poor recommendation. However, if one continues to ask enough leavers, real reasons and some consistency may emerge.

Usually voluntary or avoidable separations leave for more than one reason. Reflect back on some job that you left. It is quite likely the factors in the situation "piled up" before you made the decision to resign. Your employees are no different. For instance, a dietary aide may first find that she had to learn the job the "hard way"; then find that the supervisor has favorites when it comes to assigning undesirable hours; discovers that there is so much bickering among staff that she tries to stay aloof from the others; and finally decides to quit when the supervisor bawls her out in front of the cook for something that she had never been told about; in addition, the pay was low. When such a person is asked to give the reason for leaving, he or she may say "to seek a better job," to "earn more money" or any number of other fairly acceptable reasons. A well conducted exit interview will attempt to uncover as many reasons for leaving as possible.

Exit interviews are not necessary for every departing employee. For instance, if the dietary department has a high turnover rate regularly each quarter, problems obviously exist. When this occurs, interview at least one departing employee in depth and with honesty and candor. You might say, "I am concerned about the high turnover in our dietary department. There are obviously some problems that I should know more about in order to deal with them better." Perhaps state that you want to improve the situation so that the organization does not lose persons with this person's qualities. This approach is likely to produce a fairly honest response, as the employee will be less fearful of a poor letter of reference.

For instance, if only 16 percent leave for personal reasons, this may be a part of unavoidable turnover, but if 41 percent leave for personal reasons, one might question if the screening interview was done well or if the real reason was not obtained. If 19 percent leave because of job competition, it may be caused by upward mobility and better salary and benefits elsewhere; but if 40 percent leave for this reason, one may need to examine the organization's hour, wage and benefit schedules, personnel policies, etc. The number of persons who return to school of course indicates the number of school-age employees who are hired. In order to regulate this, one might wish to place a ceiling on the number of positions to be filled by this part of the labor pool.

Job-caused terminations and discharges are more obviously related to organizational problems. Both reasons particularly relate to the screening interview, realistic statements of job expectations, salaries, quality of induction to the organization and supervision on the job.

The first step is to look at the organization as a whole and then at each department. Monitoring absenteeism, turnover, wastage and stability of personnel is a management information tool. It can be used to diagnose certain organizational ailments. It needs to be done quarterly, not just occasionally. It must be done by department and/or unit and shift, not just for the entire organization.

What can be learned from this management data? First, it identifies trouble spots in the organization. If most problems are in one department, one section of a large department, on one shift, or among one classification of employees, it is possible to know where to begin. After that, changes can be tracked. The administrator can then share information with the appropriate department heads who will bring their observations and proceed with their responsibilities in the matter. It is at this point that the management team can problem solve together.

CALCULATING INDICATORS

How do you calculate these indicators? The following are commonly used formulas.

Turnover Rate:

$$\frac{\text{no. of leavers during the quarter}}{\text{*average no. on payroll for quarter}} \times 100 = \text{rate for quarter}$$

Example:

$$\frac{\text{no. of leavers } 10/1 \text{ through } 12/31 = 40}{200(10/1) + 196(11/1) + 198(12/1) = 594 \div 3 = 198(\text{av. no. on payroll } 10/1\text{-}12/31)}$$

$$\frac{40}{198} = .202 \times 100 = 20.2\% \text{ T.O. rate } 10/1\text{-}12/31$$

If you wish to estimate your *annual* turnover rate, multiply the quarterly rate by 4. In this case, the estimated annual T.O. would be 80.8 percent.

The reason for calculating T.O. quarterly is to find out if you have recurring seasonal changes, to evaluate any organizational changes and to help long-range staffing plans.

---

* Calculate by adding the number on the payroll at the beginning (or end, but be consistent) of each month in the quarter and divide by 3.

There are many ways of computing turnover rates. The above formula can be used when the number of employees vary only slightly during the months that are being measured. However, for large organizations with wider fluctuations of numbers of employees, the following formula is more commonly used: In this formula:

$$T.O. = \frac{c}{\frac{a+b}{2}}$$

a = no. on payroll at the beginning of the time period being measured
b = no. on payroll at the end of the time period being measured
c = no. of separations during the time period being measured

Example:

$$\frac{125\,(\text{separations})}{\frac{650(1/1)+600(3/31)}{2}} = \frac{125}{\frac{1250}{2}} = \frac{125}{625} = .20 \times 100 = 20\%$$

Stability Rate:

$$\frac{\text{no. of persons (from below) who have been there 12 mo.}}{\text{total no. on payroll on last day of a month}} \times 100 = S.R.$$

Example:

$$\frac{60\,(\text{on payroll since }12/31/01)}{100\,\text{on payroll on }12/31/02} = 60 \div 100 = .60 \times 100 = 60\%\ S.R.$$

The stability rate tells what percent of employees have been with the organization for at least one year. The stability rate is always an annual calculation. By monitoring it quarterly, one can see whether it fluctuates with the T.O. rate and see to what extent the organizational inputs change the S.R. Remember, the stability rate actually reflects what was done six to 12 months ago.

Wastage Rate: concentrates on new employees only. Because so much research in long-term care administration suggests that most employees leave during the first three to six months of employment, it can be useful. It is calculated as follows:

$$\frac{\text{no. of newly hired who leave}}{\text{no. of newly hired}} \times 100 = W.R.$$

Example:

$$\frac{10\,(\text{from }1/31\text{-}3/31)}{25\,(\text{from }1/1\text{-}3/31)} \times 100 = 40\%$$

Absentee Rate:

Absenteeism, a less final withdrawal from an organization, is closely related to turnover. In rural areas where employment opportunities are few, absenteeism rather than turnover, may express the same employee phenomenon of discontent. It can also be very costly. The cost of overtime or replacement personnel, the decline in employee morale, work disruption and decreased productivity waste time and dollars. In many instances, it also reduces the quality of care. Every organization should monitor its absenteeism rate. This is calculated by using a formula similar to the turnover and stability rate formulae. It is as follows and can be used for whatever time period you select:

$$\frac{\text{Number of days absent}}{\text{Number of days worked}} \times 100$$

It is recommended that only the first five days of an extended absence be counted in order to prevent the figure from overrepresenting one or two persons with a lengthy illness. Most organizations attempt to approach an absence rate of around 2 percent.

In addition to keeping track of the absence rate of the organization, the frequency of absences by individuals should be examined by supervisors. Obviously one ten-day absence is very different from ten one-day absences. Supervisors should not only keep a record of absences and the reasons, but look for individual patterns (before or after a day off, after payday, on the same weekday, etc.). Individuals with such a pattern should be counseled and it should be made clear that it is disruptive to the work situation and will not be tolerated if it continues.

DATA GATHERING TOOLS

Figure 12-1 is a worksheet which details each individual termination. It is recommended that this information be gathered regularly and then compiled for a quarter at a time. It can be kept by the person who maintains your personnel records. It should be noted that if T.O. is calculated quarterly, the four quarters must be summed to obtain the annual rate.

For example:

January 1 through March 31	12%
April 1 through June 30	17%
July 1 through September 30	20%
October 1 through December 31	15%
This year's T.O. rate	64%

EMPLOYEE DATA						*TENURE*		*WORKER-CAUSED*										
								Family			Health				Competition			
NAME	Job title	Department	Age	Marital status	Shift worked	Years	Months	Moved	Married	Needed at home	Ill	Injured	Retired		Seek better job	Attend school	Transportation difficult	

Figure 12-1. Worksheet.

| JOB CAUSED | | | | | | | | | | | | | | | DISCHARGES | | | | OTHER | |
| Wage & Hours | | | | The Job | | | | | | | | | Supv. | | Con-duct | | Perfor-mance | | | |
Rate of pay	Too much overtime	Poor work environment	Unsettled grievance	Change in org.	Work too hard	Too much to learn	Too much responsibility	No security	No future	Work depressing	Work unsatisfying	Dislike supervisor	Dislike employees	Inappropriate behavior	Excessive absenteeism	Unable to learn	Poor quality work		

Figure 12-1. Worksheet (continued)

Figure 12-2 summarizes the information for a quarter. Figure 12-3 summarizes information for up to two years, enabling the manager to see trends which show the results of interventions.

WHAT CAN YOU LEARN FROM YOUR DATA?

Once you have obtained your information, what assumptions can you make from it? Because every organization has individual problems, look at the quarterly summary of two organizations.

Organization A

Department Separations		T.O. Rate
10	Nursing	17% (Nursing)
7	Dietary	35% (Dietary)
4	Housekeeping	50% (Housekeeping)
3	Activities	100% (activities)
6	All others	
30	Total	30% (120% estimate annually) based on average no. of employees = 100

Age of leavers
24	24 or under
3	25–44
1	46–64
2	65 or over

Length of stay		
21	3 mo. or less	Stability rate–45%
6	4–11 months	Wastage rate–58%
1	1–3 years	Absenteeism–5%
2	3 or more years	

Causes
4	Worker caused
7	Competition
8	Job caused
8	Discharges

What does this report tell you about Organization A? It tells a great deal, indeed. Here are a few highlights that can help you to read your own summary sheets.

DEPARTMENT	TERMINATIONS			AVERAGE NO. EMPLOYEES			TURNOVER RATE		
	Part-time	Full-time	Total	Part-time	Full-time	Total	Part-time	Full-time	Total
Nursing **Unit A** **Unit B** **Unit C**									
Dietary **Housekeeping** **Laundry** **Activities** **Office** **Maintenance** **Others**									
Total Org.									
Nursing by **Days** **Evenings** **Nights**									
Reasons **Worker caused** **Competition** **Job caused** **Discharges**									

Figure 12-2. Quarterly turnover record.

CATEGORY	81 (Q1)	81 (Q2)	81 (Q3)	81 (Q4)	82 (Q1)	82 (Q2)	82 (Q3)	82 (Q4)
DEPARTMENTAL QUITS								
Nursing								
Dietary								
Housekeeping								
P.T.								
Social Service								
Activities								
Maintenance								
Laundry								
Clerical								
Other								
TOTAL								
AGE								
25 or under								
26 - 45								
46 - 64								
65 or over								
LENGTH OF STAY								
3 mos. or less								
4 - 12 months								
13 - 35 months								
3 years or more								
NURS. JOB TITLE								
R.N.								
L.P.N.								
Nurs. Asst.								
CAUSES								
Worker Caused								
Competition								
Attend School								
Job Caused								
Discharged								
TURNOVER BY DEPT.								
Nursing								
Dietary								
Housekeeping								
QUARTER'S T.O.								
QUARTER'S S.R.								

Figure 12-3. Administrator's cumulative record of turnover.

1. With a stability rate of 45 percent (only 45% of the staff having been there for a year or more) and a T.O. rate of 120 percent, a wastage rate of 58 percent and 5 percent absenteeism, you have certain jobs turning over not, once or twice but three or four times a year in some instances.
2. This seems to be happening mostly in the dietary, housekeeping and activities departments. Note, while nursing has more separations, it has the lowest T.O. rate. You are therefore sure that your wastage rate also relates to the other three departments. What causes the high turnover in these three departments? Inadequate leadership by the department head? Informal group pressure on new employees? Inadequate standards, supervision and training? Poor selection? In other words, this tells you where to look for problems and suggests certain possibilities that the administrator and department head must discuss.
3. The many young leavers suggests that it might be worthwhile to try to attract more older workers.
4. Most leavers staying less than three months suggests rather immediate dissatisfaction. Poor selection, lack of supervision and/or training are causing some of the problems.
5. Because about one third left because of the job you need to talk to leavers to find out what job factors caused them to leave. Another one third being discharged suggests that screening and selection factors are inadequate.

Organization B

Separations

20	Nursing	
1	Dietary	
10	Housekeeping	
31	Total	

T.O. Rate

20%
5%
80%
20% (80% estimate annually) based on average no. of employees = 155

Age of leavers

14	24 or under
14	25–44
3	45–64
0	65 or over

Length of stay

14	3 months or less
14	4–11 months
3	1–3 years
0	3 or more years

Causes

6 worker caused
7 competition
16 job caused
2 discharges

Stability rate–85%
Wastage rate–14%
Absentee rate–2%

Organization B has a very different set of problems even though the number of separations is almost identical.

1. With a stability rate of 85 percent, why is the turnover rate 80 percent? This means that all of the turnover is accounted for in 15 percent of the jobs. This means that turnover can be reduced by looking at a small segment of the organization, in this case, housekeeping and nursing.
2. The age of leavers is fairly well distributed so that does not seem to be a selection factor.
3. The length of stay of leavers shows rather immediate dissatisfaction and there is a high number of job-related reasons for leaving. Since the administrator must look at only two departments, housekeeping in particular, it should not be difficult to find out what is wrong.
4. The wastage rate might be lowered slightly and the absentee rate is probably about as low as it can get.

Neither of these organizations is fictitious. Therefore, the administrator findings can be described along with the actual outcomes. In the case of Organization A, the administrator found many problems and it took a year before he was able to reverse the indicators. Actually, he found a department head who was unwilling to discipline a trouble-making employee in the housekeeping department. He provided supervisory training for the department head who learned how to contain this individual. In the dietary department, he found no planned or itemized program for training new employees. He and the inservice director worked with the department head to prepare a planned orientation and training checklist for the department. The administrator was in charge of the activities department, a job that he obviously was neglecting because of time commitments. He developed one individual on the staff to direct the program, thus relieving himself of doing a task he was doing poorly.

Organization B had a much simpler task, but it was not a pleasant one. After working with the housekeeping supervisor for several months, the administrator finally asked for her resignation. This person should never have been promoted to the position and was found incapable of directing the work of others in spite of the help given. The major nursing department problem was located on the evening shift of one unit. It had to do with staff problems with two distressed families who complained regularly and disturbed the resident on many occasions. The social worker and director of nursing found ways to help the families and to assist the staff to deal with the families. The staff learned ways of handling both the families and their own behavior. This of course reduced the problem as well as gave the staff a sense of growth and new confidence.

These two organizational cases demonstrate (1) how individualized employee problems can be identified, (2) what a broad range of skills administrators and department heads must have, (3) that key indicators provide HR information that help to locate internal problems, and (4) the data itself almost identifies what the administrative actions should be.

SUMMARY

Administrators need to know both the strengths and weaknesses of their organizations in order to build on the strengths and work to eliminate or at least minimize the weaknesses. Because so many terminations from long-term care organizations are avoidable, the administrator is helpless unless he or she knows why personnel leave. What social and environmental factors are responsible? Stone observes that "the successful recruitment, retention, and maintenance of a committed, prepared, long-term care work force across a range of settings is dependent upon a variety of interactive factors that occur at different levels." Regular attention and thought to the data collected can direct managers to answers to many organizational problems.

REFERENCES

Asis, L. (1975). A study of employee turnover, as quoted in Basil Georgopoulos. *Hospital organization research: Review and source book*. Philadelphia, PA: W.B. Saunders.

Stolte, K., & Meyers, S. (1995). Reflections of recruitment and retention at the unit level. *Health Care Supervisor, 13*(3), 36.

Stone, R. (2001). Research on frontline workers in long-term care. *Generations, 25*(1), 49.

Stryker, R. (1982). The effect of managerial interventions on high personnel turnover in nursing homes. *Journal of Long-Term Care Administration, 10*(2), 21.

Tai, T. et al. (1998). Review of nursing turnover research, 1977–1996. *Social Science and Medicine, 47*(12), 1905.

Part IV

OPTIMIZING HEALTH CARE OUTCOMES

Chapter 13

REHABILITATION AND EXERCISE IN LONG-TERM CARE

RUTH STRYKER

"Good intentions and kind impulses do, not necessarily lead to wise and truly humane measure . . . meaning well is only half our duty, thinking right is the other important half." Samuel Howe said these words in 1866 at the dedication of the Institute for the Blind in Oslo, Norway. Howe's cautionary words are still relevant, even after 150 years of social and medical advances. Good intentions and meaning well without a sound knowledge base can cause elderly persons to enter into a state of hopelessness and dependency. Thinking right means combining good intentions with actions based on scientific knowledge.

If a long-term care organization plans to go beyond custodial care and minimal government standards, a rehabilitation philosophy is critical to its success. First, see what can happen to persons in a caring but purely custodial organization. In 1947, Dr. R. A. Asher, a British physician, wrote, "Look at a patient lying long in bed. What a pathetic picture he makes! The blood clotting in his veins, the lime draining from his bones, the scybala stacking up in his colon, the flesh rotting from his seat, the urine leaking from his distended bladder and the spirit evaporating from his soul." Graphic language, yes, but it accurately describes what happens to people who are inactive, whether they are left lying in bed or sitting in a chair all day long.

In less graphic language, Dr. Asher was saying that prolonged rest increases the work load of the heart, reduces cardiac reserve and increases the possibility of blood clot formation. The respiratory system is affected by reduced chest expansion (from a bed or chair back) and reduced movement of bronchial secretions, resulting in less oxygen going to the brain and other organs. People on bedrest or chair-rest are also more likely to develop constipation, urinary stones, and urinary tract infections. In addition, bones demineralize, muscles lose strength and size, and decubitus ulcers (bedsores) can occur very quickly. Finally, lack of physical and mental stimulation is known to be accompanied by depression and anxiety.

The above description of the effects of inactivity provides convincing reasons for planning activities that keep both the mind and body active. Each activity needs to be goal-oriented for an individual as well as for groups. When a philosophy of rehabilitation underlies programs of care, resident outcomes are more positive, staff act and feel more professional, and the organizational culture takes on optimism and pride. In addition, there are fewer nursigenic and iatrogenic outcomes (omissions of care or treatment that unintentionally causes harm to patients). Examples of iatrogenic and nursigenic conditions are decubitus ulcers caused by infrequent position changes, mental withdrawal resulting from a psychosocial environment devoid of stimulation, a medication error resulting in a harmful reaction or a drug response that causes confusion, and a urinary tract infection caused by improper handling of drainage tubes.

Most of us understand the concepts of inactivity because of our interest in sports, exercise, fitness, and the prevention of heart disease. For some reason, however, we do not consider them important to maintaining health in an elderly person whether at home or in an institution. This dichotomy is beginning to change, but all too slowly.

Caregivers who understand the physiology of exercise and have both a philosophy of rehabilitation and a knowledge of rehabilitative practices will prevent negative outcomes in their clients. In addition, they will be able to go a step further, to promote more positive outcomes for a better life. The alternative to rehabilitation and exercise is, of course, to allow debilitation.

CONCEPTS OF REHABILITATION

Philosophy

First of all, people who work in long-term care (at home or at an institution) deal with a very special world of reality. They do not cure, they often cannot fully restore, and not every goal may be attained. However, staff often achieve "almost miracles" when they apply rehabilitation practices. They work on the premise ". . . which concedes that, despite continuing and even catastrophic disability, a better way of life is possible." Dr. Paul Ellwood's statement balances the reality of a severe loss with the reality of an adaptive life. This optimism is basic to all definitions of rehabilitation.

Definitions

Few administrators and too few geriatric professional staff have ever learned the basic concepts and practices of rehabilitation. What increases the impact of this omission in many professional education programs is the implication that what Medicare and Medicaid payments allow defines the scope of rehabilitation. These payment systems recognize the degrees of independent performance of ADL's (activities of daily living) which include bathing, dressing, eating, grooming, moving from chair to bed or bed to chair, ambulation (walking alone or using a cane, walker, or wheelchair) and toileting. In addition to ADL's, IADL's (instrumental activities of daily living) need to be assessed. IADL's include such abilities as care of one's personal environment, using the telephone, managing one's finances, or securing personal items (groceries, clothing, newspaper, etc.). Problems in these areas indicate a person's need for home care or supervision of personal and financial affairs by a spouse, family member, and/or a legal assistant.

While being able to perform IADL's and ADL's is important, other definitions of rehabilitation describe broader aspects of living a fuller life: Each health care profession defines rehabilitation in terms of that profession's particular discipline. To provide a good rehabilitation program for the elderly, caregivers need to be acquainted with the concepts of many perspectives of rehabilitation. Because rehabilitation requires interdisciplinary teamwork, it is also beneficial to see how different professions approach the subject.

Rehabilitation is a holistic approach to care and treatment. When one considers all ages, rehabilitation includes the development of an individual to the fullest possible level of physical, mental, social, vocational, sensory and spiritual function. The areas of emphasis are determined by a specific individual's goals and needs.

For example, if a person cannot hear or see well, vocational and social rehabilitation cannot take place until something has been done about the sensory losses. Each facet of rehabilitation is interrelated and interdependent. The professions most commonly involved in geriatric rehabilitation include the physician, nurse, occupational therapist, physical therapist, social worker, dietician, recreational therapist, audiologist, psychologist, and speech pathologist. As they work together *with* the patient, the interdependency of staff becomes obvious.

One of the most important concepts of rehabilitation, that one be restored to the fullest ability of which one is capable, is often overlooked. When a young paraplegic lives in a nursing home, one must ask what kind of rehabilitation program, if any, did this person have? The late Dr. Frank Krusen, the Mayo Clinic physiatrist who was the first American physician to accept Sister Kenny's treatment methods for polio, said, "Rehabilitation is a creative process which includes the cooperative efforts of various medical specialists and their associates in other health fields to improve the mental, physical, social and vocational aptitudes of persons who are handicapped, with the objective of preserving their ability to live happily and productively on the same level and with the same opportunities as their neighbors."

While Dr. Krusen worked with young people, he adds one very important dimension to the concept, namely, the idea of rehabilitation as creativity. It is surprising how much can be learned from a patient struggling to find ways to function. For example, many adaptive aids for eating and dressing have been developed by patients. One example is the Hoyer lift which was invented by Ted Hoyer, a minister who became quadriplegic. Staff and patients need to experiment together in order to find successful ways of doing things.

Another way to view rehabilitation is as a process of decreasing dependence to the greatest extent possible. Rehabilitation stresses minimal dependence in order to support self-respect, dignity, and ego-satisfaction. It is vital that an elderly disabled person develop as much independence as possible. To focus on a **potential** ability instead of the disability is to refocus the caregiver's attention and treatment goals from the present to the future.

Mary Romano says that "rehabilitation is the process of learning rather than teaching . . . cure is not an option . . . it involves the patient's adaptation or adjustment to impairment." She also articulates the importance of family relationships. In fact, eventual treatment outcomes are often more affected by families than by health care personnel. Long-term care professionals see the effect of families, both positive and negative, every day.

Changing the psychological environment may require a loosening of rules that inhibit emotional outlets of residents. Children and animals can increase the spontaneity of institutional living. Greater decision making by a client or resident regarding choices of daily routines and activities can reduce the sense of helplessness and increase the sense of control of one's life.

The physical environment needs to be assessed, especially for elderly persons living at home. Doors may have to be widened to accommodate the width of a wheelchair. A chair lift may be needed. Visual and auditory enhancement can be built into the rooms frequented by the individual. In other words, dependency should not be caused or made worse by the physical environment.

Goals

Persons with functional deficits can be assisted either to adapt to a deficit or to recover certain capabilities. All geriatric care needs to be oriented to the goals of preserving and enhancing function. Rehabilitation in long-term care facilities needs to integrate three major goals: (1) prevention of any further deterioration or loss in the areas affected by disease, (2) maintenance of function of the areas unaffected by disease, and (3) restoration of as much function as possible. These goals are interrelated.

A diagnosis of stroke will illustrate the interrelatedness of prevention, maintenance, and restoration. The speech therapist will be working to restore as much speech as possible. The physical therapist will be working to restore as much control of the affected arm and leg as possible, to maintain the function of the unaffected arm and leg, and to decide what adaptive devices, such as a cane, walker, or wheelchair may be needed. The nurse will change bed or sitting positions on a regular basis to prevent contractures and decubitus ulcers. Both the nurse and physical therapist will do range-of-motion exercises on *both sides* to maintain function of the **unaffected** side and to prevent further deterioration of the affected side. They will also work to restore as much function as possible. Range-of-motion exercises may be passive (performed by the nurse or therapist) or active (performed by the client).

As the physical therapist teaches the patient to walk with a leg brace and quad cane, the nursing staff will make certain that he or she practices using the devices when going to the dining room or for a walk outdoors. The occupational therapist will teach dressing, grooming, and eating with adaptive devices such as a knifork, a utensil that functions as both a knife and a fork. The doctor will prescribe medication to reduce the likelihood of having another stroke. The pastor may assist with psychological and spiritual needs. The resident will need to have time to practice each new activity. Every team member, which of course includes the resident and the family, has specific responsibilities toward the goals of rehabilitation: prevention, maintenance, and restoration. In summary, elderly persons with functional deficits can be assisted to adapt to the deficits and to recover certain capabilities.

BENEFITS OF GENERAL EXERCISE FOR THE AGED

There are many misconceptions about the benefits of exercise for the aged. They include: it will not help older adults, disease and debilitation are part of aging, and the need for exercise decreases with age. Research contradicts these assumptions. Many studies present evidence that exercise, even for those in their nineties, is beneficial. In fact, there is strong evidence to suggest that the sedentary lifestyle common in elderly persons is responsible for many of their health problems as well as deterioration usually attributed to aging.

It is true that by age 70, the average adult loses 30 per cent of muscle mass which slows metabolism, increases body fat, decreases aerobic capacity, and lowers bone density. This process is called sarcopenia. However, it is well known that this process can not only be slowed but the negative effects can be reduced through exercise. Exercise also addresses two goals of rehabilitation, maintenance and prevention.

One of the more serious effects of frailty in the aged is falling. Many researchers indicate that the incidence of falls can be reduced by a routine that includes adequate sleep and dietary intake, a daily brisk walk and muscle strengthening exercises. In June 2001, the American Geriatrics Society increased its recommendations for exercise therapy to reduce pain and to increase muscle strength and joint flexibility in the treatment of osteoarthritis.

M. J. Friedrich and others have shown that regular exercise reduces the risk of osteoporosis which in turn reduces the risk of fracture. Exercises are especially aimed at increasing balance, flexibility, strength and power. Power is the force a muscle can generate when contracting at a rapid rate. Fielding finds that muscle power is critical in preventing and reducing dysfunction.

Exercise may include swimming, water exercises, walking, range of motion particularly of the arms and legs, Tai Chi, and meditation. Stretching, aerobic, isometric and isotonic exercises are used commonly along with warm-up and cool-down motions. Many can be done standing or sitting. They can be done for as little as ten to 15 minutes at a time. Benefits accumulate when routines are done regularly four to six days a week. While not common, personal trainers are beginning to be asked to do in-home teaching of exercises for specific conditions. The person can then proceed to exercise at home without further instruction.

The Jones-Harrison Residence in Minneapolis has combined the best of rehabilitation and exercise in a health program started in September 2000. In an extensive building remodeling, a warm-water swimming pool with a wheelchair lift was built in the basement. In addition, there is an exercise room with computerized weight training machines and a rehabilitation therapy room. Health club membership is part of the monthly rent for assisted living residents so a majority of residents participate. Employees can use the facilities for a nominal monthly fee and club membership is open to elderly residents in the community. The program is tracking the changes in residents and find impressive gains, particularly in strength and balance. Other benefits are social and psychological.

In summary, demonstrated benefits of exercise in older adults are (1) increased muscle strength, range of motion and flexibility resulting in improved functional abilities, (2) decreased anxiety and levels of depression, (3) improved self-esteem, (4) reduction of pain in some conditions, (5) decreased number of falls because of improved balance and better lower body strength. Researchers are agreed that many declines associated with aging can be reversed by exercise programs even for the institutionalized eld-erly. Indeed, in-home geriatric rehabilitation can often improve strength and function to a level that can prevent or postpone institutionalization.

OBSTACLES TO REHABILITATION IN LONG-TERM CARE

What are the obstacles to a rehabilitation approach to elderly persons? The first and most obvious one is that staff may never have studied it or if they did, they did not apply it to the aged. Second, nurses have learned to "help" peo-ple. With persons needing rehabilitation, "help" takes on a special meaning. The goal becomes having the resident independent of the nurse, not depend-ent upon her. "Helping" a patient requires the nurse to help the patient help herself. The key is to guard against inappropriate help. Appropriate help will change over time as a resident improves. At first, rehabilitation takes more staff time, but later on, it takes less staff time.

The success of a rehabilitation program depends in part on the expecta-tions of staff and families. Unfortunately, expectations for the elderly are fre-quently very pessimistic. Families are distraught and the elderly see themselves without hope and at the end of their lives. The idea that disabled elderly are in a cycle of inevitable and continuous decline is now recognized as false. Research shows that a substantial number of elderly can learn and regain greater independence.

Organizational routines may conflict with a resident's therapy. One often sees a person learning to walk with a cane in the physical therapy department and then sees a nursing assistant taking the same resident to the dining room in a wheelchair. A resident who loves to listen to music (with ear phones) in her room is sometimes taken to the activity room to make paper valentines which she finds boring. Somehow listening to music is not perceived to be an activity.

If a goal of rehabilitation is to improve self-esteem, then greater autonomy for residents is necessary. This means that the resident decides what activity he or she wants to do, what time to go to bed, what time to get up, what to wear, when to nap, and when to walk. Too often the routine of the facility becomes more important than a resident's control over his or her personal wishes. It is also important to realize that each resident has idiosyncratic likes, needs, and desires. Professional expertise not only recognizes this but encour-ages its expression.

Because so many residents of long-term care institutions have mild to severe dementia, the concept of rehabilitation needs to be adapted to these problems. For example, someone with dementia may not be able to make choices. If they are offered more than two choices, they may become agitated and even more confused. Therefore, the goal with severely demented residents is to provide a supportive environment with structure and predictability, allowing as much independence and decision-making as the individual person can tolerate.

Dorothy Coons expresses the essence of rehabilitation in her book on special units for persons with dementia. She talks about "wellness-fostering environments." This means that one can develop a therapeutic milieu by scanning the environment for noise, observe staff behaviors, and identify routines that cause stress, thus decreasing behavior problems. Her research-based criteria for an environment supportive to staff, family, and residents can be applied to any long-term care organization. They are:

1. The environment is most therapeutic if the population is homogeneous.
2. The organization encourages maximal autonomy and freedom.
3. The environment offers sensory and social stimulation.
4. Individuality is recognized and encouraged.
5. Activities enable continuity with the past and continued normal social roles.
6. Human dignity is fostered.

ADMINISTRATIVE RESPONSIBILITIES

While the administrator may not be a clinician, some clinical knowledge is necessary. First of all, the physical environment must assist residents to independence, both physically and mentally. In other words, dependencies should not be built in. Even with building codes and other requirements, the environment needs greater attention. One example will illustrate this point. Staff of a nursing home built with a central core for dining and social activities complained that residents were always confused getting back to their rooms which were located down three corridors coming off the center core. After a different colored stripe was painted on the wall of each corridor, residents learned their color and had less trouble finding their rooms. When a problem affects a large number of residents, the administrator and staff should assess the environment to see if it is causing or contributing to the problem.

The administrator should employ knowledgeable staff and provide opportunities for inservice education in the areas of rehabilitation, care of demented residents, and assessment of physical and psychological needs. When a problem behavior arises, staff need to try to determine the cause. Might it be a reaction to the physical environment, behavior of another resident or a certain staff-member, a perceived anxiety, or a change in physical condition? A thorough assessment must be initiated rather than have staff conclude, without any investigation, that a behavior is caused by a resident's age, personality, or condition. The latter is called attributional thinking. Attributing causes without proper assessment of possible *real* causes can deprive a person of appropriate care and interventions.

The administrator has the obligation to give residents a say in the organization. A resident may be a valuable addition to a safety committee; an admissions committee, or a decorating committee. Certainly the administrator can take seriously any issue that comes from a Residents' Council. Incidentally, in a study by Ryden (1984), the only variable found to have a significant effect on morale of "skilled" residents was perceived control. It seems that when staff are respectful of residents' rights, both control and perceived control in decision-making improves resident morale.

Finally, the administrative staff can set an example of the attitudes and behaviors expected of department heads and staff. If the psychological environment is to be therapeutic, staff need to see appropriate behaviors which they can emulate. This will not only raise the quality of care of residents but improve morale of staff.

REFERENCES

American Geriatrics Society. (2001). *Journal of the American Geriatrics Society, 49*(6), 808, June.

Asher, R. A. J. (1947). The hazards of bedrest. *British Medical Journal, 2,* 967.

Baan, C. A. (2000). Physical activity in elderly subjects with impaired glucose tolerance and newly diagnosed diabetes mellitus. *American Journal of Epidemiology, 149,* 219.

Braddom, R. L. (1996). *Physical medicine and rehabilitation.* Philadelphia: W.B. Saunders.

Butler, R. (2000). Fighting frailty: Prescription for healthier aging includes exercises. *Geriatrics, 55*(2), 20, February.

Coons, D. H. (1991). *Specialized dementia care units.* Baltimore: Johns Hopkins Press.

Friedrich, M. J. (2001). Women, exercise, aging: Strong message for the weaker sex. *JAMA, 285*(11), 1429, March 21.

Guccione, A. A. (2000). *Geriatric physical therapy.* St. Louis: Mosby.

Hoeman, S. P. (2001). *Rehabilitation nursing: Process, application and outcomes.* St. Louis: Mosby.

Kottke, F. J., & Lehmann, J. F. (1990). *Krusen's handbook of physical medicine and rehabilitation* (4th ed.). Philadelphia: W.B. Saunders.

Romano, M. D. (1990). Psychological diagnosis and social services. In F. J. Kottke et al., *Krusen's handbook of physical medicine and rehabilitation* (4th ed.). Philadelphia: W.B. Saunders.

Ryden, M. B. (1984). Morale and perceived control in institutionalized elderly. *Nursing Research, 33*(3), 130, May–June.

Smith, E. L. (1990). Exercise intervention and physiologic function in the elderly. *Topics in Geriatric Rehabilitation, 6*(1), 57, October.

Smith, E. L., & Tommerup, L. (1995). Exercise: A prevention and treatment for osteoporosis and injurious falls in the older adult. *Journal of Aging and Physical Activity, 3,* 178.

Sterling, S. A. (2000). The relationship between age, gender, disease, physical activity and functional abilities in the elderly. Master's thesis, Purdue University.

Stryker, R. P. (1977). *Rehabilitative aspects of acute and chronic nursing* (2nd ed.). Philadelphia: W.B. Saunders.

Westhoff, M. H. et al. (2000). Effects of a low-intensity strength-training program and knee-extension strength and functional ability of frail older people. *Journal of Aging and Physical Activity, 8,* 325.

Chapter 14

MEDICAL CARE AND THE ROLE OF THE MEDICAL DIRECTOR

KAREN S. FELDT

Changes in life expectancy, careful management of chronic diseases, and prolonged periods of living with multiple chronic diseases have changed the population of elderly residents in long-term care facilities. Recent analysis of federal nursing home data indicates that residents of long-term care facilities in 1997 were more dependent on assistance for activities of daily living and had higher rates of dementia and psychiatric diagnoses than residents of nursing homes in 1991 (Harrington & Carrillo, 1999). The increasing medical and psychiatric frailty and acuity of residents, new regulatory requirements, and the need for appropriate, knowledgeable direction of care has reshaped the role of the medical director for long-term care facilities (Levinson & Musher, 1995).

There are major impediments to quality medical care in long-term care facilities. There is general absence of geriatric education in medical schools, an acute shortage of physicians who have an interest in geriatric patients, and few physicians who are Board certified in geriatric medicine. A recent study using the Online survey Certification and Reporting (OSCAR) data revealed that 20 percent of long-term care facilities reported zero medical director FTEs, indicating that either medical directors are not available to those facilities or that volunteer or alternative arrangements have been made (McCarthy et al., 1999). This data suggests what may be a medical leadership crisis in long-term care at the very time when the responsibilities of medical leaders in these facilities are growing.

Recently, the American Medical Directors Association (AMDA) has developed a series of educational programs to address the specific issues that medical directors of long-term care facilities must be prepared to manage (Tarnove, 2000). This chapter will identify AMDA guidelines regarding the role and responsibilities of the medical director and identify regulations and policies which further shape this role.

Role and Responsibilities of the Medical Director

In response to a federal mandate in 1975 and the growing concern about the need for quality medical direction of nursing home care, the American Medical Directors Association (AMDA), was officially chartered in June 1978. The organization recognized the need to organize and educate physicians who would fulfill the role of the medical director for long-term care facilities. This national professional association identifies its mission as a commitment to "continuous improvement of the quality of patient care by providing education, advocacy, information, and professional development for medical directors and other physicians who practice in the long-term care continuum" (AMDA, 2001). Since its inception, AMDA has been actively working to identify curriculum for educating medical directors, developing clear roles and responsibilities for medical directors, and working to effect policy and regulation changes to improve the quality of care for nursing home residents.

Responsibilities of Medical Directors

The AMDA House of Delegates adopted a policy in 1991 which defines the specific responsibilities of medical directors in long-term care. *Resolution A91* spells out clearly the administrative, clinical, and collaborative roles of medical directors. Responsibilities identified by AMDA are listed and discussed below (AMDA, 1991).

1. "The medical director should exercise medical and clinical leadership in a multidisciplinary approach to resident care and care planning within the long-term care setting, and interact with attending staff as a colleague and a peer" (AMDA, 1991).

Nursing home settings are markedly different from hospital settings. There is a focus on maintaining functional skills of residents in a "home-like" environment, while monitoring chronic and acute medical problems. Multiple disciplines are involved in the management of care. This approach requires a different set of skills than the traditional physician-dominated medical model applied in acute care centers. The primary goal of nursing home care is to provide a living environment for the resident who needs nursing care, chronic illness management, and medical supervision. Nursing homes provide care for a variety of residents including those who are there for a temporary rehabilitation stay, a prolonged stay because of the need for physical care, supervision of care because of dementia or psychiatric illness complicated by medical problems, or palliative end-of-life care (Swagerty & Rigler, 2000).

Although accurate diagnosis, treatment, and management of chronic and acute illnesses are necessary, they do not encompass the total physical, mental, social, spiritual and personal health needs of the individuals who reside in long-term care facilities (Aaronson, 1991). Medical directors are important members of a team approach to this care. However, much of the multidisciplinary care within long-term care facilities is coordinated by the director of nursing and supervisory nursing staff with guidance and support from the medical director. Medical directors need to encourage participation and understanding of care within the nursing home for physicians who attend to the medical needs of residents.

2. *"The physician medical director should collaborate with the nursing director, the administrator, and other health professionals to develop formal patient care policies for the facility that:*

- *provide for the total medical and psychosocial needs of the resident, including admission, transfer, discharge planning, range of services available to residents, emergency procedures, and frequency of physician visits in accordance with resident needs*
- *help enhance resident's rights as identified in the federally-mandated Patient Bill of Rights*
- *show that these patient care policies are carried out, as reflected and documented in the minutes of the drug regimen review and quality assurance committees of the institution*
- *and include written designation of a registered nurse (with the guidance of the medical director as an advisory physician) as responsible for the day-to-day execution of these policies (AMDA, 1991).*

Clearly written policies are essential for providing a framework to resident care in long-term care facilities. Many nursing home residents have both medical and psychiatric complexity. Admission policies should clearly reflect the type of resident for whom care can be provided. For example, researchers estimate that 50 to 75 percent of nursing home residents have dementia. Policies need to reflect strengths and limitations of the nursing home and its ability to manage care for this population. If the nursing home does not have a secure unit for dementia patients who frequently wander and elope, admission policies and discharge policies need to identify which dementia patients are best served by the facility (Streim & Katz, 1994).

Admission policies should also reflect the complexity of care which the facility is able to provide to medically frail residents. Specific policies related to admission of patients with IVs, PEG tubes, hemodialysis, and respiratory care must be clearly delineated. Limitations of admission and criteria for discharge of these patients should be clarified.

In addition to specific admission and discharge policies, the medical director should establish a quality assurance committee which can review how the nursing home is meeting specific standards of care as established by regulatory guidelines.

3. "Perform the following roles with respect to resident care: (1) act as liaison with and coordinate the activities of other health professionals for the care of the resident; (2) in an emergency, be prepared to assume temporary responsibilities for the care of the resident in the event that the resident's own attending physician or the designated alternate physician is not available" (AMDA, 1991).

Because of the complex problems of the current population in long-term care, emergent clinical issues can arise which involve residents of other attending physicians. These issues may need immediate intervention of the medical director if the attending physician cannot be reached. The medical director needs to be willing to step in as a back-up to the primary care physician if no action is taken on acute changes (Levenson & Feinsod, 1999; Weinberg, 1999). Institutional policies should address procedures for staff when they do not receive a response from the resident's primary physician regarding treatment of an acute problem. Nursing home facilities risk being cited for neglect of a resident's medical problems if no policies and procedures are in place (MacLean, 2000).

4. "Maintain a thorough knowledge of the federal, state and local regulations and codes applicable to long-term care facilities, applicable standards of the Joint Commission on Accreditation of Healthcare Organizations (JCAHO), as well as the professional service and administrative requirements and expectations of participating public and private reimbursement programs" (AMDA, 1991).

Perhaps the most difficult responsibility of medical directors is the need to stay abreast of ongoing changes in regulations pertaining to long-term care facilities. The only industry that has more federal regulations than nursing homes is the nuclear power industry. In 1987, the Omnibus Budget Reconciliation Act (OBRA '87) set standards for nursing home reform in an effort to uniformly guide the care in nursing homes (Elon, 1995). This legislation led to the development of standardized resident assessment instrument (RAI) of all nursing home residents and the Minimum Data Set (MDS) of assessment information required. The legislation also led to the development of quality indicators, which are derived from the MDS and can identify how facilities compare to others within their state for several areas of care. These quality indicators provide data for state surveyors who conduct the annual surveys of nursing home facilities (HCFA, 1991).

Medical directors need to be acutely familiar with the MDS information and aware of areas of deficiency or concern as indicated by the quality indicator data provided to their facility. They need to be involved in the development of plans to address deficiencies noted in these data reports and monitor the work to improve the quality of care in the facility (Harrington & Carrillo, 1999; Streim & Katz, 1994; Vaca, Vaca, & Daake, 1998).

5. *"Develop, amend, recommend, and implement appropriate clinical practices and medical care policies, with the cooperation and collaboration of health professionals and administrators within the long-term care institution, which include a way to insure that each patient's medical regime is incorporated appropriately into the plan of care" (AMDA, 1991).*

Elderly residents and their families need to be assured that the overall goals for patient care and subsequent medical, nursing, and social plans are carried out. Physicians need to: provide quality health care in an economical way; provide ongoing medical evaluation and treatment of conditions; and communicate with the patient, family, and staff the nature, course and prognosis for the problems being treated (Levenson & Feinsod, 1999). This means that information from consulting physicians, clinics, therapists, and staff must be communicated to the primary physician in a timely manner. Policies should be developed and reviewed by the medical director to ensure that consultant reports are transmitted in some form to the attending physician for prompt review (Weinberg, 1999).

6. *"Act as the spokesperson of the medical staff (analogous to the chief-of-staff within a hospital), in cooperation with the administration and with the approval of the governing body, to develop rules, regulations and policies for individual attending physicians who admit their patients to the facility" (AMDA, 1991).*

Many residents in nursing home facilities have their primary medical care provided by physicians who either see them within the facility or in their outpatient offices. MacLean (2000) encourages facilities to define medically necessary primary care services and develop a policy and procedure for primary care physicians who provide care to residents within their facility. These policies can set expectations for primary physicians. The procedures linked to the policy can identify required and recommended visits, can provide guidelines for billing, and can offer guidelines for required documentation (MacLean, 2000).

There are two basic models for organizing the medical staff of a nursing home. The first, a closed model, limits the number of attending physicians to only a few physicians, or to "house doctors only." The second, an open model, allows most physicians in the service area to admit patients. The latter is the most common arrangement, but it is also the most difficult to manage for an administrator. Some physicians make it a personal policy not to see primary patients once they are admitted to a nursing facility (Levinson & Musher, 1995). Nursing facilities should have a list of potential physician providers available to new patients and family members. This list should include physicians who visit patients on site as well as those who are willing to serve patients in an office visit.

A medical practice agreement should delineate the responsibilities and obligations of the attending physician and the nursing home. This document should be signed by each admitting doctor and a verification of credentials should be made. Sample model contracts are available from the American Medical Directors Association. Education of physicians providing care to the nursing home patients should include information to help them understand regulatory compliance issues and need for accurate and complete documentation of the plan of care for residents (Levenson & Feinsod, 1999; Levinson & Musher, 1995).

7. "Monitor the activities of attending physicians and intervene as needed on behalf of patients or the administration of the facility" (AMDA, 1991).

Acute conditions such as urinary tract infections, pneumonia, venous thromboembolism and exacerbations of congestive heart failure can be managed in the nursing home if detected and treated in a timely and efficient manner. Primary care physicians who deliver quality care for vulnerable older patients can reduce unnecessary hospitalizations and improve the quality of life for nursing home residents (Ackermann, 2001). Gerontological nurse practitioners can improve care through early evaluation of subtle health status changes (Ruiz, Tabloski, & Frazier, 1995). However, medical directors need to periodically evaluate the quality of medical care within the facility. Clinical practice guidelines are potentially useful tools that can assist in guiding the evaluation of medical care (Levinson & Musher, 1995).

A review mechanism should be put in place to assure appropriate medical care compliance. In many instances, a medical review quality assurance committee, or a utilization review committee, can serve as the governing body for the medical staff. This review committee activity supports the Medical Director who functions as a physician supervisor.

8. "Review recommendations and reports of drug regimen review and quality assurance committees, and take appropriate and timely action as needed to implement recommendations" (AMDA, 1991).

Perhaps most frustrating among the current regulations for long-term care are those regarding pharmaceutical care. Many physicians regard reviews and recommendations by consulting pharmacists as a direct assault on their clinical practice, and oppose being told how to practice medicine (Levinson & Musher, 1995). However, most of the pharmacy recommendations have developed after careful review of the literature on appropriate prescribing practices for the elderly. Providing staff physicians with supporting research articles on pharmaceutical practices for long-term care can be useful in making gradual changes in the prescribing practice of staff physicians (Levinson & Musher, 1995). Well-organized pharmacy services are essential to providing high quality care to nursing home residents. Medical directors should periodically review pharmacy services for appropriate filling of prescriptions, frequency of pharmacy medication errors, and timely delivery of necessary medications (Ouslander, 1997).

9. "Routinely meet with nursing and other professional staff to discuss administrative, dietary, and housekeeping issues, specific patient care problems and professional staff needs for education or consultants, offering solutions to problems and identifying areas where policy should be developed" (AMDA, 1991).

Achievement of optimal health and function within chronic illness requires collaboration with therapists, social service workers, psychologists, dietary workers, recreational workers, and chaplains (Aaronson, 1991; Vaca, Vaca, & Daake, 1998). Although OBRA '87 only specified that medical directors must participate on the quality assurance committee of the nursing home, communication with other professional staff can be most easily facilitated if medical directors participate on other committees at the facility (Levinson & Musher, 1995).

Medical directors should also stress their availability to their directors of nursing and other key personnel for any issue involving clinical care that may potentially cause injury or be detrimental to a resident. For example, the presence of any epidemic illness in the facility needs attention by the medical director, and responses initiated should reflect the medical director's involvement (Weinberg, 1999).

10. Actively help develop ongoing inservice education programs for attending physicians and professional staff within the institution, in cooperation with the director of nursing and the administrator.

Education of medical and professional staff in long-term care facilities can occur in a variety of ways. Good educational programs may not only enhance care but may aid in the retention of employees. Teaching rounds and research activities contribute to improving education of medical and nursing staff (Levinson & Musher, 1995). The medical director can facilitate educational programs by creating affiliations with local medical and nursing schools (Ouslander, 1997). Guidance and leadership should be provided to educating attending physicians about the living-dying phase in nursing home residents to reduce unnecessary hospitalizations at the end of life (Joseph & Boult, 1998; Intrator et al., 1999).

11. "Act as a resource on patient care, new treatment modalities, and the pathophysiology of illness" (AMDA, 1991).

Regular patient rounds can provide an excellent opportunity for informal teaching of staff. These rounds can be combined with patient care, or be planned for teaching only (Levinson & Musher, 1995; Ouslander, 1997). Medical directors who make themselves available for staff questions can identify specific staff education needs and work with education coordinators to establish periodic inservices on care topics related to the patient population.

12. "Obtain the services of qualified professionals to serve as consultants to several areas of special resident need such as dentistry, podiatry, dermatology, orthopaedics" (AMDA, 1991).

Residents of long-term care facilities require a variety of specialists to attend to care needs. The complexity of their medical conditions might require access to consulting physicians in cardiology, dermatology, nephrology, neurology, oncology, psychiatry, pulmonology, rheumatology, and urology. In addition, these residents may require basic services from dentistry, podiatry, optometry, audiology, and pharmacy. The medical director has the responsibility for ensuring that necessary services are arranged for the resident (Ouslander, 1997). In larger cities, some of these medical services could be arranged to be brought on site, to reduce transportation of frail residents. In rural facilities, these specialty services may be much less frequently available and can require extensive transport to provide such services.

13. "Prepare a regular report summarizing his/her actions, concerns and recommendations as medical director" (AMDA, 1991).

Whether hired as a part-time or full-time medical director, it is essential that the facility receive an annual report of the medical director's activities. This report helps to affirm the importance of the medical director's role. The report should include: activities that have shaped changes to the care of the residents, involvement in quality assurance studies, involvement in facility committees, recommendations for improvement, interventions with attending medical staff, policies developed or revised, and educational activities provided.

14. "Represent the facility in discussions and meetings with other institutions on issues relevant to medical care" (AMDA, 1991).

In 1999, the Balanced Budget Refinement Act significantly changed how skilled nursing facilities are reimbursed for the care of post-hospitalized patients under Medicare. The prospective payment system (P.P.S.) gave skilled nursing facilities new priorities when communicating with hospitals about the types of patients that they would be willing to admit. The P.P.S. system financially linked hospitalization and nursing home stays for particular diagnostic-related groups (DRGs) and functional levels. Medical directors play an important role in the interface between the long-term care facility and acute care (Phillips-Harris & Fanale, 1995). As medical directors, they must be involved in decisions to admit medically complex patients, especially those which may require care that the facility is unable to provide, or those which place the nursing home at greater financial risk because of overall cost of care. In particular, medical directors should work with administrators and nursing directors to identify high cost medications or treatments of potential new admits. Advocating for changes to similar but less expensive treatment prior to discharge from the hospital may assist the long-term care facility in staying financially afloat while still attracting post-hospital rehabilitation patients.

15. "Conduct an ongoing program for the evaluation and management of the health of the facility's employees, by: (1) establishing policy and procedures, and (2) direct physical examination of employees, emphasizing freedom from significant infection, pre-employment physical examinations and reexaminations, and compliance with local and state health regulations" (AMDA, 1991).

Policies regarding employee health are essential. Medical directors must be involved with establishing requirements for pre-employment physical examinations. Infection control policies are particularly important. Since residents of long-term care facilities are medically frail, infected or ill employees do not serve the health care needs of the patients or the facility (Ouslander, 1997).

Medical directors must also have policies in place to prevent abuse or neglect of residents (MacLean, 2000). These should include screening of potential hires for previous criminal or abuse histories, training employees regarding abuse and neglect, and investigating any possible incidents or allegations to the facility. Medical directors should be familiar with skills of conflict resolution and negotiation with employee issues (MacLean, 2000).

16. "Help the facility administrator ensure a safe and sanitary environment for residents and personnel, including: review of incidents and accidents, identifying hazards to health and safety, and advice about possible correction or improvement of the environment" (AMDA, 1991).

In 1997, over 16 percent of the long-term care facilities were cited for failure to maintain the environment free of accident hazards. This requirement was established to prevent unexpected and unintended injuries (Harrington & Carrillo, 1999). Medical directors play an important role in the careful review of incidents and accidents. These reviews can identify areas where injuries most likely occur, patterns of falls and injuries, and residents at highest risk. Education of staff can be tailored to address some of the specific concerns identified in the review.

17. "Assist management in its review and response to any official medical review by Federal, state or local surveys and inspections" (AMDA, 1991).

The top three most frequently cited deficiencies for long-term care facilities in 1997 were: inadequate food sanitation (in storing, preparing, distributing, or serving food), failure to provide required comprehensive assessments, and failure to complete comprehensive care plans (Harrington & Carrillo, 1999). In their review of OSCAR data, Harrington and Carrillo note that there has been a significant decline in the number of deficiencies issued to long-term care facilities between 1991 and 1997, possibly reflecting that nursing homes are improving the overall quality of care that they deliver. This may be related to the standardization of resident assessment and expectations for care as established by the OBRA '87 regulations. Medical directors need to be involved with the administrator and director of nursing as they review surveyor reports and examine the citations for deficiencies. After correction of these deficiencies is met, the medical director should work with the staff on an overall plan to improve the quality of care in areas cited.

SUMMARY

Over the past 20 years the medical director in long-term care facilities has evolved from a consultant or staff physician to an integral role in the administration, planning, executing, and reviewing the care of nursing home residents. The broad scope of these responsibilities requires special preparation and education if quality care for nursing home residents is to be assured.

REFERENCES

Aaronson, W. (1991). Interdisciplinary health team role taking as a function of health professional education. *Gerontology and Geriatrics Education, 12*(1), 97.

Ackerman, R. (2001). Strategies to manage most acute and chronic illnesses without hospitalization. *Geriatrics, 56*(5), 37.

American Medical Director's Association (AMDA). 1991. *Resolution 91.*

Elon, R. (1995). Omnibus budget reconciliation act of 1987 and its implications for the medical director. *Clinics in Geriatric Medicine, 11*(3), 419.

Harrington, C., & Carrillo, H. (1999). The regulation and enforcement of federal nursing home standards, 1991–1997. *Medical Care Research and Review, 4,* 471.

Health Care Financing Administration. *Medicare and Medicaid: Requirements for long-term care facilities, final regulations.* Publication No. 48865-48921. Washington, DC: Federal Register.

Intrator, O. et al. (1999). Facility characteristics associated with hospitalization of nursing home residents. *Medical Care, 37,* 228.

Joseph, A., & Boult, C. (1998). Managed primary care of nursing home residents. *Journal of the American Geriatrics Society, 46,* 1152.

Levenson, S., & Feinsod, F. (1999). Optimizing physician and medical director roles. *Annals of Long-Term Care, 7,* 4.

Levinson, M., & Musher, J. (1995). Current role of the medical director in community-based nursing facilities. *Clinics in Geriatric Medicine, 11*(3), 343.

MacLean, D. (2000). Primary care services policy: Don't run a nursing home without it. *Caring for the Aged, 1*(12), 17.

MacLean, D. (2000). Preventing abuse and neglect in long-term care. Part II: Clinical and administrative aspects. *Annals of Long-Term Care, 8*(1), 65.

McCarthy, J. et al. (1999). Medical director involvement in nursing homes– 1991–1996. *Annals of Long-Term Care, 7*(2), 35.

Ouslander, J. (1997). The role of the medical director. In J. Ouslander et al. (Eds.) (ch. 7), *Medical Care in the Nursing Home.* New York: McGraw-Hill.

Phillips-Harris, C., & Fanale, J. (1995). The acute and long-term care interface. *Clinics in Geriatric Medicine, 11*(3), 481.

Ruiz, B. et al. (1995). The role of gerontological advanced practice nurses in geriatric care. *Journal of the American Geriatrics Society, 43*(9), 1061.

Streim, J., & Katz, I. (1994). Federal regulations and the care of patients with dementia in the nursing home. *Medical Clinics of North America, 78*(4), 895.

Swagerty, D. Jr., & Rigler, S. (2000). The physician's role in directing long-term care. Understanding the rules is important for protecting your patients and your practice. *Postgraduate Medicine, 107*(2), 217, 221, 225.

Tarnove, L. (1999). The role of the medical director: A need for definition. *Annals of Long-Term Care, 7,* 3.

Vaca, K. et al. (1998). Review of nursing home regulations. *Medsurg Nursing, 7*(3), 165.

Weinberg, A. (1999). Case report: Quality improvement. *Annals of Long-Term Care, 7*(9), 345.

Chapter 15

THE DEPARTMENT OF NURSING

CHRISTINE MUELLER

This chapter serves two purposes. The first is to acquaint managers and administrators with the nursing profession and how nurses function in order to have a basis for evaluating a nursing department. The second purpose relates to present day availability of nurses. Because many of today's administrators will not be fortunate enough to employ a fully qualified nurse administrator, tools and resources are provided to assist the nurse administrator in practice.

Between 60 and 70 percent of all personnel employed in a long-term care organization work in the nursing department. These direct caregivers have the greatest amount of interaction with residents and families because they are there 24 hours, seven days a week. Since a long-term care organization builds its reputation on the quality of care provided to its residents, it is critical that the nursing care provided to residents is based on evidence and current standards of care, and that the staff are clinically competent in caring for elderly clients with multiple, and sometimes complex, health care needs. As more residents are admitted to nursing facilities for short stays to continue their rehabilitation and convalescence from a hospital stay, the nursing department no longer has a singular focus. Rather, the department needs to be responsive to residents with a variety of medical, nursing, and rehabilitative care needs.

Integral to the care of residents in nursing facilities is the interdisciplinary plan of care that is developed from a comprehensive assessment of each resident. Under the Omnibus Budget Reconciliation Act of 1987 (OBRA '87), nursing facilities are required to use a standardized resident assessment instrument (RAI) that identifies individual needs. This forms the basis for the plan of care to ensure that services and activities attain or maintain the highest practical physical, mental, and psychological well-being of each resident (sec.

204

1919(b)(2)). The assessment and care planning process is coordinated by registered nurses. The Minimum Data Set (MDS) portion of the RAI details the resident's physical, cognitive, nutritional, functional, behavioral and emotional status. It also identifies the medical and clinical conditions of the resident and any rehabilitation needs of the resident. The individualized assessment, care plan, and implementation of the plan for residents form the core of what nursing personnel do.

ORGANIZATION OF THE NURSING DEPARTMENT

There are two key components that direct and support all activities within the nursing department: the philosophy of care and the standards of care. The philosophy of care for the nursing organization is an explanation of the systems of beliefs that determine how the mission or purpose of the organization is to be achieved (Huber, 2000, p. 496). Forming the core of a nursing organization philosophy are three components: the resident, the nurse, and nursing practice. The beliefs stated about residents could include how they are viewed (e.g., holistically) and what they are entitled to (e.g., quality nursing care, right to self-determination). Beliefs and values about the nurse and nursing practice often describe the nature of the relationship between the nurse and the resident, the role of the nurse, the type of nursing care delivery model, collaborative role of nurses with other disciplines, competence and professional development of nurses, and governance of the nursing organization. The nursing department should have a well-articulated philosophy of care. The philosophy of care is used to guide clinical and management decision-making.

Goals and objectives operationalize the philosophy of the nursing department and need to be written so their achievement can be measured. An example of a goal is: *all nursing staff will participate in the development of an individualized care plan for residents.* Goals are usually supported by objectives that are more explicit, measurable, observable and obtainable (Marquis, 2000). Objectives to support the goal provided in the example might be as follows: (1) nursing staff on all three shifts will document assessment data associated with the resident's MDS within 5 days of the resident's admission; (2) the RN care manager and primary nursing assistant will attend the resident's care plan conference following admission and quarterly; (3) resident care plans will be used to prepare assignments for nursing assistants and updated weekly.

A standard is a predetermined level of excellence that serves as a guide for practice and effective care (Marquis, 2000, p. 397). The American Nurses

Association is the professional organization that has established a set of standards for both general and specialty nursing practice. The standards for nursing practice most relevant to nursing departments in long-term care facilities are:

- **Scope and Standards for Nurse Administrators:** Defines the scope and various levels of practice; outlines qualifications for these roles across all settings; provides standards of care and professional performance for this complex nursing specialty.
- **Standards and Scope of Gerontological Nursing Practice:** These standards apply to basic and advanced practice level gerontological nurses in clinical practice across all settings and may be used in quality assurance programs as a means of evaluating and improving care. Included in the scope statement are historical perspectives and trends, and a practice definition of the basic and advanced level provider.
- **Standards for Nursing Professional Development–Continuing Education and Staff Development:** These standards and criteria describe competent practice in this specialty, regardless of the setting and role.
- **Standards and Scope of Rehabilitation Nursing Practice:** Provides standards regarding the professional nursing care and practice common to all rehabilitation nurses engaged in clinical practice. It applies to the care provided to all clients in every setting.

Other standards are clinical practice guidelines. The most well-known set of clinical practice guidelines have been developed by the Agency for Healthcare Research and Quality (AHRQ) which developed a set of 19 clinical practice guidelines between 1992 and 1996. These and other clinical practice guidelines can be found at the AHRQ website (www.ahrq.gov). Clinical practice guidelines are written for specific diseases (e.g., depression, osteoporosis) or health conditions (e.g., incontinence, pressure ulcers, hip fractures) and reflect research evidence and clinical expertise.

The types of standards and clinical practice guidelines adopted by a nursing department define the professional practice for the department and reflect the values of the nursing department. Standards of care describe an acceptable level of resident care that the nursing department strives to achieve. Standards of professional performance describe an acceptable level of professional nurse role behavior (Huber, 2000, p. 617). Nursing care policies and procedures should be based on standards of care and referenced accordingly.

Director of Nursing/Nurse Administrator

The organizational structure of the nursing department will determine the involvement nursing staff have in decision-making about nursing practice and the nursing practice environment. A key position in the nursing department is the director of nursing (DON) or nurse administrator (NA). The DON/NA should be directly accountable to the administrator, have an effective working relationship with the medical director, and have good communication mechanisms in place to work with key department heads. Four key roles have been identified for the DON/NA: (1) organization management; (2) human resources management; (3) nursing/health services management; and (4) professional nursing and long-term care leadership (Lodge, 1987). The responsibilities associated with these four roles are outlined in Appendix A.

The turnover of DONs/NAs is a common problem throughout the country and is related to the lack of preparation for the role. Less than a third of DONs/NAs have a baccalaureate degree (Arioan, 2000; Ballard, 1995; Mueller, 1998). The National Association of Directors of Nursing Administration in Long-term Care (NADONA) provides certification in long-term care nursing administration. Over 1,400 nurses hold this certification, however this is less than 10 percent of DONs/NAs in long-term care facilities. It is important that DONs/NAs have the appropriate education and preparation for this complex, challenging role. The Institute of Medicine Committee (1996) on *Nursing Staffing in Hospitals and Nursing Homes* recommended that "in view of the increasing case-mix acuity of residents and the consequent complexity of care provided, nursing facilities [should] place greater weight on educational preparation in the employment of directors of nursing" (p. 159). It is recommended that the DON/NA have a master's degree in nursing with specialized preparation and certification in nursing administration (Lodge, 1987; Mueller, 1998; Ballard, 1995; American Nurses Association, 1996). Certification in nursing administration is available through the American Nurses Credentialing Center. The National Association of Directors of Nursing Administration in Long-Term Care (NADONA/LTC) also offer certification in long-term care nursing administration.

QUALIFICATIONS AND ROLES OF NURSING PERSONNEL

The philosophy of the nursing department and accompanying goals and objectives, as well as the standards of care, are formulated through the leadership of the DON/NA and implemented by the staff in the nursing department. Thus, the education and experience of nursing staff should be considered in determining the types of staff for the nursing department.

Licensed Nurses

There are two categories of licensed nurses–the registered nurse (RN) and the licensed practice nurse (LPN) or licensed vocational nurse (LVN). Each state has a Nurse Practice Act which identifies the practice of practical nursing (LP/VN) and professional nursing (RN). Administrators should be familiar with the Nurse Practice Act in their state. Of the 2.2 million RNs employed, only 6.9 percent are employed in long-term care facilities compared to 59.1 percent employed in hospitals (Bureau of Health Professions, 2001).

Registered Nurses

Registered nurses can be graduates of a diploma (3-year hospital-based program), associate degree (2-year community college-based program) or baccalaureate degree (4-year university-based program) education program. Regardless of their educational preparation, they are eligible, upon graduation, to take the licensure examination to become a registered nurse. However, administrators should be familiar with how these educational differences can affect the practice of registered nurses. The majority (44%) of RNs in long-term care facilities have an associate degree in nursing, followed by nurses with a diploma in nursing (30%) and a baccalaureate degree (22%). It is imperative that nurses employed in long-term care facilities have education background in gerontological nursing. If gerontological nursing was not included in nursing curricula, administrators should work with the DON/NA to ensure that licensed nursing staff have opportunities to participate in gerontological nursing continuing education programs. In addition, registered nurses often function in leadership and management positions in long-term care facilities and require the accompanying leadership and management skills and knowledge to be effective.

Baccalaureate nursing education programs provide the broadest and most comprehensive education background for nurses. The core competencies for baccalaureate prepared nurses are in the areas of critical thinking, assessment, communication, and technical skills. Core knowledge areas include: (1) health promotion, risk reduction, and disease prevention; (2) illness and disease management; (3) information and health care technologies; (4) ethics; (5) human diversity; (6) global health care; and (7) health care systems and policy. Role development in baccalaureate programs focuses on the use of theory and research-based knowledge in the direct and indirect delivery of care to patients (AACN, 1998). Another important role development area is as health care designer, coordinator, and manager of patient care. Knowledge and skills in this latter area are outlined below.

- Assume a leadership role within one's scope of practice.
- Coordinate and manage care to meet the special needs of vulnerable populations, including the frail elderly, in order to maximize independence and quality of life.
- Coordinate the health care of individuals across the lifespan utilizing principles and knowledge of interdisciplinary models of care delivery and case management.
- Delegate and supervise the nursing care given by others while retaining accountability for the quality of care given to the patient.
- Organize, manage, and evaluate the functioning of a team or unit.
- Use appropriate evaluation methods to analyze the quality of nursing care.
- Utilize cost-benefit analysis and variance data in providing and evaluating care (AACN, 1998, p. 17).

Registered nurses are eligible for certification in a variety of specialties. For those employed in long-term care facilities, certification in gerontological nursing is very desirable. Certification is obtained through the American Nurses Credentialing Center. The applicant takes a certification exam in the desired nursing specialty area. To maintain certification, the RN must continue practice in the specialty area and demonstrate continued competence in the specialty area through continuing education or other scholarly endeavors.

Registered nurses have numerous roles in long-term care facilities. They function in management positions such as charge nurse, nurse manager, care coordinator, unit coordinator, assistant director of nursing. Most long-term care facilities have a registered nurse who is responsible for staff development. Federal regulations require annual inservice training for staff on safety, fire, infection control, residents rights, as well as others. Staff development directors coordinate these programs and ensure that all staff attend. In addition, they often provide orientation programs for new employees and plan education programs to keep staff updated on equipment, new standards of care, and topics relevant to care of elders.

Nursing facilities are required to have an infection control program involving the establishment and implementation of appropriate written policies and procedures to assure a safe, sanitary, and comfortable environment for residents and to control the development and transmission of infections and diseases. A registered nurse often has the responsibility for monitoring compliance with the facility's infection control policies and procedures–investigating, controlling and preventing infections in the facility, and instituting appropriate interventions.

A recent new role for registered nurses in nursing facilities is the coordinator of the resident assessment process. The title of this nurse is the registered nurse assessment coordinator (RNAC). Because the MDS portion of the Resident Assessment Instrument is used to determine payment to the nursing home as well as monitoring quality care of the nursing facility, the RN in this role is critical to the viability of the nursing facility. The technicalities of accurately completing the MDS continues to become more complex. The RNAC should be aware of state and federal rules regarding the MDS, as well as the Medicare and Medicaid payments systems that use the MDS to classify residents into a payment "group." The RNAC needs to work closely with all nursing staff to ensure that the clinical needs of residents are accurately assessed and reflected on the MDS.

Advanced Practice Nurses

A growing number of RNs are obtaining a masters degree in nursing. Approximately 11 percent of RNs have a masters or doctoral degree (Bureau of Health Professions, 2001). This advanced nursing degree usually focuses on a clinical specialization such as gerontological nursing, adult health nursing, psychiatric nursing, or maternal and child health nursing. Some graduate nursing programs also offer an emphasis in nursing administration or education. Clinical specialization in masters programs prepares nurses as nurse practitioners or clinical nurse specialists. Following completion of the graduate nursing education program, graduates can take a national certification examination in their specialty area. In many states, certification following a graduate degree in nursing entitles these nurse practitioners/clinical specialists to receive third party reimbursement and have prescription writing privileges.

Gerontological nurse practitioners (GNPs) are experts in providing primary health care to older adults in a variety of settings, practicing independently and collaboratively with other health care professionals. In this role, GNPs work to maximize functional abilities; promote, maintain, and restore health; prevent or minimize disabilities; and promote death with dignity. GNPs engage in advanced practice, case management, education, consultation, research, administration, and advocacy for older adults (ANA, 2001).

Gerontological clinical nurse specialists (GCNS) are experts in providing, directing, and influencing the care of older adults and their families and significant others in a variety of settings. Clinical specialists demonstrate an in-depth understanding of the dynamics of aging, as well as interventions necessary for health promotion and management of health status alterations. Clinical specialists provide comprehensive gerontological nursing services independently or collaboratively with multidisciplinary teams. Through theory and research, clinical specialists advance the health care of older adults and the specialty of gerontological nursing. Clinical specialists are engaged in practice, case management, education, consultation, research, and administration and typically are employed in hospitals, nursing homes, and psychiatric facilities (ANA, 2001).

A number of studies have demonstrated the clinical and cost effectiveness of GNPs/GNCNs in long-term care facilities. Ryden et al. (2000) found that when advanced practice gerontological nurses conducted focused assessments for residents and provided consultation to nursing staff about using evidence-based practice protocols for care planning, residents had improvement in urinary continence, depression, aggressive behavior, and pressure ulcers. A growing role for the GNP in long-term care facilities is to provide clinical management and oversight for residents. These advanced practice nurses make regular visits to the nursing facility and work in collaboration with a physician. Managed care health plans contract for the services of GNPs to provide advanced clinical care to residents in long-term care facilities. The GNP is more available than physicians and can quickly intervene when a resident's condition changes. Research has demonstrated reduced cost in acute and emergency care with the use of GNP/MD teams (Burl, 1998). Nursing staff value the collegial support and responsiveness they receive from GNPs (Kane et al., 2000).

Licensed Practice/Vocational Nurses

The practical or vocational nurse is a graduate of a vocational or technical school of nursing. The program includes basic fundamentals of bedside care and clinical experience in hospitals and nursing homes. This one-year program does not allow time for in-depth scientific principles to be included in the curriculum. Thus, state licensure laws require that LP/VNs work under the direction of a registered nurse, physician or dentist. Similar to the RN, upon successful completion of a practical/vocational nursing program, the graduate is eligible to take the licensure examination and subsequently become a LP/VN.

Nursing Assistants

Nursing assistants comprise the majority of nursing staff in long-term care facilities and provide 80–90 percent of the direct care to residents. All nursing assistants are required by federal regulation to have a minimum of 75 hours of training to become certified nursing assistants (CNAs). In most instances, this training is conducted at vocational or technical schools, although some long-term care organizations are approved to do their own training. In a number of states, nursing assistants can obtain additional training certifying them to administer medications to residents–trained medication assistants (TMAs). A specialized role for nursing assistants that includes additional training is the restorative nursing assistant. They do range of motion, mobility programs, and have specialized training with feeding skills. Restorative nursing programs are coordinated by a registered nurse and carried out by restorative nursing assistants. The minimum required training for CNAs is hardly adequate to provide quality, individualized care to residents. Thus, both continued education opportunities and effective professional nursing supervision are essential for nursing assistants employed in long-term care facilities.

There are national organizations for CNAs including the National Association of Geriatric Nursing Assistants and the National Network of Career Nursing Assistants. In addition, several states such as Florida and Iowa have organizations for nursing assistants.

NURSE STAFFING

Nurse staffing has recently become a controversial issue. Advocates for improving the quality of care in nursing facilities have called for mandated minimum staffing ratios. While many States have legislated staffing standards, the standards are barely adequate. Current minimum federal standards require that all Medicare or Medicaid certified nursing facilities have an RN director of nursing; an RN on duty for eight hours a day, seven days a week; and a licensed nurse (either an RN or LP/VN) on duty on the other shifts. The federal law also requires sufficient nursing staff to provide nursing services for residents to attain or maintain the highest practicable level of physical, mental, and psychosocial well being of each resident.

The evidence that higher nurse staffing levels, especially RN staffing, is related to better quality of care outcomes for residents compels administrators to consider strategies to ensure the appropriate number and type of nursing staff in the facility at all times. Yet, determining the appropriate number and type of nursing staff to meet the needs of residents is one of the more challenging administrative roles for both the administrator and the director of nursing.

Nurse staffing is a process that involves determining, allocating and delivering the nursing resources to provide a certain standard of care to residents (Mueller, 2000). Ratio staffing has been used to determine staffing for a nursing unit or a nursing facility. Typically, this involves prescribing a specified number of residents per nursing care provider. For example, on the day shift, the CNA to resident ratio might be one to eight and the RN to resident ratio might be one to 24. Another strategy for staffing is simply establishing fixed staffing for each unit. For example, a 40-bed nursing unit might have six CNAs, one LPN and one RN on the day shift. Neither of these commonly used staffing strategies take into account different and varying care needs of residents.

A framework for nurse staffing in long-term care facilities (Figure 15-1) provides an overview of the complex variables associated with determining, allocating, and delivering nursing resources to meet the needs of residents and delineates the crucial links between the components of the framework (Mueller, 2000).

Nurse staffing should be based consistently on the values and beliefs of the nursing staff about residents and nursing care. The standards of nursing practice should reflect the current state of knowledge of gerontological nursing practice and subsequently provide guidance on identifying and meeting the nursing care needs of residents.

The residents' needs or clinical factors reflect the holistic nature of human beings–physical, emotional, educational, technical, social, and rehabilitative needs. These needs vary in complexity and amount of time required to meet them. Accurately identifying each resident's multidimensional needs is integral to the staffing framework. Patient classification systems, acuity systems, case-mix classification systems, and nursing workload management systems have been used to identify patient/resident needs for the purpose of staffing, budgeting, and evaluating productivity. The Resource Utilization Group-Version III (RUG-III) case-mix classification system was developed as part of a federal demonstration project to determine the Medicare payment nursing facilities should receive for individual residents. A number of states use this system for Medicaid payment. The RUG-III classification system uses items on the MDS as the resident care indicators and classifies a resident into one of 44 or 34 case-mix groups (depending on the version of the RUG-III classification system being used). Nursing time, by nursing skill level (RN, LP/VN, CNA), is associated with each of the RUG-III groups. Thus, nurse staffing on a unit may vary on a daily or weekly basis depending on changing nursing care needs of residents. This nursing resource driven case-mix classification system should serve as a guide for making daily staffing decisions as well as budgeting for staffing. Appendix B provides an example using the RUG-III nursing time to determine nurse staffing.

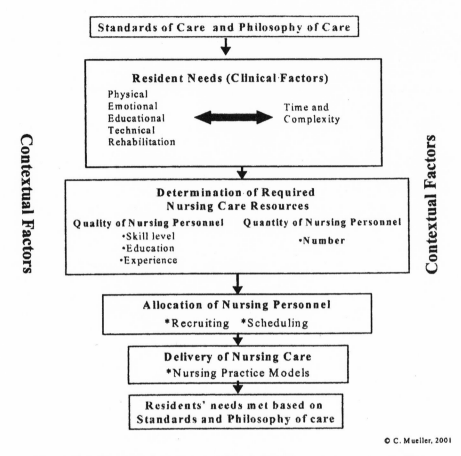

Figure 15-1. Framework for nurse staffing in long-term care nursing facilities.

The nursing care needs of residents are the critical indicators to determine the number and type of nursing staff needed on any shift. If the needs of residents remain stable, which might be the case on a Special Care Dementia Unit, staffing for the unit can be stable. If the needs of the residents are either unstable or vary (e.g., residents with complex, changing health conditions; frequent admissions and discharges), staffing needs will likely change more frequently. Need for professional nursing care is important to consider when making staffing decisions. In the case of a nursing unit in which residents' needs are complex and unstable, registered nurses may be needed to provide all or most of the care for those residents. An acuity classification system, such as the RUG-III classification system, can be very useful to help make those daily staffing decisions.

When the amount and type of nursing staff to meet the needs of residents are determined, then nursing staff need to be recruited. Issues related to recruitment and retention of nursing staff are addressed in another chapter. The education, experience, and skill level of nursing staff are crucial aspects to consider when recruiting nursing staff. For example, nursing staff with experience in caring for cognitively impaired older adults would be highly desirable for staffing a Special Care Dementia Unit. As noted earlier, a higher complement of registered nurses may be necessary for a Medicare skilled unit that has residents with complex, medical health conditions. Another Medicare skilled unit that focuses on rehabilitation might benefit from registered nurses with certification in rehabilitation nursing and nursing assistants who are trained as restorative nursing assistants.

The next challenge in the allocation of nursing staff for a facility or a nursing unit is scheduling staff. This involves the intricate balance of meeting the residents' needs with the needs of nursing staff. Although scheduling staff can be a time-consuming and often stressful activity, it is an activity that can promote and improve job satisfaction of staff. Providing staff opportunities to have control over scheduling, shift options, and staffing policies can lead to staff satisfaction.

There are many creative scheduling options and each have positive and negative aspects. For example, 12-hour shifts provide much more personal time off, but can also potentially cause errors in clinical judgment due to fatigue.

Some of the most frequently used scheduling options include:

1. Using different shift lengths (e.g., 8 hours, 10 or 12 hours, 4 hours)
2. Part-time staffing pool for weekend shifts
3. Job sharing
4. Flextime
5. Staff self-scheduling
6. Allowing nursing staff to exchange hours of work among themselves
7. Cyclical scheduling

Block scheduling or cyclical scheduling is an effective way to meet the requirements of equitable distributions of hours of work and time off. The basic time pattern for a certain number of weeks is established and then repeated in cycles. Often policies regarding scheduling determine how block or cyclical scheduling is operationalized. These policies could address scheduling for weekends and holidays, making changes to the schedule, rotation to different shifts, use of part-time personnel, use of float personnel, exchangeability of staff, the work week, vacations, and sick leave and so on. Appendix C provides two examples of a creative cyclical staff schedule. The staffing needs for both schedules were based on the residents' needs as determined by the RUG-III classification system. The first cyclical staff schedule is for a 24-bed skilled nursing unit that has residents with complex medical needs. Staff are scheduled for 12 and eight-hour shifts.

The second cyclical schedule is for a 20-bed Special Care Dementia Unit. On this unit, staff are scheduled for six and eight-hour shifts. Staffing needs were again based on the needs of residents as determined by the RUG-III case-mix classification system. The staffing and scheduling policies for this unit are as follows:

1. All nursing staff work every other weekend unless specifically hired to work every weekend.
2. Staff do not rotate shifts.
3. A cyclical schedule is used for scheduling staff.
4. The same number of staff by skill level are scheduled 7 days a week.
5. Staff work 8 hour shifts unless specifically hired to work shorter shifts.
6. Part-time staff work 32 hours a week or less.

On this schedule, some staff are scheduled to work another unit. For example, RN 2 works two shifts on the Special Care Unit and four shifts on another unit to make up a 0.6 full time equivalent. Another strategy used to ensure that staffing is consistent seven days a week is scheduling staff to work less than eight-hour shifts. This type of flexible scheduling provides the opportunity to schedule staff at peak work times (e.g., meals, bedtime). Experimenting with flexible staffing is both a challenge and a step toward retaining staff who might not otherwise be in the work force or who might otherwise be in someone else's work force.

There are a number of factors that can affect the allocation of nursing personnel to meet the needs of the residents. For example, perhaps it has been determined that the needs of residents require hiring a gerontological nurse specialist, but no one in the community meets those qualifications. Or, perhaps vacant positions cannot be filled due to a work force shortage. Or 75 percent of the nursing staff are needed to work 12-hour shifts, but only 25 percent want to work 12-hour shifts. Each nursing facility has unique factors that impact staffing and scheduling. Creative management strategies are needed to address these factors. The bottom line is that systematic determination of the needs of the residents serves as the basis for recruitment and scheduling decisions and actions.

NURSING PRACTICE MODELS

Administrators need to become acquainted with models for organizing the delivery of nursing care to meet residents' needs. Nursing staff are a limited resource, thus ensuring that they are used in the most effective and efficient manner is a critical administrative concern. Nursing practice models are the manner in which nursing staff assemble to accomplish the clinical goals. They provide a framework for the design and delivery of nursing care to residents (Anthony et al., 2000). Key aspects to nursing practice models are accountability, continuity of care, communication, and collaboration.

Nursing practice models have traditionally been categorized or defined as primary nursing, team/modular nursing, or functional nursing. However, these nursing practice models are operationalized very differently in nursing organizations and most of the information about how they have been operationalized has been described in acute care settings. Table 15-1 provides the definition and outlines the characteristics of each category of nursing practice models (Mueller, 2001).

Assignments or work allocation is an important aspect to a nursing practice model. Some long-term care nursing facilities have used permanent assignments with their certified nursing assistants to facilitate continuity of care. This involves having the same nursing assistant assigned to the same group of residents for at least one month or longer. The few studies that evaluated permanent assignments found there were improvements in resident outcomes (e.g., behavior) and staff were more satisfied (Teresi et al., 1993; Cox, 1991; Anderson et al., 1995; Haff, et al., 1988; Patchner et al., 1993; Skima, 1999). Registered nurses have also been used as primary nurses and case managers in long-term care facilities. While it is the most challenging model to implement due to so few RNs in long-term care facilities, it is the model that enables the RN to have the most accountability for the residents.

There is some disagreement about the value of permanent assignments for nursing assistants. Those that would argue against it say it is difficult to implement due to turnover and absenteeism. They might also argue that the CNAs could have uneven assignments or that some residents are too difficult to care for day after day. Those that advocate for permanent assignments would say that it saves time each shift in doing the assignments for CNAs, the residents like to have the same care provider on a consistent basis, and the CNAs get to know the residents better and can provide better input into the care planning process (Mueller, 2001).

Work allocation for licensed personnel also needs to be carefully considered. A common practice in nursing facilities is to use registered nurses and licensed vocational/practical nurses interchangeably. That is, in the role of staff nurse, either an RN or LP/VN is used to carry out the responsibilities outlined in a job description for a staff nurse. Such practice is potentially risky and should be carefully considered within the context of the state's nurse practice act and the educational preparation differences between RNs and LP/VNs (Mueller, 2001).

TABLE 15-1
CHARACTERISTICS OF NURSING PRACTICE MODELS

	Primary Nursing	Team/Modular Nursing	Functional Nursing
Definition	24-hour accountability by a nurse for specific clients from admission through discharge	Care to a group of clients by a mixed-staff team, sometimes using geographic modules to facilitate convenience	Assignments by function or tasks for a large group of clients
Clinical Decision-Making	Continuous; 24-hrs/day	Shift based	Shift based
Work Allocation	Client-based assignments	Task-based assignments	Task-based assignments
Communication	Primary nurse to associate nurse and unlicensed staff who perform delegated activities	Team leader to team member	Charge nurse to care provider assigned to tasks
Responsibility/authority of registered nurse	Responsibility to manage all nursing care for a consistent and manageable (in size and acuity) group of clients 24 hrs/day	Responsibility for care given to a large group of clients by other staff during a shift.	Responsibility for specific care tasks given to a large group of clients during a shift.

Mueller, C. (2001). *Developing a Comprehensive Staffing Program.* University of Minnesota, School of Nursing. (http://ltcntirseleader.umn.edu/)

The nursing process can be used as a framework to analyze and evaluate the knowledge and skills obtained in the two different education programs. Education programs to prepare someone to be a registered nurse provide comprehensive knowledge and skill in all phases of the nursing process (assessment, diagnosis, planning, implementing and evaluating). Practical/vocational nursing programs prepare someone to collect assessment data and to implement plans of care (that have been developed by an RN) that are within the scope of their practice. Further, LP/VNs need to be under the supervision of an RN or an MD (Mueller, 2001).

The Resident Assessment Instrument (RAI) process is the basis for providing information about the needs of the residents. The RAI consists of the:

1. Minimum Data Set (MDS) which is completed on admission and at least quarterly for each resident;
2. Items on the MDS which 'trigger' the Resident Assessment Protocols (RAPs);
3. RAPs which continue the assessment process to determine if this is a care area that needs to be addressed for the resident.

An interdisciplinary plan of care is then developed for the care areas triggered from the resident's MDS assessment. The interdisciplinary care plan consists of goals/objectives for each care area and corresponding interventions designed to meet the goals/objectives. The RAI and care planning process are designed to ensure that each resident's needs are individually addressed and the plan of care is individualized to meet the residents' "highest practicable level of functioning and well-being."

Ideally, all nursing staff involved in providing care to the residents should have input into the RAI and care planning process. If a facility has RNs assigned as primary nurses or case managers to residents, the RN should do the MDS and other assessments for the resident and attend care planning conferences. If a facility uses permanent assignments with nursing assistants, the nursing assistants should attend the care planning conferences. These are important strategies to ensure continuity of care and information that care providers need to know about the resident.

After the plan of care has been developed, the information has to be communicated and delegated to the nursing staff providing care to the residents. Developing an efficient way to extrapolate information from the care plans to an assignment sheet for CNAs is a key component to facilitate continuity of care for residents. Nursing assistants should be able to carry written information about the care needs of their assigned residents with them. Three by five stock cards are an ideal size to put into a pocket and can include resident care information on the front and back of the card. Write the resident care need information (e.g., cognitive needs, needs with function, bladder and bowel needs, nutritional needs) in pencil so that as needs change, information can be updated (unless there is the capacity to have the information generated on the cards by computer). Punch a hole in the upper left-hand corner of each card and reinforce the hole. The resident assignment cards for each CNA's assignment can be hooked together by a metal ring and will fit in their pocket.

In summary, the premise of the *Framework for Nurse Staffing in Long-term Care Facilities* is that nurse staffing should be based consistently on the values and beliefs about residents and nursing care (philosophy of care). The standards of nursing practice to which the nursing organization subscribes should reflect the current state of knowledge of gerontologic nursing practice and subsequently provide guidance on identifying and meeting the nursing care needs of residents. Thus, if the philosophy of the nursing organization and the standards of care permeate the components of the nurse staffing framework (e.g., identifying needs of residents, matching needs of residents with adequate and appropriate nursing resources, scheduling, assignments, nursing practice model), then the needs of the residents should be met. Outcomes will be measured in the facility's quality assurance program (see Chapter 19).

EXCELLENCE IN NURSING SERVICES

The nursing department should strive to attain excellence in the services it provides to residents and their families. Excellence should also be noted in the competence, professional development, involvement in governance, and job satisfaction of nursing staff. The American Nurses Association *Scope and Standards for Nurse Administrators* specifies the criteria for achieving this level of excellence. The American Nurses Credentialing Center (ANCC) sponsors the Magnet Nursing Services Recognition Program which recognizes excellent nursing organizations in hospitals and long-term care facilities. The program is based on years of research which demonstrated that nursing organizations in some hospitals had no difficulty recruiting and retaining nursing staff because they were distinguished by sustained professional nursing practice, flat organizational structures, decision making at the unit level, creative scheduling to maximize patient continuity and personal needs of nurses, effective nurse leaders, and investments in the education and development of nurses. These nursing organizations were referred to as "magnet" organizations. Research comparing magnet and nonmagnet nursing organizations found that magnet nursing organizations had better patient outcomes and higher nurse satisfaction.

The administrator should support and encourage the nursing department in working toward becoming a "magnet" nursing organization. While meeting the standards and associated criteria for magnet status is rigorous, the benefits include recognizing the importance of nurses to the success of the organization, diminishing recruitment and retention problems, having a competitive advantage in recruiting staff and attracting residents to the facility, creating a dynamic and positive milieu for professional nurses, and improving resident outcomes.

SUMMARY

The nursing department is certainly the largest, and perhaps the most complex department in a nursing facility. The administration and management of this department demands effective nurse leaders that are committed to excellence in resident care and nursing management. This chapter has provided an overview of key components of the nursing department addressing issues related to staffing, qualifications of staff, and organization and delivery of nursing care. Creativity, innovation, and promoting and managing change are essential administrative skills needed by nurse leaders in the nursing department.

RECOMMENDED RESOURCES FOR NURSES

Nursing Administration

American Nurses Credentialing Center. *Magnet Nursing Services Recognition Program.* http://www.nursingworld.orglancclmaknet.htm

Bradley, M., & Thompson, N. (2000). *Quality management integration in long-term care: Guidelines for excellence.* Baltimore: Health Professions Press.

Health Education Network. *Nursing Administration Manual for Long-term Care Facilities.* [http://healthed.net]

Health Education Network. *Staff Development Handbook for Long-term Care Facilities.* [http://healthed.net]

Lodge, M.P. (1987). *Professional education and practice of nurse administrators/directors of nursing in long-term care.* Kansas City: American Nurses Foundation.

Long-term Care Nursing Leadership and Management [http://Itcnurseleader.unm.edu/index.html]

Mitty, E. (1998). *Handbook for directors of nursing in long-term care.* Albany: Delmar Publishers.

Wisconsin Director of Nursing Council Manual. (2000). [262-375-1976].

Journals

Journal of Nursing Administration
Nursing Management

Nursing Administration Quarterly
The Director (Journal of the National Association of Directors of Nursing Administration in Long-Term Care)

Gerontological Nursing

Easton, K. (1999). *Gerontological rehabilitation nursing.* Philadelphia: Saunders.
Ebersole, P., & Hess, P. (1998). *Toward healthy aging* (4th ed.). St. Louis: Mosby.
Eliopoulos, C. (2001). *Gerontological nursing* (5th ed.). Philadelphia: Lippincott.
Gerontological Nursing Interventions Research Center [http://www.nursing.uiowa.edu/gnirc/index.htm]
Hartford Institute for Geriatric Nursing [http://www.hartfordign.org/]
Hogstel, M. (2001). *Gerontology: Nursing care of the older adult.* Albany: Delmar Publishers.
Luekenotte, A. *Gerontological Nursing.* St. Louis: Mosby.
Maas, M. Buckwalter, K., Harcy, M., Tripp Reimer, T., Titler, M., & Specht, J. (2000). *Nursing care, of older adults. Diagnosis, outcomes and interventions.* St. Louis: Mosby.
March, C. (1997). *The complete care plan manual for long-term care.* San Francisco: Jossey-Bass.
Stone, J., Wyman, J., & Salisbury, S. (1999). *Clinical gerontological nursing: A guide to advanced practice* (2nd ed.). Philadelphia: Saunders.

Journals

Journal of Gerontological Nursing
Geriatric Nursing

REFERENCES

American Association of Colleges of Nursing. (1998). *The essentials of baccalaureate education for professional nursing practice.* Washington, D.C.: AACN.
Anderson, C. L., & Hughes, E. (1995). An evaluation of modular nursing in a long term care setting. *Canadian Journal of Nursing Administration, 8*(2), 63–87.
Anthony, M. K., Casey, D., Chau, T., & Brennan, P. F. (2000). Congruence between registered nurses' and unlicensed assisstive personnel perception of nursing practice. *Nursing Economics, 18*(6), 285–293.
Arioan, J., Patsdaughter, C., & Wyszynski, M. (2000). DONs in long-term care facilities: Contemporary roles, current credentials and educational needs. *Nursing Economics, 18*(3), 149–156.
American Nurses Association. (1996). *Scope and standards for nurse administrators.* Washington, DC: American Nurses Association.
American Nurses Association. (2001). *Scope and standards for gerontological nursing.* Washington, DC: American Nurses Association.
Ballard, T. M. (1995). The need for well-prepared nurse administrators in long-term care. *Image: Journal of Nursing Scholarship, 27*(2), 153–154.

Bureau of Health Professions. (2001). *The registered nurse population: National sample survey of registered nurses–Preliminary findings.* Rockville, MD: HRSA.

Burl, J., Benner, A., Rao, M., & Khan, A. (1998). Geriatric nurse practitioners in long-term care: Demonstration of effectiveness in managed care. *Journal of the American Geriatric Society, 46,* 506–510.

Cox, C., Kaeser, L., Montgomery, A., & Marion, L. (1991). Quality of life nursing care: An experimental trial in long-term care. *Journal of Gerontological Nursing, 17*(4), 6–11.

Haff, J., McGowan, C., Potts, C., & Streekstra, C. (1988). Evaluating primary nursing in long-term care: Provider and consumer opinions. *Journal of Nursing Quality Assurance, 2*(3), 44–53.

Huber, D. (2000). *Leaders and nursing care management.* Philadelphia: W.B. Saunders.

Kane, R.L., & Huck, S. (2000). The implementation of the Evercare demonstration project. *Journal of American Geriatrics Nurses, 48,* 218–223.

Lodge, M.P. (1987). *Professional education and practice of nurse administrators/directors of nursing in long-term care.* Kansas City, KS: American Nurses Foundation.

Marquis, B., & Huston, C. (2000). *Leadership roles and management functions in nursing: Theory and application* (3rd ed.). Philadelphia: Lippincott.

Institute of Medicine. (1996). *Nursing staff in hospitals and nursing homes. Is it adequate?* Washington, DC: National Academy Press.

Mueller, C. (1998). Education for nurse administrators: A need or a demand. *Nursing Management, 29*(11), 39–42.

Mueller, C. (2000). A nurse staffing framework for long-term care facilities. *Geriatric Nursing, 21*(5), 262–267.

Mueller, C. (2001). *Long-term Care Nursing Leadership and Management.* [http://ltc-nurseleader.umn.edu/]

Patchner, M.A., & Patchner, L.S. (1993). Essential staffing for improved nursing home care: The permanent assignment model. *Nursing Homes, 42*(5), 37–39.

Ryden, M., Snyder, M., Gross, C., Savik, K., Pearson, V., Krichbaum, K., & Mueller, C. (2000). Value-added outcomes: The use of advanced practice nurses in long-term care facilities. *Gerontologist, 40*(6), 654–662.

Skima, S. (1999). An innovative model for long-term care nursing delivery. *Research Nursing Registry: Sigma Theta Tau International.*

Teresi, J., Hohnes, D., Benenson, E., Monaco, C., Barrett, V., & Ramirez, M. (1993). A primary care nursing model in long-term care facilities: Evaluation of impact on affect, behavior, and socialization. *The Gerontologist, 33*(5), 667–673.

Chapter 16

SOCIAL SERVICES IN LONG-TERM CARE

JAMES R. REINARDY

A major goal of the 1987 Nursing Home Reform Act and subsequent federal regulations has been to place greater emphasis upon services that address the quality of life as well as the medical and personal care needs of nursing home residents. Social workers, who have been trained to address the psychosocial needs of clients, are a key component in helping to realize that goal. Although the responsibilities of social workers vary from facility to facility, their major tasks include admissions, assessment and care planning, and direct services/interventions with residents and families. They also play an important role in supporting residents' autonomy and in advocating on their behalf. In carrying out their tasks, they work closely with other staff within the nursing home and serve as a member of an interdisciplinary team. The following pages describe these social service functions, and provide a brief discussion of federal regulations and the hiring of social services personnel.

SOCIAL SERVICES PERSONNEL

The 1987 Omnibus Reconciliation Act (PL 100-203, *The Nursing Home Reform Act*) requires skilled nursing facilities to provide social services that reach or maintain the highest practicable physical, mental, and psychosocial well being of residents. It also requires that facilities with 120 or more beds have a social services director. The Centers for Medicare and Medicaid Services (CMS, formerly the Health Care Financing Administration) interprets a qualified social services director to be someone from an accredited school of social work with a master's or bachelor's level degree (MSW or BSW). It also allows others, who are deemed social service designees, to serve as directors. A social service designee includes those with a bachelor's degree in other related fields who have had a year's experience working under a social worker or those without degrees who have been "grandfathered" into the position. Finally, nursing homes may employ consultants, often with MSW, to supervise designees or provide part-time services.

The federal rules on personnel and staffing also require nursing homes to follow all state laws regulating licensing or registration of social workers. Some states require licensed social workers; others do not. Licensing laws can be complex, defining several levels of social work practice from licensed independent clinical social workers to social workers at the bachelor's level.

Recently, professional organizations such as the National Association of Social Workers have formally complained to CMS about the broad variance found from state to state in the enforcement of regulations on the qualifications of social service personnel—some nursing homes hiring clinical MSW social workers and others hiring persons with almost any degree. They also argue that no profession within the nursing home industry other than social work—physicians, nurses, or therapists—is allowed untrained, unlicensed designees. The need for qualified practitioners is an important consideration if nursing homes are to achieve the quality of well being mentioned in OBRA '87. This is particularly evident when one considers that the majority of nursing home residents experience mental health or cognitive problems in addition to the normal challenges faced with aging and institutional living.

SOCIAL SERVICE FUNCTIONS

Admissions and Discharge Planning

Nursing home admissions have changed significantly over the past several years. More residents are admitted directly from hospitals or other facilities, fewer from the community. On one hand, given the growth of long-term care alternatives, more of the long-stay residents have serious mental and physical disabilities. On the other hand, there are also more short-term residents. The prospective payment system for hospitals has had a major impact, resulting in earlier discharges of these patients to nursing homes for post-acute care. Social workers may at times find themselves, particularly at intake, relying almost solely upon the input of the family or other sources rather than on that of the new resident. Since the Prospective Payment System has also increased the number of residents who are admitted for short-term stays, a greater part of the social services work load is now devoted to discharge planning as well as to admissions. Another change, due partly to state concerns about rising costs, is that a large percentage of persons entering nursing homes will have undergone pre-admission screening to determine whether their placement is appropriate. Although this is an important component of the relocation process, surveys continue to show that many nursing home residents indicate that they have had little input or control in the decision to move to a facility. Given all of the above, social workers face many challenges in admitting and orienting new residents.

The admissions process includes one or more intake meetings in which the facility's policies and programs are shared with the resident and family, and in which information on the resident's background and preferences is obtained. The process is much broader than intake, however, and social service personnel will have frequent contacts with a new resident in the first few weeks of her stay to introduce her to the nursing home, its staff and residents, and to promote a smooth transition into the facility. Covering too much information on the first meeting–consider, for example, the challenge of helping someone determine preferences on advance directives–will overwhelm the new resident. The overall goal of the process is to move towards a plan of care that promotes daily living that is as consistent as possible, within the constraints of the nursing home setting, with the identity, values, and life style that the resident brings to the home.

During the admissions process social workers collect information on multiple dimensions, although this varies among facilities according to the work arrangements of the nursing home interdisciplinary team. Information is collected on the social history of new residents and on their emotional and cognitive status. The social worker identifies physical and medical problems, particularly as they relate to psychosocial needs. Of equal importance are the interests and strengths of the residents, as well as their daily routines prior to admission. Social workers also determine the preferences of the residents in a broad array of areas of daily living–preferences about advance directives to religious activities to bath routine. Finally, in addition to explaining nursing home policies and programs, and addressing financial issues, social workers help make residents and families aware of their rights, in particular, those articulated in the Nursing Home Bill of Rights.

Despite efforts to welcome new residents and maintain life continuity (e.g., retaining furniture and possessions, and adapting the nursing home routine to personal needs), moving to a nursing home is a major adjustment that involves significant personal loss. Social workers need to build a trusting relationship with new residents and allow them as much control and participation in decision-making as is possible. Families also are participants in this process. They have the potential to become partners with the social worker throughout the residents' stay in the home. Admissions include assessing the strengths and concerns of the family, using it as a major resource in learning about the resident, and determining what role family members are able to play in care planning and in the life of the resident. In a less formal sense, admissions work with the family continues beyond admission to the facility–the social worker, for example, may help a family work through the decision to move their parent or spouse to an Alzheimer's unit.

Social workers are often responsible for discharge as well as for admissions. This process, which is a growing responsibility for social workers in all major sectors of health care, involves arranging for the most appropriate setting, whether at home or in an alternative living facility. It includes assessing the resources of the family and others to support the discharged resident, helping with financial assistance and insurance, and arranging for needed services such as home health care. There may be differences in expectations between the resident and family members, or residents may have an unrealistic view of their abilities to get along by themselves once discharged: all of these potential conflicts demand considerable interviewing and mediating skills.

Assessment and Care Planning

Social workers are involved in resident assessment and care planning from the point of admissions to discharge. Assessments combine information from secondary sources such as hospital and pre-admission screening reports with information obtained directly through interviews with the resident and family. They often involve the use of standardized tools to assess emotional and cognitive status, such as the Geriatric Depression Scale and the Mini Mental Status Exam.

Assessment and care planning is an interdisciplinary process, involving all members of the nursing home interdisciplinary team. CMS requires nursing facilities to use the Resident Assessment Instrument, a clinical instrument developed to identify residents' strengths, weaknesses, and needs in key areas of functioning. The tool, administered early on and periodically throughout the resident's stay, collects data that trigger the need for further evaluation and the use of protocols that lead to care plans. Members of the team, which often consists of a floor nurse, social worker, dietitian, activity director, and therapist, complete sections that relate to their expertise. Social workers typically complete the sections on mood and behavior problems, and on psychosocial well-being. Teams that are truly interdisciplinary integrate many perspectives on a problem to produce a plan superior to what each profession would be able to do on its own. It is one thing, for example, to obtain a depression score on a resident; another thing to untangle the resident's feelings of hopelessness with interconnected experiences of personal loss and current behaviors such as a decrease in activities, problems in diet, and failures to respond to staff.

Residents have a right to take part in their care planning, and it is the responsibility of social workers to encourage residents and their families to participate. Families can be of particular help, especially when residents are incapacitated. Families help to identify needs and preferences, and are an important link in monitoring the resident's ongoing experiences in areas such as quality of food, and the impact of the routine and personal care. They are an essential part of the care plan, providing the resident with links to the past and present, and maintaining relationships with relatives, friends, and the community.

Direct Services to Residents and Families

Social workers serve residents and their families in many different ways. They provide both counseling services and education, and strengthen lines of communication among residents, families, and staff. They mediate between residents and their families, or between residents and staff. They assist residents and relatives in using the nursing home's resources, and refer them to additional resources, such as financial and legal services, in the community. They also play a role in maintaining and developing linkages between the nursing home and the community, helping to create greater opportunities for social interaction between residents and members of the community. In addition to working individually with clients, they lead a variety of groups.

Much counseling is directed to helping the resident and family adjust to the nursing home, and to deal with loss and changes in functioning while at the same time helping the resident to adapt and maintain the best possible quality of life. Families need help in learning to cope with their own guilt, anger, or loss, or they won't be able to offer effective support to the life and care of their parent or spouse in the nursing home. They also, may bring with them long-standing problems in their relationship with the resident that is suddenly exacerbated by the relocation and the challenges of a new environment. Social workers will sometimes support groups of relatives to help them address these issues.

Although social workers play different educational roles, a key one is educating staff to appreciate the backgrounds and qualities that residents bring to the nursing home, and to understand the problems they face. A resident, for example, wants to spend a little time each day sweeping his room—he once was a janitor. Staff, particularly nursing aids, will be better able to treat residents with care and understanding to the extent that they know them as persons.

Psychosocial and behavioral assessment and intervention is another important social work function, although the extent of the responsibility will depend upon the social worker's training and qualifications. Residents may refuse assistance from the staff or, on the other hand, regress and become overly dependent. Inappropriate sexual activity, hostile actions towards roommates and staff, major changes in style of social interaction and activities: social workers need to work with the family and staff to determine the underlying causes and appropriate interventions for such changes in behavior. Again, educating staff is of key importance since misunderstood behavior is often misinterpreted as simply attempts to annoy or irritate others.

Social workers also lead or promote several different kinds of group activities. These can be for the purpose of therapy, education, or social support–all foster meaningful social involvement. Reality orientation and remotivation groups, for example, may help to modify residents' confusion; reminiscence or life review groups encourage socialization and promote a sense of self-worth. Other groups may help plan events and give residents input into other aspects of nursing home life such as meal planning or changes in routines and procedures.

Advocacy and the Support of Resident Autonomy

Although autonomy is often used to mean independence, it has a broader meaning when applied to life in nursing homes where residents are in many ways dependent. Although it involves freedom of choice and participation in decision-making, it also implies living within a caring environment that affirms the resident's past, and is consistent with his or her current values and life goals. Maintaining autonomy and life continuity is a major axiom of social work practice in nursing homes. Those who achieve success listen carefully to the client, understand her needs and preferences, and, as mentioned throughout this chapter, collaborate closely with the family, staff, and interdisciplinary team. One key area of autonomy is medical decision-making and planning for health care in the event of mental incapacity. Here social workers or nurses or both, depending upon the facility, help residents think through decisions on advance directives. These decisions can be a source of conflict between the resident and family, and require skill in upholding the resident's choice while maintaining a supportive family relationship.

Advocacy skills are a major component of social work training and social workers, like other professionals, consider themselves accountable not only to the administrator but to standards of practice and to their profession's Code of Ethics. They advocate for individual residents as well as for improvements in the facility and long-term care system. Issues include substandard care, failure to respect legal rights, financial exploitation, oversedation, and lack of respect for the right to privacy and for conjugal rights. Conflicts in rights often call for the use of mediation rather than advocacy skills. Social workers find themselves mediating between roommates, for example, with the goal of respecting the autonomy of both parties.

Social workers are often responsible for forming and maintaining the nursing home resident council. This gives them an opportunity to work with residents in advocating for changes in the facility's policies, organizational routines, and procedures.

IMPLICATIONS FOR ADMINISTRATORS

It is important for nursing home administrators to understand the federal and state regulations that govern the hiring and practice of social workers—particularly their state's licensing statutes and rules. For example, a social worker with a BSW, although capable of addressing many of the psychosocial needs of residents, is not trained or typically allowed by law to diagnose and treat mental illness. However, licensed clinical social workers, usually not part of the staff of the nursing facility, may do so. But even here, to carry the example further, matters can be complex and in a state of flux. Currently, some Medicare fiscal intermediaries will reimburse these practitioners as separate providers; others consider their services already covered under the Prospective Payment System reimbursement.

Relevant training and educational background are essential if the social worker is to be an effective member of the nursing home staff. Although a degree in social work does not in itself guarantee skills in geriatric practice, there currently exists a strong effort among bachelor and graduate social work programs to enrich geriatric social work content and practical experience. In addition to educational qualifications, administrators need to hire social workers who are able to be interdisciplinary team players, and should make certain that the social worker's psychosocial role on the team is clearly defined. The ability to collaborate with staff; to educate, and to mediate among residents, families, and staff (multicultural issues are growing more prominent, particularly with the employment of New Americans as nursing assistants); to navigate community resources quickly in the fast pace of discharge planning; to adequately document services to residents; to promote resident autonomy; and to advocate on behalf of those unable to express their needs and rights: these are all attributes that administrators should look for and support in social work personnel.

Each nursing home should have an organized social services department under the direction of a social worker, with adequate staff, space, and equipment to support its role. Administrators should make sure that the department maintains and periodically updates a written plan for social work services in the facility. It should include a statement of the philosophy and goals of the department, its relationship and that of its personnel to other departments and personnel in the facility, and a clear and detailed articulation of measurable objectives. Understanding and endorsing the department's vision and plan, and systematically evaluating its progress, the director can make a significant step in promoting the quality of life and social service needs of nursing home residents.

REFERENCES

Department of Health and Human Services. (2001). *Nursing Home Resident Assessment Quality of Care*. Office of Inspector General. OEI-02-99-00040, January.

Gamroth, J. et al. (1995). *Enhancing autonomy in long-term care*. New York: Springer.

Garner, J. (1995). Long-term care. *Encyclopedia of Social Work*. Washington, DC: NASW Press.

Gleason-Wynn, P., & Mindel, C. (1999). A proposed model for predicting job satisfaction among nursing home social workers. *Journal of Gerontological Social Work, 32*(3), 65–78.

Mellor, J., & Lindeman, D. (1998). The role of the social worker in interdisciplinary teams. *Journal of Gerontological Social Work, 30* (3/4), 3–7.

Nathanson, I., & Tirrito, T. (1996). *Gerontological Social Work: Theory into Practice*. New York: Springer.

National Association of Social Workers. (1981). *NASW Standards for Social Work Medicare Equity Act*. News Brief, November.

O'Neill, J., & Rosen, A.L. (1998). *Survey of Current Practice and Recommendations. Professional Social Work Services in Skilled Nursing Facilities*. National Association of Social Workers, July. Retrieved January 21, 2002 from http://www.naswdc .org/practice.

Peak, T. (2000). Families and the nursing home environment: Adaptation in a group context. *Journal of Gerontological Social Work, 33*(1), 51–66.

Reinardy, J. (1999). Autonomy, choice, and decision-making: How nursing home social workers view their role. *Social Work in Health Care, 29*(3), 59–77.

Stahlman, S., with Kisor, A. (2000). Nursing homes. In R. Schneider, N. Kropf, & A. Kisor (Eds.), *Gerontological Social Work*. Belmont, CA: Brooks/Cole.

Chapter 17

THERAPEUTIC ACTIVITY

CARLA E.S. TABOURNE

The aim of this chapter is to offer a framework for understanding the essential role of meaningful activity in the lives of older adults, particularly in long-term care. The intent is to assist in the process of creating and administrating programs that yield outcomes that make life worth living into advanced years. Four tenets provide the keystone. First, health is more than the absence of illness (WHO, 1980). Second, being alive is more than merely breathing (Baltes & Baltes, 1990). Third, a person is an integrated whole, not just the sum of parts (Kivnick, 1993). Fourth, at the end of life, what do people value most and how do healthcare providers include these values in their plans for delivering services?

BACKGROUND

While there is little agreement among gerontologists about the experience of aging, the biological process and final outcome is known. It is during the years preceding death when older adults increasingly require services and products. Although these years may be marked with physical and social losses, they may also be profiled by the ability to balance losses and gains and the realization that this ability can continue to develop until death. The ability to maintain this balance is certainly an important dimension of quality of life and a measure of success in the process of aging.

The Surgeon General issued a series of reports called "Healthy People" in 1979, 1980, and in 2000 (U.S. DHHS, 1990). "Healthy People 2010" is now available from the Public Health Service on-line (U.S. DHHS, 2001). The reports shifted the focus of healthcare to preventive interventions that: (1) promote health and independent functioning; (2) minimize the effects of con-

232

ditions and reduce the risks for additional or secondary impairments; (3) maximize individual capacity in the nondisabled areas of functioning; and (4) maximize quality of life. Chapter 13 expands on these goals.

This model of service delivery is holistic and requires an integrative multidisciplinary team approach to healthcare rather than the traditional medical approach. To deliver services according to this model, providers of health services need new knowledge and skills and a new vision for management. These concepts are stressed in Chapters 2 and 13.

Projections of the population of the United States made by the U.S. Department of Commerce, Bureau of the Census, adjusted between the 1989 and 2001 census, revealed the growth and diversity of the American population. The fastest growing age group is over 85 years of age, the oldest old (Spencer, 1989). In 1987, older adults incurred more than one-third of healthcare services and will reach 50 percent or more in 30 years (Aday & Shortell, 1988).

The Department of Health and Human Services (DHHS) expressed concern as early as 1989 over the projected shortage of trained professionals needed to provide care to the burgeoning populations of older adults (U.S. DHHS, 1990). In particular, there was concern that there was going to be a critical lack of trained professionals who could move the prevention focused healthcare agenda forward and with it, attention to mitigating disability and maximizing the quality of life over the long term.

Gerontologists report differences between criteria for quality of life identified by consumers of long-term care and the criteria cited by industry and policymakers. Consumers, their family members, and advocates emphasize the need to ensure meaning in aging. The winter issue of *Generations* 1999–2000 was dedicated to sustaining identity, personal significance, and supporting individual reasons of old and frail residents to want to grow older. Kaufman (1986) aptly describes the clash between quality and quantity, biomedical, and existential values.

To summarize, efforts to guarantee that nursing home care is of high quality miss the boat when the focus is only on biomedical and environmental criteria. While these aspects are essential to good care, older adults and their families verbalize the importance of caring relationships and activities that enhance meaning in their lives and that promote continuity of self. Residents want to be recognized and respected as individuals distinct from other residents, with contributions yet to make.

The federal government assumed increasing responsibility for the enormous expenditure of public money for institutional long-term care and for overseeing the quality of that care. The Nursing Home Reform Act of 1987 (OBRA, 1989) gave birth to the Minimum Data Set in an attempt to ensure that each nursing home knew the needs of each resident and was making efforts to meet those needs. However, these efforts are focused on biomedical needs. Psychosocial and spiritual needs are given less attention. A prevention model of care, particularly in the context of caring for the elderly, needs cost-effectiveness analysis using formal data obtained through efficacy research and clinical trials to compare relative benefits of services competing for resources. Chapter 26 discusses some of the problems related to this issue.

THERAPEUTIC RECREATION SERVICES (a.k.a. RECREATION THERAPY DEPARTMENT OR THERAPEUTIC ACTIVITY UNIT)

The following section offers a structure for comprehensive therapeutic recreation services in long-term care, the bridge between addressing bio-medical need and the needs of the whole person. To be comprehensive, the direction of the department should be clear and the connections between the different aspects of service should be logical. The design of the department should be conceptualized systematically beginning with the interrelationships of program design and delivery, and documentation of client outcomes, stability, flexibility, and accountability. The purpose for having a comprehensive therapeutic service is two-fold: (1) to deliver therapy, and (2) to lead activities.

The purpose of recreation therapy is to integrate or complement purposeful interventions in the form of activities that are resident-centered, goal-directed, and outcome-based with other specialized therapies (U.S. Dept. of Labor, 1996–97). The goals are to restore functioning, mediate disabling effects of impairment, and mitigate risk for developing new conditions. Recreation therapy interventions are prescribed, often physician-ordered, and may be included in the three-hour rule for active treatment; therefore, a part of case-mix prospective payment (HCFA, 1984). Under some circumstances, and depending on the parameters of the nursing home, therapy interventions may be charged as acute rehabilitation (e.g., therapy with a patient in coma from a traumatic brain injury) (CARE, 2001).

The intent of recreation service is to provide resources to residents, families, and attending staff and to offer activities that maximize strengths and the ability to enjoy life. Activities should be planned to enrich life and diminish institutional depersonalization. Activities can promote leisure behavior and community integration to prevent boredom and isolation. They ought to help residents avoid feelings of helplessness or pessimism, sustain individual identity, and retain mastery over their environment. Programs in which older adults are leaders or role models (e.g., intergenerational, peer support, and staff-resident therapeutic relationships) encourage generativity and affirm their self-worth because they are contributing to others in the face of dependency and deterioration.

Organized recreation activities that are diversional offer the sheer enjoyment of being alive, are entertaining and engaging, or are unstructured opportunities to relax and to socialize and are freely chosen. They offer a change of routine, different scenery, and something to do that might be fun. These activities may be educational, mentally stimulating, a chance to socialize, exercise, or participate in the arts; one can try something new or rekindle old interests and revitalize the spirit. These services are included in the room rate and are considered to be a routine part of the general care of the residents.

A comprehensive program design, therefore, may include treatment/therapy in the form of rehabilitation and habilitation interventions for physical and mental functions, counseling and leisure education for decision and choice making, control and increased independence, opportunities for contemplation and religious expression for the emotional and spiritual aspects of life, and occasions to engage in psychosocial behaviors of friendship and reciprocity.

Comprehensive therapeutic recreation services (i.e., therapist directed, educational, and opportunities to participate by choice or for diversion) must be spelled out in detail in the department's written plan of operation. Content, process, intent, and evaluation of the program need to complement the efforts of other departments. Additionally, the process for assessing residents' need, interest, and performance in programs is explained, documented, and evaluated in terms of outcomes.

The Written Plan of Operation: Agency and Departmental

The mission and philosophy of the department are stated first in the written plan. They reflect the mission and philosophy of the facility and define responsibilities. The mission also interprets the minimum requirements and minimum standards of mandated governmental regulations and standards of voluntary accrediting bodies like the Council for Accrediting Rehabilitation Facilities (CARF). The stated philosophy of the department directs the ordering of priorities and the way each priority should be approached. Professional standards for the design and delivery of services are expounded in the written plan and divided into program and patient management.

Following preliminary assessment and screening of residents using the Minimum Data Set v. 2.0 (MDS), a more in-depth analysis is made using the Residents Assessment Protocols (RAPS) of any problems targeted in the initial screening. Other standardized assessment or facility specific appraisals may also be employed. The intent is to determine the best way to deliver the most care with the least redundancy, misuse, or unnecessary number of resources.

Utilization reviews determine effective administration of the facility in terms of appropriate allocation of resources (space, materials, efficient expenditure of monies, and use of staff). For budgeting cycle reviews and requests, the departments must project fiscal needs in terms of anticipated benefits from the expenditure. Utilization reviews seek information through the Resource Utilization Guidelines (RUGS) about the overuse or underutilization of resources and the impact on resident care. Of the seven major categories, therapeutic activity is implicated in five: rehabilitation, special care, impaired cognition, behavior, and physical function. In other words, the purpose for utilization review is to evaluate the relationship between patient outcomes and resources used to deliver the care.

As described in Chapter 19, monitoring patient care is a major administrative function and involves input from all departments including the department responsible for therapeutic activity. Therefore, a system for monitoring patient progress and outcomes is an essential part of the written plan of operation for the department. Additional program management responsibilities are staff growth and development, research, and ensuring patient rights.

The Department's Plan

The therapeutic activity department's plan begins with a stated purpose and goals for each *type* of service. One way to ensure that the breadth of services is adequate is to make sure that at least five domains of life are addressed in some way. The five domains most often considered for therapeutic activity are cognitive (mental), motor (physical), psychological (emotional), social, and spiritual (including religious expression). A good plan has an array of programs to meet the needs of the residents.

For example, therapy services might be divided into three categories: prevention, early intervention and rehabilitation programs, and leisure education. These types of interventions require detailed protocols that detail the purpose, content, and process for implementation, and the desired outcomes. These services are prescriptive and may be physician ordered. They can be delivered as co-treatment and patient performance is evaluated according to outcome measures. The characteristics of the physical environment (e.g., free of distractions or interruptions), the safety demands for materials to be used, and leadership style and strategies are included in protocols for each intervention. The individual programs should be flexible in design and easily modified as needed. Leisure education can include activities that are outside of rehabilitation goals and focus more on pure leisure skill development and would not be part of therapy services. However, these programs should still be selected and implemented thoughtfully in order to be meaningful.

Prevention programs might include strength, gait, and balance training to retain independent ambulation and to reduce the risks of falling. One intervention might be Tai Chi; another, simply walking heel to toe on a broad, painted line. Early intervention and rehabilitation programs might include writing cue cards for one person with early signs of dementia to keep in his pocket or completing crossword puzzles for someone who had brain surgery. Lastly, leisure education programs renew old, valued experiences and introduce new ones connecting individuals to the immediate environment and to the rest of society.

To increase awareness of the need for leisure, information is presented about the countless choices of things there are to enjoy throughout life. Strategies for decision-making and choice-making are useful skills for other aspects of their lives. They are more likely to be applied if the resident feels efficacious (Bandura, 1986; Seligman, 1975). Feelings of mastery and accomplishment emerge from learning new skills, and with practice, comes enough competence to experience success. The content of leisure education programs must reflect the culture and interests of all who might participate and be appropriate to the range of their abilities. A point at which to begin, perhaps, is to help participants recognize that they each have inner strengths and resources that they can tap into. Motivation to continue this work is more likely to occur if participants believe that they are not helpless and they have something to share with others.

For a nursing home in which the residents are very diverse in age and ability, a range of programs might include meditation, bird-watching or feeding, and a drama club. Meditation is an activity that requires no interaction with a person or object, bird watching or feeding involves only one person and something in the environment but not a person, whereas a drama club involves several residents working together to present a play for the other residents. The next decision in the program design process involves appropriate staffing. The number and qualifications of professional and paraprofessional staff needed to execute the written plan reflect the mission and philosophy of the department.

Professional Staff, Assistants, and Volunteers

Who provides what programs? Prior to 1987, the role of activities in a nursing home was to provide diversion and fun to residents to pass the time each day. The activities often included birthday parties, board games, puzzles, simple art projects like decorating paper cups, or sing-alongs. Activities were provided by the "Activity Department" led by someone who needed no formal education beyond high school. In part, this arrangement was prior to regulation of the long-term care industry. The intent was to keep old people busy, out of bed, and out of trouble (i.e., engaged in behaviors disturbing to others or creating more work for staff). During the past 30 years, the focus has increasingly shifted to therapeutic interventions that are outcome-based and measurable, as well as activities that meet the interests of residents and that are enjoyable.

In 1989, the Department of Health and Human Services also expressed concern over the projected shortage of trained professionals needed to provide care to the burgeoning populations of older adults. In particular, there was concern that there was going to be a critical shortage of trained professionals who could move the prevention-focused healthcare agenda forward and, with it, attention to mitigating disability and maximizing the quality of life over the long term. However, despite federally funded projects to increase the availability of specialists, there is still a shortage of prepared personnel.

The therapeutic recreation field was slow to prepare professionals with specialized backgrounds in gerontology. Concurrently, therapeutic recreation students began to focus their education on preparing to work in gerontology. Activity providers have organized, developed standards, and constructed certification on three levels, activity assistant, activity director, and activity consultant. Occupational therapy assistants have also been hired to deliver activity services.

In sum, certification as an activity assistant requires a high-school diploma or GED, plus 90 hours of training or activity experience. Requirements for certification as activity director include a bachelor's degree, activity experience, and evidence of continuing education in specified areas. The highest level is activity consultant requiring a college degree, master's degree preferred, along with the requirements for director plus consulting experience. Each level allows other ways to balance academic education, special learning, and activity experience.

Occupational therapy assistants are sometimes hired to work activities. Training for occupational therapy assistant requires an associate academic degree including the basic concepts of occupational therapy, interpersonal skills, group dynamics, group leadership skills, and the use of human occupation strategies. Supervised fieldwork and a national exam are required for certification. Many states also have some form of regulation in order to practice. Generally, state regulations are based on the results of the certification examination. The requirements for certification as a therapeutic recreation specialist (CTRS) are considerably more stringent.

The basic preparation for a therapeutic recreation specialist is a bachelor's degree with a major focus or an academic minor in therapeutic recreation.

Supervised fieldwork includes pre-internship experience and a formal supervised 480-hour consecutive full-time minimum internship with academic and clinical supervision and evaluation. The culminating certifying step is passing the three-hour national examination managed and administered by the Educational Testing Service in Princeton, New Jersey. There are also formal requirements for a certified therapeutic recreation assistant. Some states have some form of regulation in order to practice.

The mission and written plan of operation of the organization guide decisions about the kind of services that are to be provided. The scope of service dictates the qualifications needed by the staff. The director of the department is responsible for patient and program management and should have specialized knowledge of gerontology, managerial skills, and the credentials to conduct staff training and continuing education. The director should have requisite skills and experience delivering purposeful interventions in long-term care and be able to organize and lead staff, students, and volunteers.

Specialized knowledge that allows for appraisal of pathological symptoms distinguished from aspects of normal aging is critical to safe and effective program design. The ability of activity staff to interface and coordinate patient care with nursing, social services, and other health care providers for optimal outcomes is invaluable.

Managerial duties include responsibility for overseeing the comprehensive program of services needed by residents. The director is responsible for the quality assurance plan and monitoring process in the department, as well as the criteria for appropriate staffing, orientation, and establishing clinical supervision when needed. The director must assign staff to patients and/or programs according to their expertise and credentials to provide specific types of services. The department schedule should allow adequate time for staff to chart progress and review protocols for the interventions they implement so as to get the best patient outcomes. The director is also responsible for holding regular departmental meetings around particular patient or program issues and for routine review of how resources are being used according to policies and procedures concerning professional performance, time, budget, logistics, materials, equipment, and space, safety, and availability.

Staffing Patterns

One-person therapeutic recreation departments exist in small organizations. However, this organizational structure is unlikely to meet either OBRA regulations or the spirit of the laws governing most long-term care organizations. Overuse and misuse of resources are inefficient. One therapeutic recreation specialist with no professional peer with whom to collaborate and exchange ideas cannot be expected to grow professionally unless there are opportunities to mingle with peers. Burnout and staff turnover are inevitable when staff feel isolated, overextended, and hindered from practicing as their profession dictates.

Staff burnout is costly to the facility and to residents as described in Chapter 7. Therefore, a second therapeutic recreation specialist should be on staff to provide purposeful interventions to appropriate patients and to share management duties with the director and be able to carry out the director's duties during vacation, sick leave, or professional conferences. Paraprofessionals, pre-professional students, and trained volunteers complete the staff. The latter group make it possible for the more-credentialed, higher-paid professionals to deliver the prescribed and/or physician-ordered therapies. The ratio of staff to patients should be a measure of efficiency in quality review, and should not include pre-professional students and volunteers in the count.

Patient/Client Management: Outcome-Based and Goal-Directed

The older population in the United States is in reality many populations of varied education, economics, experience, power, and expectations of living a life with quality. The demographic characteristics have also changed dramatically in terms of diversity of race, ethnicity, gender, age, and culture. Therefore, the criteria used in measuring quality in peoples' lives have also changed. To maximize patient outcomes according to the mission and philosophy of the facility and department, and to satisfy external regulations, the design and process for delivering therapeutic activities must adapt accordingly.

Appropriate assessment in long-term care goes well beyond the interest finder and record of past behaviors, not that this information is not important, but this is inadequate information on which to determine appropriate type and intensity of interventions. Functional assessment of abilities across all domains is indispensable, particularly with regard to motor skills, cognitive abilities, social emotional behaviors and possible constraints to leisure. Data must be detailed enough and broad enough to give an accurate picture of each resident's strengths, vulnerabilities, and what ignites a zest for living. Moreover, therapeutic relationships that can develop are, in and of themselves, purposeful interventions that support individual identity, self-worth, and empower older adults in institutional environments.

The individual program plan is probably the single best way to personalize each nursing home resident. Attention to individual strengths and potential contributions of each resident prevent an amorphous profile for an individual. Focus on sustaining meaning in life for residents is an essential part of both the work of therapeutic activity and of social services.

Approach, implementation strategies, and methods for delivering therapeutic activity to improve patient outcomes result from quality, detailed assessments, and individual planning. Similarly, success results from both formative and summative evaluations of the content of program offerings and interventions, as well as the process of program delivery. Obviously, prescriptive programming for therapy requires greater specificity.

Activity and Task Analysis

Analysis of the components of tasks needed to perform a particular activity is important for leisure education and the activities available for resident selection. Careful evaluation of typically offered programs is necessary to improve the likelihood that residents will be motivated to attend, become engaged, experience leisure, and find joy in participating. There must be a match of functional abilities with requisite behaviors necessary to the activity. Residents should have the right to refuse participation and should not be arbitrarily escorted into activities. An activity may or may *not* be the best choice for the person at that time. If current offerings do not meet the interests of particular residents, they may prefer isolation or bed. New choices should then be offered individually or in small groups.

REPRESENTATIVE GENERAL ACTIVITIES

A comprehensive activities program includes opportunities to engage in a wide variety of normal social relationships, which range from being alone to large assembly-type activities. There are many daily tasks that are normally done *alone* such as reading, writing letters, watching TV, listening to music, or sewing. Most people look forward to some period of privacy each day to review their thoughts, pray, or simply do nothing. This is particularly difficult in a nursing home setting. One way to provide more privacy is to encourage roommates to participate in activities at different times, allowing each individual some time to be alone in his/her room.

In the normal course of a day, residents spend much time with others just visiting and taking meals. These activities are routine and familiar. Planned small interest group participation, however, is more likely to elicit social interactions and promote friendships. Large group activities (such as movies, concerts, church, etc.) can be stimulating and enjoyable but they require little social interaction.

Common activities include:

- discussion groups–current events, special topics
- playing cards and games
- gardening
- exercise groups
- music–resident players, sing-alongs, dancing
- book and poetry readings and discussions
- bird-watching and playing with pets
- community visits–shopping, art museums, zoos, restaurants
- holiday and special occasion parties

It is important that activities be available to residents seven days a week and afternoons and evenings. To accomplish good programming, one might look to community resources such as schools, universities, churches, libraries, hobby groups, political interest groups, or small theater groups. The possibilities are endless. Other resources might be found in the facility itself. Consultants, social workers, music therapists, staff with special talents, families with special talents, and residents will have ideas and be able to increase the variety of the activity program.

SUMMARY

Few would argue that people wish to complete the life cycle with dignity, meaning, and with the highest quality possible. Helplessness and hopelessness are deadly to the spirit and to that which makes us who we are. If sustaining life includes retaining value as human capital, health must be interpreted as being more than the absence of illness.

To borrow from the address of Martin Luther King, Jr., on the steps of the U.S. Capitol, "[If], somehow you lose the vitality that keeps life moving, you lose that courage to be, that quality that helps you go on in spite of it all (King, 1963). And as Stair wrote, "If I had my life over, I would pick more daisies" (Martz, 1992).

RESOURCES

American Art Therapy Association
1980 Isaac Newton Square, S.
Reston, VA 22090

American Association of Community Theatre
8402 BriarWood Circle
Lago Vista, TX 78645
www.aact.org

American Association for Leisure and Recreation
1900 Association Drive
Reston, VA 22091

American Association for Music Therapy
66 Morris St.
P.O. Box 359
Springfield, NJ 07081

American Association for Rehabilitation Therapy
Box 93
North Little Rock, AK 72216

American Dance Therapy Association
2000 Century Plaza, Suite 108
Columbia, MD 21044

American Library Association, Inc.
Association of Specialized and Cooperative Agencies
50 E. Huron Street
Chicago, IL 60611
www.ala.org

American Occupational Therapy Association, Inc.
4720 Montgomery Lane
P.O. Box 31220
Bethesda, MD 20824-1220
www.aota.org

American Therapeutic Recreation Association (ATRA)
1414 Prince Street, Suite 204
Alexandria, VA 22314
www.atra-tr.org

CARF–The Rehabilitation Accreditation Commission
4891 East Grant Road
Tuscon, AZ 85712
www.carf.org

National Association of Activity Professionals
P.O. Box 724
Park Ridge, IL 60068

National Association of Activity Therapy and Rehabilitation Program Directors
Box 111
Independence, IA 50644

National Association for Music Therapy
910 Kentucky Avenue
Lawrence, KS 66044

National Coalition of Arts Therapies Associations (NCATA)
c/o ADTA, 8455 Colesville Rd., Ste. 1000
Silver Spring, MD 20910
www.ncata.com

National Council for Therapeutic Recreation Certification (NCTRC)
7 Elmwood Drive
New York, NY 10956

National Therapeutic Recreation Society (NTRS)
National Recreation and Parks Association
2237 Belmont Ridge Road
Asbum, VA 20148-4501
www.nrpa.org

Therapeutic Recreation Directory
www.recreationtherapy.com

REFERENCES

Aday, L.A., & Shortell, S.M. (1988). Indicators and predictors of health service utilization. In S.J. Williams & P.R Torren (Eds.), *Introduction to Health Services* (vol. 3). New York: Wiley.

Atchley, R.C. (1989). A continuity theory of aging. *Gerontologist, 29,* 137–144.

Baltes, P.B., & Baltes, M.M. (Eds.). (1990). *Successful aging: Perspectives from the behavioral sciences.* Cambridge: Cambridge University Press.

Bandura, A. (1986). *Social foundations of thought and action.* Englewood Cliffs, NJ: Prentice Hall.

Binstock, R.H., & Post, S.G. (Eds.). (1991). *Too old for healthcare? Controversies in medicine, law, economics, and ethics.* Baltimore, MD: The Johns Hopkins University Press.

Byock, I.R. (1999). Conceptual models and the outcomes of caring. *Journal of pain and symptom management, 17*(2), February, 83–92.

CARF. (2001). *Standards Manuals.* Tucson, AZ: The Rehabilitation Accreditation Commission Publication.

Csikszentmihalyi, M. (1996). *Creativity: Flow and the psychology of discovery and invention.* New York: Harper-Collins.

Guyatt, H., & Cook, D. (1994). Health status, quality of life and the individual. *JAMA.* *272*(1), 630–631.

Health Care Financing Administration. (1994). *HCFA intermediary & carrier directory.* DHHS Publication No. 342-238-73466. Washington, DC: U.S. Department of Health and Human Services.

Health Care Financing Administration. (1988). Expenditures and percent of gross national product for national health expenditures by private and public funds, hospital care, and physician services: Calendar years 1960–87. *Health care financing review,* 10,2. Washington, DC: Office of the Actuary, Winter.

Health Care Financing Administration. (1984). *Medicare hospital manual.* DHHS No. 10, Section 212.1 {A} {2}. Washington, DC: U.S. Department of Health and Human Services.

Joint Commission (JAHCO). (2001). Taking a look at the staffing assessment model. *Joint commission perspectives.* June.

Joint Commission (JAHCO). (2001). *Accreditation manual for long term care.* Oakbrook Terrace, IL.

Kaufman, S. (1986). *The ageless self.* Madison, WI: University of Wisconsin Press.

Kivnick, H.Q. (1993). Everyday mental health: A guide to assessing life strengths. *Generations. Winter/Spring.*

Lawton, M.P. (1991). A multidimensional view of quality of life in frail elders. In J.E. Birren et al. (Eds.), *The concert and measurement of quality of life in the frail elderly.* (pp. 3–27). San Diego: Academic Press.

National Center for Health Statistics. (1990). *Health, United States, 1989 and prevention profile.* DHHS Pub. No. (PHS) 90-1232. Hyattsville, MD: U.S. Dept. of Health and Human Services.

Ory, M.G., Abeles, R.A., & Lipman, P.D. (Eds.). (1992). *Aging, health and behavior.* London: Sage.

Pegels, C.C. (1988). *Healthcare and the older citizen: Economic, demographic, and financial aspects.* Rockville, MD: Aspen Publishers.

Seligman, M.P. (1975). *Helplessness: On depression, development and death.* San Francisco, CA.: W.H. Freeman & Co.

Spencer, G. (1989). Projections of the population of the United States, by age, sex, race: 1988 to 2080. *Current populations reports, population estimates, and projections.* Series P-25, No. 1018. Washington, DC: U.S. Department of Commerce, Bureau of the Census.

Stair, N. (1992). If I had my life over, I would pick more daisies. In S.H. Martz (Ed.), *If I had my life to live over, I would pick more daisies.* Watsonville: CA. Papier-Mache Press.

U.S. DHHS. (2001). *Healthy people 2010: Volumes I & II* (2nd ed.). from http://web.health.gov/healthypeople/publications.

U.S. DHHS. (1989). Omnibus reconciliation act of 1987 rules and regulations. *Federal register.* Health Care Financing Administration, 54:21, 53 16-5373. Washington, DC: U.S. Government Printing Office.

U.S. DHHS. (1990). *Healthy people 2000: National health promotion and disease prevention objectives.* Washington, DC: U.S. Government Printing Office.

U.S. DHHS. (1980). *Healthy, people: Surgeon, general's report on health promotion and disease prevention*. Public Health Service, Washington, DC: U.S. Government Printing Office.

U.S. DHHS. (1980). *Promoting health preventing disease: Objectives for the nation*. Public Health Service, Washington, DC: U.S. Government Printing Office.

U.S. DHHS. (1979). *Healthy people: Surgeon general's report on health promotion and disease prevention*. Public Health Service, Washington, DC: U.S. Government Printing Office.

U.S. Department of Labor. (1996–97). Professional specialty occupations. Recreational Therapists. *Occupational Outlook Handbook*. (D.O.T. 076. 124-014, pp. 172–173). Washington, DC: U.S. Bureau of Labor Statistics.

World Health Organization. (1980). *International classification of impairment, disabilities and handicaps*. Geneva: World Health Organization.

Chapter 18

ENHANCING ORGANIZATIONAL PERFORMANCE THROUGH ENVIRONMENTAL DESIGN

LESLIE A. GRANT

The field of environmental design as it relates to long-term care is undergoing dramatic change in nursing facilities and assisted living facilities. Architects, interior designers, and other environmental designers working with innovative provider organizations are beginning to think "outside the box" to look for new solutions that better meet the needs of seniors, their families, and the long-term care work force. This imperative to be more creative and find better solutions is driven by a number of factors including increased market competition from alternative models of care such as home health care; problems in current approaches in addressing concerns about the quality of life, quality of care, and quality of the workplace; and changing demographics which portend the coming of the baby boomers who will have more financial resources than previous generations and far greater expectations about what the long-term care system should offer.

New models are emerging within nursing facilities and assisted living facilities. Traditional approaches are rooted in the organizational model taken from acute care hospitals. Innovative models are built on a different "organizational chassis" and incorporate features taken from hotels, restaurants, resorts, or other segments of the hospitality industry. Still others have features of a social model that emphasizes a "normal" lifestyle in a setting that emulates living with a family at home. There is a growing trend toward more specialized models of care for specific client groups. Some models encompass specialized care such as for persons with Alzheimer's disease and related dementia, developmental disabilities, terminal illness, AIDS, alcohol or drug problems, traumatic head injuries, spinal cord injuries and so forth, but many more are intended for frail elders at large. More and more, we are seeing a movement away from "institutionalized" and "medicalized" models of care toward "residential" and "normalized" settings. As this chapter will show, these trends have major implications for architectural, landscape, interior and even urban design. Increasingly, provider organizations are moving away from large undifferentiated nursing units based on the medical model towards specialized units and small households in family-like settings. Different terminology is used to describe these new types of living arrangements within nursing facilities and assisted living facilities. Words such as "neighborhoods," "clusters," "households," "homes," and "houses" are used to describe them.

THE ENVIRONMENTAL SYSTEM

The environments in which we live have a profound impact on the way we experience the aging process. This is the thesis of M. Powell Lawton, a pioneering gerontologist and prominent theorist in the field of aging and environment. His theory known as the "social ecological model" describes how the aging individual adapts to his or her environment. The theory provides the basis for the "environmental docility hypothesis" which states that the lower the level of competence of the aging individual, the greater the influence of the environment on behavior (Lawton and Nahemow, 1973). For the aging individual who faces cumulative, progressive declines in functional competence, the physical environment plays an increasingly important role over time. Broadly speaking, the physical environment encompasses almost everything that is part of the man-made or built environment as well as the natural environment in which we live. Within long-term care facilities key features of the environmental design system include landscape design, architectural design, and interior design.

Key components of the environmental system within a nursing facility can be described starting from the micro-environment going to the macro-environment. Each resident has a room with furnishings and personal belongings. Each room is located on a nursing unit. Each facility is comprised of one or more buildings made up of one or more nursing units. Each building sits on a piece of property or site that is located within the fabric of a larger urban, suburban, or rural neighborhood. Each neighborhood is located in a community within a city, county or other jurisdiction. The basic point here, is simple: Design professions with differentiated roles and overlapping responsibilities are involved in the design process that ultimately shapes the physical environment that we experience in our daily lives. Urban designers work at the scale of communities or neighborhoods; landscape architects at the scale of real estate lots or sites; architects at the scale of buildings and rooms;

interior designers at the scale of rooms, interior finishes, and furnishings; and engineers at the scale of structural, mechanical, and electrical systems. This division of labor among design professionals poses a major challenge to many provider organizations who want to improve their facilities and services. The design process itself is fractured across professional disciplines with different disciplines competing for resources. On any design project, the administrator must assemble or find a design team that can work collaboratively across disciplinary boundaries to optimize the environmental design system. Ultimately, this process requires close collaboration among design professionals who are willing to make the "right" tradeoffs.

THE ROLE OF DESIGN PROFESSIONS

Urban and regional planners work at the macro-environmental scale, that of entire regions, cities, or neighborhoods. They develop regional plans that guide the development of infrastructure such as roads, water, sewage, gas, electricity, communication, and transportation systems. Urban and regional planners develop zoning ordinances and regional plans that affect land use patterns for parks and other open spaces, and for commercial, residential, and industrial developments. There are numerous examples that illustrate ways in which urban planners could improve the physical environment to make it more accommodating to the needs of a greying society. Seniors often lack access to effective transportation systems when they no longer can drive safely. Indeed, the design of our cities and roads promote the use of automobiles, and most public transit systems are not well-suited to the needs of frail elders. The timing of pedestrian lights at crosswalks is an environmental hazard for many seniors. Strictly enforced zoning ordinances can interfere with the development of new models of long-term care, for example, when granny "flats" and "group homes" are not allowed within certain types of residentially zoned neighborhoods. Zoning ordinances directly affect site selection criteria for long-term care facilities since variances to city zoning ordinances are frequently required to build senior housing, assisted living facilities, or nursing facilities. Among real estate developers, neighborhood and site selection criteria are often cited as essential to market success. Facilities in vibrant communities providing access to basic services (e.g., banks, libraries, medical offices, churches, stores, restaurants and entertainment centers located within high visibility transit corridors) are more marketable than facilities sited in isolated, less desirable locations. Unfortunately, the cost of land often makes it difficult to build affordable units in the most desirable neighborhoods. An alternative strategy is to incorporate some of these services on-site depending on the market a facility targets.

Landscape architects work at the scale of an individual site or campus. They develop plans for outdoor spaces. Site plans delineate the location of buildings, access roads, parking, outdoor structures, walkways, courtyards, plants (trees, shrubs, and flowers), and other amenities. Poor landscape design does little more than provide parking for cars. Another mistake is to use landscape design merely to create an aesthetic backdrop for the building, rather than provide useable outdoor space for residents. The design of outdoor spaces should enable therapeutic recreation staff to make use of the outdoors as part of an ongoing activities program, for example, by providing raised gardens or flower beds. Sheltered spaces (e.g., a gazebo or other outdoor structure) large enough to accommodate group activities should be provided to offer shelter from direct sun and wind.

Poor landscape design presents environmental hazards. Berries on plants may be ingested by persons with Alzheimer's disease, so toxic plants must be avoided. Outdoor areas accessible to persons with Alzheimer's disease must be secured so that residents do not elope. Falls and other accidents may occur due to poorly designed walkways. Walkways should provide a hard, stable, nonslippery surface with a nonglare finish. Many walkways are made from poured concrete without any color treatment. On sunny days the light-gray color of the concrete makes light reflecting off the surface too bright for the aging eye. Walking paths should be wide enough to allow two wheelchairs to pass in opposite directions. Walkways or ramps with inclines greater than a ratio of one to 20 should be avoided. Outdoor seating should be provided along outdoor paths at 20 to 40 feet intervals. When outdoor spaces are poorly designed, they become inaccessible, unusable, and potentially hazardous.

The architect is the most important member of the design team since this person usually plays the role of the team leader responsible for coordinating activities of all other members on the team, be they city planners who approve building documents for code compliance; landscape architects who develop outdoor spaces to work effectively with interior spaces; interior designers who specify furnishings to make sure each room can accommodate the right chairs, tables, couches, beds, and other furnishings; or engineers who develop technical specifications for structural, mechanical, and electrical systems. The architect integrates the expertise of all of these specialists into a coherent whole. For a building to be successful it must come in on budget and on time. All design parameters (architectural, interior, landscape, and engineering design) must meet the needs of all end-users. At the macro-environmental scale the building and site must fit into the fabric of the surrounding community.

Architects work at the scale of site, buildings, and rooms. The architectural design process has been likened to "successive approximation." It starts with conceptual or schematic design, goes through design development, and finally results in working drawings. At each stage of building design, there is greater specificity and detail about how the building should be built. Architects develop building elevations to show exterior building features (e.g., roof, walls, windows, and doors). They develop construction drawings to show how these building components fit together. Construction drawings are needed to solicit bids from building contractors. Until construction drawings have been developed it is often difficult to arrive at precise estimates of construction costs. Architects develop floor plans to show the overall layout of various functional areas within the building (e.g., entry, lounges, dining rooms, activity areas, nursing units, resident rooms, and bathrooms). The building floor plan determines what types of services can be provided by the facility. It drives operational and programmatic factors that affect staffing patterns and operational costs. It affects the overall workability and functionality of the building. And, it has major consequences for the daily lives of staff and residents. A well-designed floor plan enhances operational efficiency for staff and supports the quality of life for residents.

An innovation called the "Swedish Service House" illustrates this point. A nursing facility in Minnesota renovated an existing 15-bed wing into a service house with nine residents. Resident rooms were renovated into studio apartments with Swedish-style showers and toilets. The redesigned showers improved efficiency in bathing because residents could be given assisted showers without leaving their rooms. The redesigned toilets made it safer for staff assisting residents with toileting because two person lifts on and off the toilet were accommodated. Residents were afforded a higher degree of privacy in daily living especially in bathing and dining. The morning and evening meals were prepared in the resident's own kitchenette and eaten in the resident's own dining area. Residents were given much more autonomy in mealtimes and choice of food than was possible before the renovation. Well-designed buildings (e.g., nursing units, dining areas, common spaces, resident rooms, and bathrooms) can decrease staff workload due to improved efficiencies in job design. Good architectural design solutions enhance quality of life for residents by promoting privacy and autonomy.

Interior designers specify interior details, such as the selection and placement of lighting, signage, and furniture. They specify finishes on floors, walls, counters, and ceilings. They select fabrics, fixtures, hardware, and artwork. Interior design decisions (e.g., carpeting versus vinyl tiles in corridors) are often based on the singular goal of minimizing cost of maintenance and upkeep. All too often interior designers do little more than coordinate choice of "decor" to create esthetic appeal and ambiance. While these considerations are important, interior design potentially has a far more profound influence. By its very nature, interior design is focused on the micro-environment. This is where the "rubber meets the road." Good interior design enhances functional competence among residents.

A combination of technical competence and artistic creativity characterize good interior design solutions. On the technical side, the designer needs to understand age-related changes in sensory systems. These are important considerations because the micro-environment can be modified or adapted to accommodate these age-related changes to maximize functional competence. On the artistic side, the designer needs to coordinate interior design elements (e.g., lighting, colors, fabrics, carpets, window treatments, furnishings, and so forth) into an esthetic statement that says: "This is a great place to live and a fun place to work."

Age-related sensory changes occur in vision, hearing, and other systems. An administrator or interior designer with a basic understanding of these age-related changes can make simple environmental modifications to improve the lives of residents. Margaret Christenson is an occupational therapist who has developed a broad ranging set of recommendations about environmental adaptations to support the needs of the aged (Christenson, 1990). Some recommendations with direct relevance to interior design are highlighted below.

As the individual ages, structural changes in the eye affect vision. Environmental adaptations related to vision include use of visual aids, lighting, colors to accommodate changes in color perception, and flooring materials to accommodate poor depth perception. A large proportion of residents in long-term care facilities have visual impairments. One study found that 24 percent of residents were legally blind and another 35 percent had low visual acuity (Snyder et al., 1976). The development of small opacities and vascularities in the eyeball make the older person susceptible to glare. Matt finishes should be used on counter surfaces, table tops, floors, and walls. Carpet in corridors and indirect lighting help reduce glare. Window treatments, especially on west-facing windows are important in controlling glare from direct sunlight when the sun is low on the horizon.

Presbyopia is an age-related difficulty in accommodation of the eye due to loss of elasticity in the lens which makes it harder for the older person to focus on the detail of objects at close distance or at varied distances. Large print books with high contrast print would benefit the older person in later stages of presbyopia when corrective lenses for near vision no longer work. Signage should use large contrasting lettering with letters at least 5/8 inch in height. These letters should be recessed or raised 1/32 inch for readability through touch (Bowersox, 1979). Light colored letters on a dark background make it easier for the older person to read letters on signage (Reznikoff, 1979).

Adequate levels of lighting are critical for comfort and safety. The typical older person needs four to five times more light to distinguish a figure from the background than a younger person with normal vision. As the eye ages the lens becomes less transparent and thicker. As the lens of the eye loses transparency and becomes opaque, a cataract results. By the time a person reaches age 70, signs of cataract formation are commonplace (Colavita, 1978). Sight recovery due to sudden changes in levels of illumination between light and dark spaces takes longer in the older person. Spaces should be designed to allow for gradual transitional zones (e.g., between indoor and outdoor spaces) to facilitate sight recovery.

Color perception is altered in the older individual due to a yellowing of the lens. Certain colors such as green, blue, or purple take on a different hue and appear more grayish. Dark shades of navy, brown, and black are hard to distinguish except under intense light. Pastel colors are also difficult to distinguish. One goal for using colors when designing for the elderly is to create clear contrasts between surfaces and objects so they are more easily seen. For example, walls should contrast clearly from floors where they meet. In selecting fabrics for chairs or other furnishings, colors should stand out clearly from background finishes on floors and walls. These considerations are equally important in the selection of dinnerware. The designer should specify dishes that stand out from the background (e.g., light colored plates on dark tablecloths). The color of the plates should contrast well with different types of foods. Highly patterned tablecloths or dishes confuse the eye and make it difficult to see.

Depth perception is affected by the level of illumination and degree of figure ground contrast. Older persons with poor depth perception may perceive bold two-dimensional patterns on floors as three-dimensional objects. Boldly patterned floors should be avoided especially in corridors, lounges, and dining rooms.

The most common source of hearing problems in the aged is presbycusis which results in a loss in the ability to hear high pitches. It is caused by damage to nerve endings and auditory hairs cells in the inner ear. Properly adjusted hearing aids, portable listening devices, and closed captioning on televisions can assist older persons with hearing loss. Background noise from phones, television sets, call lights, and public address systems can increase confusion among residents with Alzheimer's disease. Acoustical treatments such as ceiling tiles, textured wall coverings, and carpeting are important in dining areas. Noisy functions such as kitchens and mechanical rooms should be separated from adjacent areas with sound insulated walls. Other important environmental adaptations have to do with floor finishes and handrails to assist with ambulation, proper chair selection for safety and comfort, and special environmental adaptations for persons with Alzheimer's disease (Christenson, 1990; Cohen and Weissman, 1991; Cohen and Day, 1993).

Structural engineers develop technical specifications for major building components such as foundations, structural walls, and other load-bearing systems. Structural systems have a major impact on construction costs. Building codes concerning seismic safety can add significantly to the cost of construction in parts of the United States that are seismically active. Nursing facilities (like hospitals, fire stations, and police stations) are considered essential structures that must withstand major earthquakes and other natural disasters.

Mechanical engineers design heating, ventilation and air conditioning (HVAC) systems. Older persons are more sensitive to temperature extremes, and they adapt more slowly to temperature changes than younger persons. Mechanical systems should have multiple zones, so that temperatures can be controlled separately in different parts of the building.

Electrical engineers specify electrical and fire annunciation systems. Fire annunciation systems should have a high and low pitch auditory alarm and a visual alarm such as a strobe light for persons with presbycusis who have difficulty hearing high pitches. Backup electrical generators and emergency lighting that activate during power failures are required by code in some types of long-term care facilities. All building systems (structural, mechanical, and electrical) are critical because they affect physical comfort and safety of residents.

ENVIRONMENTAL DESIGN AND ORGANIZATIONAL PERFORMANCE

Environmental design plays a critical role in organizational performance. All design elements ranging from macro-environmental features to micro-environmental features need to be integrated into an environmental design system that addresses the needs of staff, residents and family caregivers. Environmental design is one of five core organizational systems that affect organizational performance in long-term care facilities (Grant, Potthoff, and Olson, 2001). Aligning the environmental design system with other organizational systems improves organizational performance. A poorly designed physical environment can impede the performance of other systems. Environmental design features can affect organizational performance across a broad range of parameters.

Figure 18-1 shows a conceptual model that identifies five core organizational systems and key indicators of organizational performance in nursing facilities. This model was developed to evaluate quality management prac-

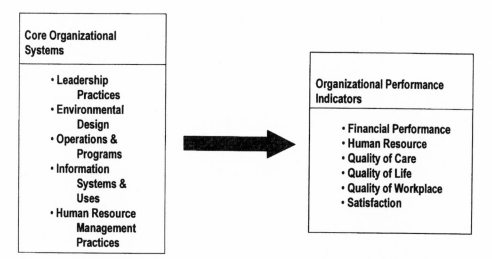

Figure 18-1. Conceptual Model Linking Organizational Systems to Performance Indicators.

tices within nursing facilities using a framework adapted from the Malcolm Baldridge Quality Award Program (National Institute of Standards and Technology, 2002). It was developed through a study funded by a research grant from the National Science Foundation to evaluate quality management practices.

Organizational performance within long-term care facilities can be defined by a variety of criteria. Financial performance indicators are things such as lease-up rates, operating margins, and occupancy rates. Human resource indicators include staff recruitment, retention, turnover, absenteeism, and stability. Quality of care indicators include measures of clinical performance in areas such as behavior management, medications errors, nutritional status, and hospitalization rates. Quality of life indicators are such things as functional competence, resident autonomy, privacy, involvement in meaningful activities, and having meaningful social relationships. Quality of the workplace refers to job design, work routines, job stress, burnout, and workplace injuries. Satisfaction refers to job satisfaction among staff members, and satisfaction with services among residents and their family caregivers.

Five core organizational systems influence these performance indicators. Ideally, all five core organizational systems are aligned because deficiencies in one system can impede performance of other systems. Each of the five core organizational systems is described below.

Effective organizational leadership is critical because it tends to drive all other systems. As discussed in Chapter 4, top management's vision and strategy affect programs, facility design, information systems, and human resource management practices. Executive leadership sets the agenda, supports change, and develops effective communication. Without effective executive leadership, improvement in other systems becomes difficult.

Environmental design includes architectural, interior, and landscape design as discussed above. The physical environment affects many, if not all of these performance indicators directly or indirectly through their influence on other systems. As noted earlier the physical environment affects the quality of life of residents. It affects the quality of the workplace for staff. It affects financial performance. Facilities with good environmental design features have greater market appeal to residents and their families than facilities without such features. A poorly designed building can undermine safety and physical comfort among residents and contribute to job stress and workplace injuries among staff. In turn, injuries and accidents can lead to higher worker's compensation claims, added litigation, and higher insurance premiums. Effective leadership aligns the environmental design system with other core organizational systems to enhance organizational performance.

Programs and operations affect costs and have a direct impact on the quality of life and quality of the workplace. Some innovative models have adapted practices from the hospitality industry. Others are reminiscent of home and family with emphasis placed on familiar activities that offer continuity with a resident's past by engaging them in "normalized" social roles.

Many facilities have information systems focused primarily on basic financial data (e.g., payroll, accounting, and billing). As will be discussed in Chapter 26, more sophisticated information systems are needed to track nonfinancial performance indicators such as quality of life, clinical outcomes, human resource outcomes, and satisfaction among residents, staff, and family caregivers. Better information systems are needed to provide the critical feedback loop to leadership to drive improvement on each of the performance indicators.

Human resource management practices refer to such things as hiring practices, staff training and development, supervision, job design, and performance evaluation as discussed in Chapters 7 through 12. Within some organizational models (e.g., Swedish Service House), environmental design and human resource management practices are changed simultaneously through renovation and job redesign. Instead of having large groups of residents live together and share centralized services (e.g., for dining, activities, and bathing), some provider organizations are moving towards smaller, more family-like communities with permanently assigned staff and self-directed work teams. "Universal" or cross-functional workers with blended roles that cross-cut the division of labor across nursing, activities, housekeeping, social service, and food service functions are also being introduced. Innovative organizations are moving away from hierarchically arranged departments with centralized authority structures toward decentralized organizational models. In some of these models, closer more meaningful interpersonal relationships among family members, residents, and staff have been observed.

CONCLUSION

This chapter highlights basic principles that can be used to create better physical environments in long-term care settings. Organizational performance can be enhanced through thoughtful architectural, interior, and landscape design. Many of these principles apply whether the senior lives in a nursing facility, assisted living facility, senior housing, or a single family home. Because building design is integral to organizational performance, it is unfortunate that many existing physical plants in nursing facilities are outdated. Improvements to the quality of life for nursing home residents and enhancements to the quality of the workplace for staff, require an upgrade of obsolete systems including the physical environment. This is an area where creative environmental designers and visionary leaders can make significant improvements in coming years.

What we are witnessing in the field of environmental design today is an early exploration of ways to renovate existing facilities and build new facilities to implement innovative organizational models with more effective organizational systems. Needless to say, the replacement of obsolete systems (particularly outdated physical plants) will probably require major capital investments, although some organizations have successfully completed renovations at very modest cost. Without a new set of environmental and organizational design specifications, significant gains in organizational performance will be difficult (if not impossible) to achieve.

Forward thinking provider organizations with visionary leaders are working successfully with environmental design professionals to improve the way long-term care services are delivered. Administrators don't have to become "overnight" design experts. They must, however, work with creative designers who know how to derive the best design solutions possible given a multiplicity of impediments to innovation. Regulatory issues, site constraints, financial and economic constraints, and operational or logistical issues need to be addressed creatively. For any organization to be successful it must work with designers who are competent in their disciplines, who understand the vision of the organization, and who are willing to develop design solutions that can best achieve that vision.

RESOURCES AND REFERENCES

American Institute of Architects. (1985). *Design for aging: An architect's guide.* Washington, DC: AIA Press.

Bowersox, J. (1979). Architectural and interior design. In L.J. Wasser (Ed.), *Long term care of the aging: A socially responsible approach.* Washington, DC: American Association of Homes for the Aging.

Christenson, M.A. (1990). *Aging in the designed environment.* New York: Haworth Press.

Cohen, U., & Day, K. (1993). *Contemporary environments for people with dementia.* Baltimore, MD: The Johns Hopkins University Press.

Cohen, U., & Weisman, G.D. (1991). *Holding on to home: Designing environments for people with dementia.* Baltimore, MD: The Johns Hopkins University Press.

Colavita, F. (1978). *Sensory changes in the elderly.* Springfield, IL: Charles C Thomas.

Grant, L.A., Potthoff, S.J., & Olson, D.M. (2001). Staffing and administrative issues in special care units. *Alzheimer's Care Quarterly, 2*(3), 22–27.

Illuminating Engineering Society of North America (IESNA). (1998). *Lighting and the visual environment for senior living.* (RP-28-98). New York: IESNA.

Lawton, M.P., & Nahemow, L. (1973). Ecology and the aging process. In C. Eisdorfer & M.P. Lawton (Eds.), *The psychology of adult development and aging.* Washington, DC: American Psychological Association.

National Institute of Standards and Technology (NIST). 2002. http://www.quality.nist.gov.

Reznikoff, S.C. (1979). *Specifications for commercial interiors.* New York: Whitney Library of Design, Watson-Guptill Publications.

Snyder, L., Pyrek, J., & Smith, K. (1976). Vision and mental function of the elderly. *Gerontologist, 16,* 491–495.

Chapter 19

MONITORING CLINICAL OUTCOMES

Christine Mueller

INTRODUCTION

Every profession is guided by standards set by state laws and professional organizations. In addition, professions set their own code of ethics, educational criteria, and broad goals for the practice of that profession. In the field of long-term care, the most frequently encountered professional employees and consultants include physicians, nurses, social workers, physical therapists, occupational therapists, speech therapists, dieticians, and clergy. In addition, long-term care facilities are regulated by many state and federal laws.

What is missing from all of this relates to the resident/patient. What happens to the individual? Is he or she better, the same, or worse from all of the clinical interventions? Does a particular capsule, intervention, activity, or therapy achieve its goal? Quality assurance and improvement programs answer these questions, both for individuals and groups of clients. Without such monitoring of clinical practices, it is impossible to improve and assure quality of care.

ASSURING AND IMPROVING QUALITY CARE

Every department needs to have some way of measuring quality. Departmental quality assurance and improvement (QA/I) plans must be consistent with the organization's QA/I plan. To assure and improve quality, organizational outcomes and indicators are identified and subsequently used in the QA/I system.

259

Because so many quality indicators are related to nursing care, some facilities have a registered nurse responsible for its quality assurance and improvement program. This role involves coordinating the facility's quality assurance plan. Through that plan, data collection systems and associated quality indicators (e.g., clinical, resident satisfaction, human resources, financial) are identified. The quality assurance coordinator facilitates the collection, organization, and analysis of these data. Quality improvement efforts are based on the results of the ongoing collection and analysis of data.

Clinical outcomes or indicators are related to residents or the recipients of care. The most well-known clinical indicators are the nursing home quality indicators (QIs) developed by the University of Wisconsin's Center for Health Services Research and Analysis (CHSRA). The 24 QIs are defined from the items on the Minimum Data Set (MDS) (Table 19-1). For example, the QI for prevalence of urinary tract infections is determined by the number of residents in the facility with the urinary tract infection item checked on the most recent MDS assessment divided by all the residents in the facility who have a recent MDS assessment. Nursing facilities can monitor the prevalence and incidence rates of the 24 QIs. They are provided reports, usually from their State's department of health, which profiles their prevalence and incidence rates on the 24 QIs and also provides the rates for all nursing facilities in the State and nation.

Other clinical outcomes or indicators relevant to residents may include pain management, food and fluid intake, risk for falls, mobility, activities of daily living, attendance and participation in activities, and appearance and grooming. Process indicators relevant to residents may include the completion of a skin risk assessment, safe administration of medication, proper assessment and application of physical restraints, proper positioning in bed and chairs and so forth.

Another category of outcomes or indicators relevant to residents is satisfaction. Satisfaction with answering call lights, courtesy of staff, providing privacy, respect and dignity, and overall satisfaction with nursing care can be assessed by surveying or interviewing residents and their families.

Outcomes or indicators relevant to the nursing care providers is their satisfaction with various aspects of their job, the nursing department and the overall organization. Staff satisfaction surveys, focus groups, complaint/suggestion boxes are strategies that can be used to collect data to determine if there are areas of improvement that need to be addressed regarding staff satisfaction. Several of the more relevant organizational outcomes/indicators for the nursing department include staff turnover and staff absenteeism.

A QA/I plan (Figure 19-1) for the nursing department should include the components outlined in the diagram.

TABLE 19-1
NURSING HOME QUALITY INDICATORS

	QI Domain	Quality Indicator
1	Accidents	Incidence of new fracture
2		Prevalence of falls
3	Behavioral/Emotional	Prevalence of behavioral symptoms affecting others
4	Patterns	Prevalence of depressive symptoms
5		Prevalence of depression without antidepressant therapy
6	Clinical Management	Use of 9 or more medications
7		Incidence of cognitive impairment
8	Elimination/Continence	Prevalence of bladder or bowel incontinence
9		Prevalence of occasional or frequent bladder or bower incontinence without a toileting plan
10		Prevalence of indwelling catheters
11		Prevalence of fecal impaction
12	Infection Control	Prevalence of urinary tract infections
13	Nutrition/Eating	Prevalence of weight loss
14		Prevalence of tube feeding
15		Prevalence of dehydration
16	Physical Functioning	Prevalence of bedfast residents
17		Incidence of late loss decline
18		Incidence of decline in range of motion
19	Psychotropic Drug Use	Prevalence of antipsychotic use in the absence of psychotic and related conditions
20		Prevalence of antianxiety/hypnotic use
21		Prevalence of hypnotic use more than two times in last week
22	Quality of Life	Prevalence of physical restraints
23		Prevalence of little or no activity
24	Skin Care	Prevalence of stage 1–4 pressure ulcers

ESTABLISH STANDARDS AND CRITERIA. In chapter 15, it was noted that standards of care are a key component for directing and supporting all activities within the nursing department. The clinical, staff and organizational outcomes/indicators deemed essential for defining quality of care/services in the nursing department can serve to develop and/or identify standards of care. For example, some standards of care might be related to the nutritional status of residents. Table 19-2 provides some examples related to the nutritional status of residents.

DETERMINE THE TYPE OF INFORMATION TO BE COLLECTED AND HOW IT WILL BE COLLECTED. Strategies to collect data to determine if the standards have been met can include concurrent and retrospective audits of resident care records, observational audits of care provided by nurses to residents (e.g., administration of medications), MDS data (e.g., quality indicators), sur-

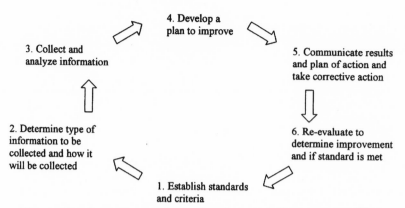

Figure 19-1. Components of a Quality Assurance/Improvement Plan

veys, interviews, and focus groups. Table 19-3 provides examples of the types of data or indicators that might be collected for the different standards associated with the nutritional status of residents. Setting up an annual calendar for QA/I data collection is imperative to ensure there is a systematic way to evaluate compliance with all the standards of care. Chart audits and observational audits do not need to include all the residents. Usually a sample is selected. For example, ten percent of all resident charts might be randomly selected on each nursing unit to determine if food intake was documented.

COLLECT AND ANALYZE THE INFORMATION. The collection of data may involve the development of data collection forms or the collection of data using an electronic format. A data collection form (Table 19-3) to complete a chart and observational audit of the nutritional status of residents is provided as an example.

Once the data are collected, the challenge is to organize and analyze the data. Using the example for nutritional status of residents, chart and observational audit data can be aggregated to determine the overall percent compliance with the standard and compared to the established threshold for the standard (Table 19-4). In this example, compliance was not achieved for any of the standards.

The QI reports, which are sent to the facility on a quarterly basis, should be reviewed to determine how the facility compares to other facilities and to previous quarterly reports. Bar graphs can be very useful to visualize these data.

Analysis of the data also includes comparing the collected data with established criteria. For example, data regarding the nutritional status of residents can be compared with established facility thresholds and other facilities. In addition, data can be compared with previous data collected to determine facility trends regarding the standards and associated criteria. Comparing col-

TABLE 19-2
STANDARDS, INDICATORS, AND THRESHOLDS RELATED TO
NUTRITIONAL STATUS OF RESIDENTS

Criterion	Indicator	Threshold
Residents will not have unintended weight loss.	Prevalence rate for weight loss	≥95% will not have a ≥5% weight loss
Residents will have ample opportunity to complete three daily service meals.	Resident satisfaction rate time to finish their meals	100% satisfaction rate
Food will be served at the appropriate temperature.	Resident satisfaction rate with temperature of food	100% satisfaction rate
	Temperature check of food	100% of food checked is at appropriate temperature
Residents will have a nutritional assessment completed on admission and every three months or more often if weight loss is noted.	Chart audit of nutritional assessments	100% resident charts have nutritional assessments
Food intake of residents will be documented in residents' charts after each meal.	Chart audit of food intake documentation	100% resident charts have documentation of food intake

lected data with established criteria and trends enables the nursing or other department to make a judgment about the quality of care for care areas. As noted in the examples provided, improvement efforts are needed in the care area of nutritional status for residents as demonstrated by being at or below the established compliance thresholds established by the facility.

DEVELOP A PLAN TO IMPROVE AND/OR CONTINUE TO MONITOR QUALITY OF CARE AREA. While the data collected may indicate there is a quality of care concern, the collected data may not provide insight into what is causing the care area to be problematic. Thus, one of the most crucial aspects to this step in a QA/I plan is doing further investigation to determine the cause of the quality of care problem. This usually involves the collection of additional data. For example, further investigation is needed to determine why the residents' food is not served at the appropriate temperature before a plan for improvement can be developed. Involving the appropriate persons in determining the cause of the problem is likely to assure that the correct cause(s) of the problem will be identified and the plan to improve care will be appropriate. In many situations, staff who provide direct care to residents should be involved in this aspect of the quality assurance/improvement process.

TABLE 19-3
SAMPLE DATA COLLECTION FORM FOR COMPLIANCE WITH STANDARDS
RELATED TO NUTRITIONAL STATUS OF RESIDENTS

Unit: A				Resident ID: 02468
Standard	Met	Not met	Exception	Comments
Nutritional assessment completed on admission and every three months or more often if weight loss is noted.	√			
Food intake recorded in resident's chart after each meal.	√			
Resident's weight recorded in resident's chart weekly.		√		
Nutritional supplements recorded in resident's chart.			√	No food supplements ordered for resident
Food served at appropriate temperature.	√			
Ample time provided to complete meal.	√			

**COMMUNICATE RESULTS AND PLAN OF ACTION TO STAFF AND TAKE COR-
RECTIVE ACTION.** This key step in the QA/I process requires effective leadership and creative communication strategies. Communicating the results of
the numerous QA/I audits and reports can be challenging when staff work
part-time, different shifts, weekends only, and are scheduled to work on different nursing units. A monthly QA/I newsletter or a QA/I bulletin board in
a prominent place for all staff to see may be effective strategies to communicate results and the proposed plan of action.

Corrective action may include strategies such as staff education programs,
changes in policies and procedures, adopting new clinical practice guidelines,
repairing or purchasing new equipment, strengthening supervision, developing or changing documentation practices. It may involve the development of
new programs (e.g., recruitment and retention; restorative nursing). It may
involve changes in management and administrative practices (e.g., scheduling
staff, interviewing potential employees, budgeting). Identifying the cause(s) of
the quality of care problem is the key to selecting the appropriate corrective
action(s). For example, it may be that the food isn't at the appropriate temperature because the dietary staff set up the meal trays too early and the meals
stay sitting on the cart an extra 15 minutes or there aren't enough staff avail-

TABLE 19-4
EXAMPLE FOR AGGREGATION OF DATA TO DETERMINE COMPLIANCE
WITH STANDARDS RELATED TO NUTRITIONAL STATUS OF RESIDENTS

Standard	Established Threshold	Percent Meeting Threshold			
		Unit A	Unit B	Unit C	Entire Facility
Nutritional assessment completed on admission and every three months or more often if weight loss is noted.	100%	95%	92%	99%	95.3%
Food intake recorded in resident's chart after each meal.	100%	77%	80%	90%	82.3%
Resident's weight recorded in resident's chart weekly.	100%	90%	98%	97%	95%
Nutritional supplements recorded in resident's chart.	100%	100%	97%	97%	98%
Food served at appropriate temperature.	100%	80%	75%	70%	75%
Ample time provided to complete meal.	100%	88%	72%	90%	83.3%

able to assist residents with their meals and many residents have to wait to eat their food. The corrective action for these two causes would obviously be very different.

RE-EVALUATE TO DETERMINE IMPROVEMENT AND IF THE STANDARD IS MET. Corrective action is intended to improve compliance with the standards of care and associated criterion and indicators. Compliance with the standard of care should be re-evaluated at a pre-determined date. The process is cyclical as noted in Figure 19-1.

Departmental QA/I plans may be integrated and implemented with the overall organization's QA/I plan. Some standards of care for one department may also have interdisciplinary involvement. However, it is important for each department to clearly identify the standards of care and criteria that provide a comprehensive picture of each aspect of quality relevant to management and clinical practice and to develop and implement a strategy for assuring and improving quality.

SUMMARY

More than ever, with the increasing public scrutiny of nursing home care, administrators need to ensure that care and services are of the highest quality. Information on quality care indicators for nursing home residents is publicly available over the Internet through the Centers for Medicare and Medicaid Services.

Quality assurance/improvement programs are an important administrative tool to ensure that the care and services provided to residents are according to established standards. The objective of QA/I programs is to determine whether the actual services provided matches predetermined criteria (Swanburg and Swanburg, 2002). Information obtained through the QA/I program enables administrators to make wise and sound management decisions.

REFERENCES

Swanburg, R., & Swanburg, R. (2002). *Introduction to management and leadership, for nurse managers* (3rd ed.). Sudbury, MA: Jones and Bartlett.

RECOMMENDED RESOURCES

Quality Indicators and Improvement for Long-Term Care

Book/Journal Resources

Bradley, M., & Thomson, N. (2000). *Quality management integration in, long-term care: Guidelines for excellence.* Baltimore: Health Professions Press.

Karon, S., & Zimmerman, D. (1996). Using indicators to structure quality improvement initiatives in long-term care. *Quality Management in Health Care, 4*(3), 54–66.

Rantz, M. et al. (1997). Setting thresholds for MDS quality indicators for nursing home quality improvement reports. *JCAHCO Journal on Quality Improvement, 23*(11), 602–611.

Rantz., M. et al. (2000). Setting thresholds for MDS quality indicators for nursing home quality improvement reports: An update. *JCAHCO Journal on Quality Improvement, 26*(2), 101–110.

Rantz, M. et al. (1998). Nursing home care quality: A multidimensional theoretical model. *Journal of Nursing Care Quality, 12*(3), 30–46.

Zimmerman, D. et al. (1995). Development and testing of nursing home quality indicators. *Health Care Financing Administration, 16* (4), 107–128.

Website Resources

Center for Health Services Research and Analysis (CHSRA) Nursing Home Quality. Indicators http://linear.chsra.wisc.edu/

National Quality Forum. http://www.qualityforum.org/

Centers for Medicare and Medicaid Services Nursing Home Quality Initiative. http://cms.hhs.gov/providers/nursinghomes/nhi/default.asp)

Centers for Medicare and Medicaid Services Sharing Innovations in Quality. http://www.hcfa.gov/medicaid/siq/siqhmpg.htm

Centers for Medicare and Medicaid Services Nursing Home Compare. http://www.medicare.gov/NHCompare/Home.asp

Centers for Medicare and Medicaid Services MDS Quality Indicator Reports. http://www.hcfa.gov/projects/mdsreports/default.asp

Statewide Continuous Quality Improvement Project in Pain Management. http://www.chcr.brown.edu/commstate/STATEWIDE_CQI_PROJECT_IN_P AIN_MA.HTM

National Guideline Clearing House (Agency for Healthcare Research and Quality). http://www.guideline.gov/index.asp

Part V

CREATING A SUPPORTIVE LIVING ENVIRONMENT

Chapter 20

MANAGING THE EFFECTS OF INSTITUTIONALIZATION

George Kenneth Gordon and Leslie A. Grant

This chapter describes social institutions such as nursing homes that are labeled as *total institutions*. It highlights physical, social, and psychological effects commonly associated with life in a total institution. It describes ways to "desinstitutionalize" the nursing home to reduce the "totality" of the setting, and thereby, improve quality of life for residents.

What makes being a long-term care administrator different from other healthcare managers or managers in the hospitality industry? One difference lies in the fact that long-term care administrators are managers of communities in which people live for extended periods of time often for years. Few of us can afford the luxury of living in a hotel or on a cruise ship for more than a few weeks or months at a time. Yet, in some upscale assisted living communities, staff have complained about residents who develop a "cruise ship" mentality. These residents see themselves as "guests" who are supposed to be catered to until they return safely home. Sometimes these same residents expect "first-class" services at "coach" prices. Regardless of how unrealistic expectations about service quality are managed, such misperceptions can undermine adjustment to living in the new setting if residents never come to accept the reality that this is their new home.

Long-term care administrators run communities where residents live and die, and where people work and play. These organizations must keep functioning nonstop during the day, the night, and all the time. In nursing homes, administrators are legally accountable and responsible for the lives of residents 24 hours a day, seven days a week, 365 days a year.

Compare this organizational model to a hospitality model. A hotel is not considered a total institution. The management of a hotel in New Orleans is not responsible and accountable for what the hotel guests do on Canal Street during Mardi Gras. The employees of the hotel are not likely to be interviewed on national TV and asked how come they were not aware when one of the hotel's guests was being mugged on Rampart Street, or where they were when one of the hotel residents was making lewd overtures to passersby on Bourbon Street; or how come they were not aware of it when one of the residents slipped out a back entrance at 1:00 AM dressed only in pajamas.

Hotel management is not responsible and accountable for the behavior of the guests. In contrast, management of a nursing home is responsible and accountable for the activities of residents 24 hours a day. If a nursing home resident dressed only in pajamas were to walk away from a nursing home at 1:00 AM in subfreezing weather, it would not be a good thing. The organization would be held accountable for the consequences of the resident's behavior.

Similarly, one's home or apartment in the community is not considered a total institution. A home as a domestic unit comprises a family unit bound together by emotional bonds that are formed by kinship or marriage. It is a small unit containing individuals with a long-term commitment to one another. The family unit is linked to other institutions in society, as family members work, attend school, go to church, or socialize and engage in other external contacts. A person living at home maintains a high degree of control over the physical and social environment. One can get up in the morning and go to bed in the evening when one pleases. The home is a private place of residence with a high degree of flexibility in how personal lifestyles and daily routines are experienced.

The typical nursing home, on the other hand, provides an extreme contrast to living with a family at home, or living independently in an apartment or hotel. Some residents, upon entering a nursing home, do not expect to leave it. They are entering because they are no longer able to live independently except at great risk. Their disabilities have outstripped the capacity of family, friends, and formal services to sustain safe independent living within the broader community. For an older person who is forced under these circumstances to enter a nursing home, adverse institutional effects can be predicted. The move will invariably increase distance from family and friends. The move will cause a sharp break with accustomed social activities. By its very nature, the nursing home will be inferior to home, an apartment, or hotel in quality of life due to loss of independence, privacy, and autonomy. When a person enters a nursing home, the resident loses the familiarity of one's own home or apartment. Nursing homes can't offer the conveniences of staying in a luxury hotel, at least not at the current rates at which they are typically reimbursed.

TOTAL INSTITUTIONS

The average American nursing home as it is organized today is a *total institution*. It provides a place of residence for a group of similarly situated individuals who are cut off from wider society who together lead an enclosed, formally administered round of life for an appreciable length of time. According to the sociologist, Erving Goffman life in a total institution has a profound impact on residents. Goffman (1961) identifies five types of total institutions that are designed to fulfill differing functions in modern society. First, are those that care for people who are harmless but incapable of caring for themselves (e.g., nursing homes and homes for the indigent). Second, are those that care for people who are incapable and seen as a threat to the community (e.g., tuberculosis hospitals, mental hospitals, and leprosaria). Third, are those that protect the community from dangers (e.g., jails and prisoners of war camps). Fourth, are those that pursue common work-like tasks (e.g., army barracks and boarding schools). Fifth, are those that provide retreat from the world (e.g., abbeys and convents).

While these total institutions have widely differing social functions, they share common features that affect their inhabitants in similar ways. These settings also have a number of organizational similarities. There is no segregation between settings, for work, play, and sleep. Every phase of life is carried out in the immediate company of many others: The day's activities are tightly scheduled, with one activity leading to another at a prearranged time. The sequence of activities is imposed through a system of explicit formal rules and enforced by staff in official roles. The enforced rules are brought together into a rational plan, purportedly designed to fulfill the aims of the institution. Contact with other institutions and links to individuals on the outside are usually limited.

A series of changes have been observed in residents when they move into a nursing home (Townsend, 1962). In adapting to loss of privacy, residents may construct a defensive shell of isolation. Their social experiences become even more limited if they are deprived of intimate family relationships and close friendships. Residents may experience difficulty in finding substitute relationships that are comparable in intimacy and emotional support to what they had experienced in the community. As mobility becomes more limited, residents do not have as much access to the broader community. As residents are subjected to an orderly and restrictive daily routine, the capacity for mastery and self-determination declines. Such institutional effects have been described as "learned helplessness."

Moving into a nursing home has also been described as a process of *depersonalization* similar to what happens to a new recruit in a military boot camp

(Townsend, 1962; Johnson and Grant, 1985). Becoming a resident in a nursing home often undermines a positive sense of self. The resident is stripped of past concepts of self. Assaults on the self begin with the admission process, when the resident is stripped of most personal belongings from home, subjected to a new set of behavioral expectations, and denied usual sources of self-esteem that were available in the community. Upon admission to the nursing home, the resident becomes dependent, and with the decreasing capacity for self-assertion, a regression to a more childlike status may occur. Residents are often forced to accept the authority of staff and thus lose the ability to control one's environment. The resident's ability to make decisions is compromised. If the resident is not given opportunities to use remaining abilities, personal talents wither with disuse. Without a future orientation in time, residents gradually become resigned to the situation. Depression, withdrawal, apathy, and lack of initiative are common results (Townsend, 1962; Johnson and Grant, 1985).

Over the years, researchers have studied the effects of institutionalization. The effects vary depending on the "totality" of the institution (Coe, 1965). Things such as the amount of privacy, rigidity of the scheduling and controls, access to personal property, and extent of isolation from the outside world affect the way people adapt to life in a total institution. Institutional effects common among nursing home residents include the following (Sommer and Osmond, 1961).

- The individual may lose the capacity for thought, action, and self-direction due to deindividuation which results from dependence on the institution. There is frequently a loss of adult competence, for example, among residents with cognitive impairment. As individual differences among residents become less noticeable to staff, an impression of sameness among residents is observable.
- Lifelong rules and behaviors that provided the individual with sources of self-affirmation may be lost due to disculturation. Over time residents acquire institutional values and attitudes that are markedly different from those the resident had before entering the nursing home.
- Psychological effects include agitation, depression, unhappiness, intellectual ineffectiveness, low energy, negative self-image, feelings of personal insignificance, docility, and submissiveness. Social effects include a low level of interest and activities, living in the past rather than the future, withdrawal from and unresponsiveness to others, and increased concerns about death.
- Physical effects are evidenced in increased mortality rates after admission. A nursing home with poor clinical management has heightened

iatrogenic effects such as urinary tract infections, upper respiratory infections, and bedsores.

Most nursing home residents are institutionalized at a point in their life when they are functionally impaired and dependent. Upon entering, they face a drastic change from the community and must adapt to life in a total institution. Reports about the difficulty of re-entering society after institutionalization are not uncommon. A prisoner refuses to return to the community after serving a long prison sentence. A mental patient cannot adjust to independent community living. Nursing home residents returning to the community may face similar challenges. Deleterious social, psychological, and physical effects can persist even after the resident is discharged home from the nursing home. Losses in status, security, and self-affirmation are often not recouped, and readjustment to a "normal" environment is difficult. The outside world can change during a protracted stay. Because of isolation from this world, skills, knowledge, and abilities may become obsolete. One's home and family may no longer exist. For the older person leaving the nursing home, the death of a spouse, or the breakup of a household may be especially difficult to rectify due to declining personal resources.

The longer a resident remains in the nursing home, the greater the isolation from society in general. Isolation can foster a feeling of being different from those who have not experienced life in a nursing home, and therefore, cannot fully appreciate the situation one has endured. Stimulus deprivation refers to a deadening of the senses in an individual who has grown accustomed to the institutional environment. Sensory deprivation can be heightened by poor environmental design (as discussed in Chapter 18). Isolation from society at large makes it even more difficult for the resident to readjust to community living because social isolation adds to stimulus deprivation.

Nursing homes face an ongoing dilemma due to a conflict between two fundamental competing ethical principles. Non-malfeasance (the goal of doing no harm) implies that nothing bad should happen to the resident through any act of commission or omission by the organization. The organization should eliminate all sources of potential risk to the resident, even if it means limiting opportunities for individual initiative among residents. In contrast, the value of autonomy (that of maximizing resident choice and control) implies that the organization should give residents as much freedom and independence as possible. Balancing these two conflicting values presents a constant source of ambivalence and contradiction for both management and frontline staff. Nursing homes constantly walk a fine line between being overly protective of residents and thereby eroding their physical and psychological independence, on one hand, while on the other hand, being open to charges of negligence if they do not take reasonable precautions to protect residents from undue risk of harm.

As total institutions responsible for the welfare of residents around the clock, nursing homes risk liability when residents who are intermittently more and less capable in making decisions about their own behavior, are given complete freedom of self-determination and autonomy. On the other hand, even greater risks can arise when organizations systematically are too cautious about risk of liability and impose too many limits on the choices available to residents. The point is that when a nursing home systematically limits residents' choices and initiatives in order to minimize the home's liability, that home has, in fact, diluted or undermined the residents' quality of life in favor of maintaining order. Such organizational practices can add to the totality of the institution, contribute to adverse social and psychological effects, and undermine the residents' quality of life.

MANAGING CAUSES AND EFFECTS

For long-term care administrators, key questions remain: What causes these adverse institutional effects? What can be done to better manage the effects of institutionalization? At least four explanations have been identified in the literature for the negative effects associated with institutionalization of the aged in nursing homes: (1) selection bias; (2) pre-admission effects; (3) environmental effects; and (4) environmental discontinuity (Kasl, 1972; Tobin and Lieberman, 1976).

Some researchers maintain that the adverse consequences of institutionalization stem from selection biases or *who* is being institutionalized rather than *what* the institution does to the person when nursing home placement occurs. Individuals entering long-term care facilities are largely those already in a seriously debilitated or incapacitated state. They share common adverse life changes that undermine social and psychological well-being and increase morbidity and mortality (e.g., illness, death of significant others, physical deterioration, erosion of economic resources, or a traumatic hospital stay). According to this view, differences between persons living in an institution and those remaining in the community result, not from the organization of the nursing home, but from differences in population characteristics between persons who are institutionalized and persons who choose to remain in the community.

Pre-admission effects are changes to the prospective resident that occur before the person actually enters the nursing home. The process of depersonalization and other psychosocial changes begin long before the person moves into the facility. The individual may be changed by the process of becoming a nursing home resident–reaching the decision to seek institutional care, applying for admission, and being on a waiting list. Once a decision has been made to seek institutional care, the person may be changed by the process itself and come to resemble residents already living in the nursing home. This decision can set into motion a series of self-redefinitions by the individual and cause the family to re-evaluate the person's capacity to continue living in the community. Some seniors associate the impending move to the nursing home with a loss of independence, rejection by their children, or a prelude to death. Thoughts about the imminence of death certainly are not irrational given the high mortality rates during the first year after nursing home placement.

Another view maintains that institutional effects result from exposure to noxious aspects of the organization (e.g., inadequate nutrition, poor sanitary conditions, sensory deprivation, and lack of adequate geriatric or physical care). The iatrogenic effects associated with poor clinical management play a prominent role according to this view. Understaffing among nursing professionals, physician neglect, poor medication management, and immobility make residents deteriorate after admission. Some of these institutional effects could be rectified if more economic resources were available to pay for improved clinical, rehabilitative, nutritional, environmental, and other services.

The fourth explanation views changes in the environment following relocation to a nursing home as leading to adverse consequences due to the stress of environmental change. Discontinuities between pre- and post-relocation environments have been associated with deleterious results in terms of increased morbidity, mortality, and social and psychological decline. Rather than stemming from noxious organizational factors, per se, declines in resident well-being result from the relocation process and the subsequent environmental change or discontinuity that occurs when a person moves into a nursing home.

Relocation is commonly viewed as a stressful life event for the elderly. It has been associated with excess mortality, increased incidence of illness, and adverse psychological changes. Several factors intervene or mediate the effects of relocation. The degree of risk for adverse outcomes has been traced to the degree of environmental change or discontinuity, the personality of the individual being moved, and the voluntary versus involuntary nature of the move. The greater the choice an individual has, the less the negative effects of relocation. Voluntary moves are less stressful than involuntary moves. The more predictable a new environment is, the fewer the adverse effects. Predictability also depends on the degree of change between the old and new environments.

An individual's response to relocation is also influenced by the enduring aspects of his or her personality and past experiences in similar institutions. Persons who view themselves as in control of their fate are usually less devastated by the move. However, when those who are accustomed to controlling their environment are forced into a total institution where they are unable to control the environment, adverse effects may be worse. In comparison, those who are more passive and less prone to exert controls over their environment will experience fewer institutional effects. These risks have also been found to vary according to whether a person is moving within the community (e.g., from one apartment to another apartment), from home to an institution such as a nursing home, or from one institution to another institution (e.g., from one nursing home to another nursing home) (Schultz and Brenner, 1972).

In reviewing causes of institutional effects, it is likely that several factors are involved simultaneously. Research suggests that the stress of moving into a nursing home is mediated by at least three factors: continuity, predictability, and controllability (Schultz and Brenner, 1972). A number of strategies might be used to better manage the effects of institutionalization.

As much continuity as possible should be maintained between the pre-relocation and post-relocation environments. One solution is the creation of new organizational models that provide a more homelike setting. Permitting residents to keep as many personal possessions as possible—meaningful artifacts from the resident's past such as furnishings, photographs, and other objects from home. More personalized rooms permit residents to keep more of their personal belongings to maintain continuity with the past. Creating opportunities for residents to maintain contact with friends and family would also be helpful. Redesigning nursing units to allow residents to experience more "normalized" lifestyles where they can stay engaged in familiar social activities is a strategy that is being used in more and more facilities. This approach seems to be especially helpful for persons with Alzheimer's disease and related dementia. For persons experiencing memory loss, continuity with one's past is especially critical.

With regard to predictability, preparing the older person for the changes associated with moving to and living in a nursing home would be beneficial. Encouraging an older person to volunteer in a nursing home or to visit the nursing home may ease the stress of relocation. Educational programs or counseling services to teach the resident and family more about programs and services offered in a nursing home are another strategy. It is also vital to allow the potential resident to participate in decision making throughout all phases of the preadmission period. In this way, the resident can stay well-informed about any impending move to a nursing home.

In order to maximize self-direction and control of the environment, the resident should be provided with opportunities to make decisions, to participate in meaningful activities, to retain old skills and develop new ones, and to form relationships with other residents and staff. These objectives can be fulfilled by activities programs and recreational therapies that are better tailored to resident needs and individual preferences. Even seemingly insignificant activities can have beneficial effects. For example, one study found that residents who were approached by staff in ways that gave them a greater sense of control and choice and who were given the responsibility of care of houseplants fared better than did residents who were not afforded a similar sense of control, autonomy, or purpose.

New organizational models are emerging within nursing homes with the goal of lessening the institutional effects commonly associated with life in a total institution. Many new models change the organizational culture to "deinsititutionalize" the settings in which long-term care services are delivered. Although each model is unique, they often incorporate new environmental design features and new organizational structures. Environmental features such as private rooms, personalized rooms with more personal belongings and artifacts from home, smaller decentralized dining rooms, and small groupings of rooms so that residents live in smaller households are used to create a more "normal" and homelike setting. Interdisciplinary team models of service delivery are used to break down traditional departmental barriers and to maximize cost effectiveness of staff. These models frequently support resident choice and independence, maintain resident ties to the community, and provide a family-oriented atmosphere that encourages personal growth of residents, families, and staff. As more and more organizations implement changes to "deinstitutionalize" the nursing home, the negative institutional effects of life in a total institution should diminish. The range of settings in which long-term care services are being delivered is expanding with the development of alternative models of care. Providing services in alternative settings is another strategy for lessening adverse institutional effects.

REFERENCES

Coe, E. (1965). Self-Conception and institutionalization. In A. Rose & W. Peterson (Eds.), *Older people and their social world*. Philadelphia, PA: F.A. Davis.

Goffman, E. (1961). *Asylums*. Garden City, NY: Anchor Books.

Johnson, C.L., & Grant, L.A. (1985). *The nursing home in American society*. Baltimore, MD: The Johns Hopkins University Press.

Kasl, S.V. (1972). Physical and mental health effects of involuntary relocation and institutionalization of the elderly—A review. *American Journal of Public Health, 62,* 377–384.

Schultz, R., & Brenner, G. (1977). Relocation of the aged: A review and theoretical analysis. *Journal of Gerontology, 32,* 323–333.

Sommer, R., & Osmond, H. (1961). Symptoms of institutional care. *Social Problems, 8,* 254–262.

Tobin, S.S., & Lieberman, M.A. (1976). *Last home for the aged.* San Francisco, CA: Jossey-Bass.

Townsend, P. (1962). *The last refuge: A survey of residential institutions and homes for the aged in England and Wales.* London: Routledge and Kegan Paul.

Chapter 21

FAMILIES: THE SECOND CLIENT

WAYNE CARON

INTRODUCTION

Caring for each other at time of illness or disability is a distinctly human characteristic. It is our highest calling and most uplifting activity. We depend on care when we are young. And we often depend on care when we are old. The family provides primary care for children. Often families and professionals share care for elders. This shared care often occurs in nursing homes.

Caregiving is an expression of deep cultural values. Everyone wants the best possible quality of life for elderly persons. Because they share the same goal, families and professionals ought to form strong bonds of cooperation. However, family and staff relations are often distant and strained. Why should this be so? Families and staff have much to offer each other. Collaboration offers so much more than conflict. It is easier to work together than against each other. But the nature of long-term care carries inherent barriers to family-staff collaboration. These are structural barriers arising out of the dynamics of family caregiving and the organization of nursing home care.

In this chapter, the human ecological perspective will be used to examine the relationship between families and nursing home staff. Human ecology offers new insights into the dynamics of family and staff interactions. It provides new clues into causes for family and staff strain. And it provides direction for change bringing new vitality to the partnership between those who provide intimate care and those who provide professional care.

The Human Ecological Perspective

Nursing homes are too often more nursing than they are home. We struggle with how to merge these two very different environments. One is a professional context. It is a place for specialized care. Procedures, protocols, and duties organize daily life. The other is an intimate context. It is a place where lives are lived. Relationships organize daily life. The vision of long-term care is the delivery of technical medical care in homelike settings. The professional context should co-exist with the intimate. However, often the professional culture dominates.

Human ecology alerts us to the ways in which social systems are organized through different types of discourse. Discourse structures interaction through the types of words and symbols that get used. Professional discourse is technical while intimate discourse uses everyday language. In professional discourse, elders are described in terms of their medical conditions and treatment needs. In intimate discourse, elders are described in their unique personalities and interests. Professional discourse is depersonalizing while intimate discourse celebrates the individual. Professional discourse is the language of the workplace. Intimate discourse is the language of the home. (Caron, Hepburn, Luptak, Grant, Ostwald, & Keenan, 1999).

When professional discourse dominates, the focus is on the work of nursing care. The most important activities are those of the staff. Daily life is structured around their activities resulting in routines and rules which promote efficient delivery of cares. The nursing home is primarily a place to work more than it is a place to live (Nystrom & Segesten, 1996).

In this context, the family's contribution is secondary to that of the staff. They are the secondary caregivers, to the extent that they are caregivers at all. Yet, prior to nursing home placement, family is foremost in guarding the elder's well-being. This shift creates inevitable tensions between family and staff.

Human ecology shows us how the structure of the nursing home organization may contribute to staff-family strain. To gain deeper understanding of these dynamics, the family experience from the beginning of nursing home placement must be reviewed.

The Experience of Families in Placing an Elder

There are two trajectories that bring an elder to long-term care—acute and chronic. Many elders enter nursing homes after some acute incident—a broken hip, a serious infection, or a stroke. They require intensive nursing care. For these families, nursing home placement is a crisis. Their elder may go quickly from a healthy and independent member of the family to one who is injured, ill and dependent.

More often, families come to nursing homes not after some acute injury but after chronic and long-term illness. Family members have provided care often for years before placement. These families come to the nursing home exhausted. They have traveled the caregiving journey—dealing with the ambiguity of emerging impairments, the trauma of receiving serious diagnoses, stepping into the elder's life to help them face the loss of independence, and managing the constant demands of chronic caregiving (Caron, Pattee, & Otteson, 2001).

Nursing home placement is the last choice for families (Kelly, Knox, & Gekoski, 1998; Ryan & Scullion; 2000). It represents a breakdown in the capacity of the family to provide care. Changes in the elder's condition (especially difficult to manage behavior problems) can lead to placement (Morris, Rovner, & German, 1996). But exhaustion of family caregiving resources is more often the culprit. Placement is more likely when there are fewer community services (Jette, Tennstedt, & Crawford, 1995; Boaz & Muller, 1994) or few family members to help provide care (Kelly, Knox, & Gekoski, 1998; Russel, Cutrona, & Wallace, 1997; McClaran, Berglas, & Franco, 1996; Freedman, 1996). And placement is more likely when family relations are more distant or conflicted (Kesselring, Krulih, Bichsel, Minder, Beck, & Stuck, 2001; Fisher and Lieberman, 1999; Freedman, Berkman, Rapp, & Ostfeld, 1994).

Whether families come to placement exhausted or in crisis, the process of placement takes it own toll. Families are often highly ambivalent about placement, plagued by feelings of guilt and regret (Ryan & Scullion, 2000; Kellett, 1999; Mcauley, Travis, & Safewright, 1997; Bell, 1996). The process of finding a nursing home creates tremendous strain. Families feel a sense of urgency (Lundh, Sandeberg, & Nolan, 2000) and most often report getting little useful help from health care professionals (Nolan and Dellasega, 2000).

By the day of placement, families and staff are in very different places. For staff, it is a beginning. The elder resident is a new member of their community. They present new challenges. For families, it is an ending. It represents their failure to meet the challenges of care.

The Family Experience After Placement

Perhaps not surprising, almost half of families decrease their involvement with their elder after placement (Port, Gruber-Beldini, Burton, Baumgarten, Hebel, Zimmerman, & Magaziner, 2001). For the other half, involvement remains high, with families providing up to 30 percent of caregiving services (Keating, Fast, Dosman, & Eales, 2001). Families who stay closely involved tend to have had closer ties to the elder before placement (Port, Gruber-Beldini, Burton, Baumgarten, Hebel, Zimmerman, & Magaziner, 2001; Friedemann, Montgomery, Rice, & Farrell, 1999). They experienced less caregiving stress prior to placement (Gaugler, Leitsch, Zarit, & Pearlin, 2000).

Caregiving stress itself does not decrease with nursing home placement (Lieberman & Fisher, 2001; Bowman, Mukherkee, & Fortinsky, 1998). Nursing home placement is not a "hand off" from family to staff. Families remain concerned and affected by the condition of the elder (Dupuis & Norris, 1997). Caregiving does not end, only the nature of it changes (Caron, Pattee, & Ottesen, 2001).

In addition to dealing with the elder's medical conditions that compelled nursing home placement, the family must also deal with the staff. Caregiver distress is linked not only with how well the elder manages in the facility (Whitlach, Schur, Noelker, Ejaz, & Looman, 2001) but also the number of hassles they experience with the staff (Almberg, Grafstrom, Krichbaum, & Winblad, 2000).

The Relationship Between Families and Staff

Families and staff must figure out a way to share care of the elder. For families who have been providing direct care prior to placement, adjustment to their new role is a major challenge (Krause, Grant, & Long, 1999). Families often see themselves as taking responsibility for social and personal well-being of their elder family member, leaving physical and medical care to the nursing staff (Ryan & Scullion, 2000; Keefe & Fancey, 2000; Fleming, 1998; Ross, Rosenthal, & Dawson, 1997). They also see themselves as acting as advocates protecting the interests of their elder (Stull, Cosbey, Bowman, & Menutt, 1997).

Nursing home staff reports do not agree with family descriptions. They rate families as less involved in elder care than families see themselves (Ryan & Scullion, 2000). And nursing staff may be ambivalent about family involvement. Since nursing staff are legally responsible for care, they may see family involvement as threatening interference (Ryan & Scullion, 2000; Tilse, 1997).

These differences set the stage for poor relations. Family members report staff as being distant and uncommunicative (Finnema, de Lange, Droes, Ribbe, & van Tilburg, 2001; Hertzberg, Ekman, & Axelsson, 2001; Sandberg, Lundh, & Nolan, 2001). For their part, staff members describe families as uninvolved in the lives of their elder and overly critical of care (Setterlund, 1998; Sandberg, Lundh, & Nolan, 2001; Nolan & Dellasega, 1999). Tension can become so high that verbal and even physical assaults occur. Vinton and Mazza (1994) documented over 1,000 verbal assaults and 13 physical attacks of family members on staff over a six-month period in Florida nursing homes.

Interventions to Bring Families and Staff Closer

As this review of the recent literature shows, the structural barriers that distance families and staff are real. Families encounter the nursing home exhausted and disempowered. The strains and worries of their elder's care remain strong. Families struggle to find their place in the nursing home system—to find their proper role.

But the recent literature also contains reports of interventions that successfully bring families and staff together. Peak (2000) reports on an eight week program supporting families in visiting elders. Through educational programming and group discussions, families reported increased satisfaction in their visits. Especially useful was having a staff member work with the resident and incorporate their own experiences of interacting in helping the family members improve their visits.

Pillemer and associates (1998) describe the Partners in Caregiving program that brings families and staff together in communication workshops. Simultaneously training families and staff in communication and conflict resolution techniques garnered enthusiastic support from participants and improved relations within the facility. The Family Stories program (Hepburn, Caron, Luptak, Ostwald, Grant, & Keenan, 1997) took a different approach to education. Families were recruited to become the teachers, not the students. Their job was to teach staff about the residents for whom they cared. Through the construction of life history narratives, families shared with staff the rich histories of their elders and helped staff see the person behind the disability. Although the program faced challenges in fitting into the structure and routines of nursing home life, the stories were well received by staff and promoted new appreciation of the individuality of the residents (Caron, Hepburn, Luptak, Ostwald, Grant, & Keenan, 1999).

Towards a Future of Family Centered Long-Term Care

These initiatives have shown that families and staff do respond to efforts to bring them together. But the challenges are daunting. The structure of long-term care embedded in professional and technical models empower staff while disempowering residents and families (Caron, 1996). The culture of surveillance and restraint (Powers, 2001) and the discourse of medical care (Caron, Hepburn, Luptak, Ostwald, Grant, & Keenan, 1999) result from the same mindset. The nursing home is more nursing than it is home. Changing the discourse of nursing home care can impact on these structural barriers.

Alternative visions of nursing home life have been developed. Thomas (1996) promotes in his Eden Alternative, the vision of a nursing home as "human habitat." Central to this vision is daily life devoted to spontaneity, growth and nurturance. The nursing home is not a medical facility–sterile and routinized. It is full of growing things–children, plants, and animals. Everyone shares in the nurturance of the human habitat–elders, staff and family.

Envisioning nursing homes as places of history rather than illness and disability provides another change of perspective. Our children's schools are often described as holding our society's future. Our elders in nursing homes hold our society's past. Their individual stories form our history. Valuing these stories creates a new sense of meaning and purpose in the everyday life of facilities. The elder resident is more than a nursing patient. They are a resource connecting us directly to where we have been. Staff and family can equally share the riches of the elders' stories and guard their legacy (Caron, 1996; Caron, Hepburn, Luptak, Ostwald, Grant, & Keenan, 1999).

By changing perspectives, families emerge as central rather than peripheral to the nursing home environment. Nursing staff come and go. But the family remains a stable presence, providing continuity in the life of the elder. When nursing homes become family centered, their intimate knowledge of the elder is as important as the technical medical knowledge of professional staff.

CONCLUSION

The literature on families and nursing homes raises many concerns. Families enter the nursing home experienced in crisis and exhausted. Many drop away, in effect handing their elder over to the care of professionals. For those who stay involved, stresses from the nursing home itself represent a major source of burden. Families would like to be more involved with staff, but find many barriers to connecting. Staff often find family members foes rather than friends. Family members take on the role of advocacy resulting in interactions with the staff that center around complaints and problems. Family and staff tensions can run high, to the point of open conflict.

But there is hope. Studies show interventions successfully bring staff and family together. They form partnerships in caring for the elder and honoring their legacy. Bringing these lessons to the day-to-day life of long-term care requires we change how we think about nursing homes. The preeminence of staff and staff work must be replaced with new visions. In seeing nursing homes as more than places of care, we open ourselves to seeing elders in new ways–beyond their illness and disability.

In this re-envisioning, families are key. They complement professional caregivers in the continuity and intimacy which their relationship with the elder holds. Bringing families together to form communities supporting each other and the staff is a central step to bring nursing homes closer to family centered care.

REFERENCES

Almberg, B., Grafstrom, M., Krichbaum, K., & Winblad, B. (2000). The interplay of institution and family caregiving: Relations between patient hassles, nursing home hassles and caregivers' burnout. *International Journal of Geriatric Psychiatry, 15*(10), 931–939.

Bell, J. (1996). Decision making in nursing home placement. *Journal of Women & Aging, 8*(1), 45–60.

Boaz, R.F., & Muller, C.F. (1994). Predicting the risk of permanent nursing home residence–The role of community help as indicated by family helpers and prior living arrangements. *Health Services Research, 29*(4), 391–414.

Bowmen, K.F., Mukherjee, S., & Fortinsky, R.H. (1998). Exploring strain in community and nursing home family caregivers. *Journal of Applied Gerontology, 17*(3), 371–392.

Caron, W. (1996). Systemic approaches to nursing home care. In T.D. Hargraves & S.M. Hanna (Eds.), *The aging family: New visions in theory, practice, and reality*. New York: Brunner-Mazel.

Caron, W., Hepburn, K., Luptak, M., Grant, L., Ostwald, S., & Keenan, J. (1999). Expanding the discourse of care: Family constructed biographies of nursing home residents. *Families, Systems & Health, 17,* 323–335.

Caron, W., Pattee, J., & Otteson, O. (2001). *Alzheimer's disease: The family journey*. Plymouth, MN: North Ridge Press.

Dupuis, S.L., & Norris, J.E. (1997). A multidimensional and contextual framework for understanding diverse family members roles in long-term care facilities. *Journal of Aging Studies, 11*(4), 297–325.

Finnema, E., de Lange, J., Droes, R.M., Ribbe, M., & van Tilburg, W. (2001). The quality of nursing home care: Do the opinions of family members change after implementation of emotion-oriented care? *Journal of Advanced Nursing, 35*(5), 728–740.

Fisher, L., & Lieberman, M.A. (1999). A longitudinal study of predictors of nursing home placement for patients with dementia: The contribution of family characteristics. *Gerontologist, 39*(6), 677–686.

Fleming, A.A. (1998). Family caregiving of older people with dementing illnesses in nursing homes–A lifeline of special care. *Australian Journal on Ageing, 17*(3), 140–144.

Freedman, V.A. (1996). Family structure and the risk of nursing home admission. *Journals of Gerontology Series B–Psychological Sciences & Social Sciences, 51*(2), S61–S69.

Freedman, V.A., Berkman, L.F., Rapp, S.T., & Ostfeld, A.M. (1994). Family networks–predictors of nursing home entry. *American Journal of Public Health, 84*(5), 843–845.

Friedemann, M.L., Montgomery, R.J., Rice, C., & Farrell, L. (1999). Family involvement in the nursing home. *Western Journal of Nursing Research, 21*(4), 549–567.

Gaugler, J.E., Leitsch, S.A., Zarit, S.H., & Pearlin, L.I. (2000). Caregiver involvement following institutionalization: Effects of preplacement stress. *Research on Aging, 22*(4), 337–359.

Hepburn, K.W., Caron, W., Luptak, M., Ostwald, S., Grant, L., & Keenan, J.M. (1997). The family stories workshop–Stories for those who cannot remember. *Gerontologist, 37*(6), 827–832.

Hertzberg, A., Ekman, S.L., & Axelsson, K. (2001). Staff activities and behaviour are the source of many feelings: Relatives' interactions and relationships with staff in nursing homes. *Journal of Clinical Nursing, 10*(3), 380–388.

Jette, A.M., Tennstedt, S., & Crawford, S. (1995). How does formal and informal community care affect nursing home use? *Journals of Gerontology Series B–Psychological Sciences & Social Sciences, 50*(1), S4–S12.

Keating, N., Fast, J., Dosman, D., & Eales, J. (2001). Services provided by informal and formal caregivers to seniors in residential continuing care. *Canadian Journal on Aging, 20*(1), 23–45.

Keefe, J., & Fancey, P. (2000). The care continues: Responsibility for elderly relatives before and after admission to a long term care facility. *Family Relations, 49*(3), 235–244.

Kellett, U.M. (1999). Transition in care: Family-carers' experience of nursing home placement. *Journal of Advanced Nursing, 29*(6), 1474–1481.

Kelly, L.E., Knox, V.J., & Gekoski, W.L. (1998). Womens views of institutional versus community-based long-term care. *Research on Aging, 20*(2), 218–245.

Kesselring, A., Krulik, T., Bichsel, M., Minder, C., Beck, J.C., & Stuck, A.E. (2001). Emotional and physical demands on caregivers in home care to the elderly in Switzerland and their relationship to nursing home admission. *European Journal of Public Health, 11*(3), 267–273.

Lieberman, M.A., & Fisher, L. (2001). The effects of nursing home placement on family caregivers of patients with Alzheimer's disease. *Gerontologist, 41*(6), 819–826.

Lundh, U., Sandberg, J., & Nolan, M. (2000). 'I don't have any other choice': Spouses' experiences of placing a partner in a care home for older people in Sweden. *Advanced Nursing, 32*(5), 1178–1186.

McAuley, W.J., Travis, S.S., & Safewright, M.P. (1997). Personal accounts of the nursing home search and selection process. *Qualitative Health Research, 7*(2), 236–254.

McClaran, J., Berglas, R.T., & Franco, E.D. (1996). Long hospital stays and need for alternate level of care at discharge–Does family make a difference for elderly patients? *Canadian Family Physician, 42,* 449 ff.

Morris, R.K., Rovner, R.W., & German, P.S. (1996). Factors contributing to nursing home admission because of disruptive behaviour. *International Journal of Geriatric Psychiatry, 11*(3), 243–249.

Nolan, M., & Dellasega, C. (2000). 'I really feel I've let him down': Supporting family carers during long-term care placement for elders. *Journal of Advanced Nursing, 31*(4), 759–767

Nystrom, A.E.M., & Segesten, K.M. (1996). The family metaphor applied to nursing home life. *International Journal of Nursing Studies, 33*(3), 237–248.

Peak, T. (2000). Families and the nursing home environment: Adaptation in a group context. *Journal of Gerontological Social Work, 3*(1), 51–66.

Pillemer, K., Hegeman, C.R., Albright, B., & Henderson, C. (1998). Building bridges between families and nursing home staff–The partners in caregiving program. *Gerontologist, 38*(4), 499–503.

Port, C.L. Gruber-Baldini, A.L., Burton, L., Baumgarten, M., Hebel, J.R., Zimmerman, S.I., & Magaziner, J. (2001). Resident contact with family and friends following nursing home admission. *Gerontologist, 41*(5), 589–596.

Powers, B.A. (2001). Ethnographic analysis of everyday ethics in the care of nursing home residents with dementia–A taxonomy. *Nursing Research, 50*(6), 332–339.

Ross, M.M., Rosenthal, C.J., & Dawson, P.G. (1997). Spousal caregiving in the institutional setting–Task performance. *Canadian Journal on Aging, 16*(1), 51–69.

Russell, D.W., Cutrona, C.E., & Wallace, B.B. (1997). Loneliness and nursing home admission among rural older adults. *Psychology & Aging, 12*(4), 574–589.

Ryan, A.A., & Scullion, H.F. (2000). Nursing home placement: An exploration of the experiences of family carers. *Journal of Advanced Nursing, 32*(5), 1187–1195.

Sandberg, J., Lundh, U., & Nolan, M.R. (2001). Placing a spouse in a care home: the importance of keeping. *Journal of Clinical Nursing, 10*(3), 406–416.

Setterlund, D.S. (1998). Dementia care staff and family carers–Their relationships in the context of care. *Australian Journal on Ageing, 17*(3), 135–139.

Stull, D.E., Cosbey, J., Bowman, K., & Menutt, W. (1997). Institutionalization–A continuation of family care. *Journal of Applied Gerontology, 16*(4), 379-402.

Thomas, W. (1996). *Life worth living: How someone you love can still enjoy life in a nursing home–The Eden Alternative in action.* Acton, MA: VanderWyk & Burnham.

Tilse, C. (1997). Family advocacy roles and highly dependent residents in nursing homes. *Australian Journal on Ageing, 16*(1), 20–23.

Vinton, L., & Mazza, N. (1994). Aggressive behavior directed at nursing home personnel by residents family members. *Gerontologist, 34*(4), 528–533.

Whitlatch, C.J., Schur, D., Noelker, L.S., Ejaz, F.K., & Looman, W.J. (2001). The stress process of family caregiving in institutional settings. *Gerontologist, 41*(4), 462–473.

Chapter 22

INTERGENERATIONAL PROGRAMS

Ruth Stryker

The mobility of contemporary American families and the lifestyle of retired persons conspire to separate many children from their grandparents except for occasional visits. As a result, young people miss the nurture, support, and sense of roots that closeness to grandparents provides. By the same token, older persons miss the joy of knowing youthful perspectives and the gratification that comes from the role of generativity.

If this is a loss for grandparents living in the community, it is even more exaggerated for persons living in nursing homes where there is also a loss of many former psychological supports. Research in long-term care has helped to identify characteristics that improve quality of life and the presence of children in the environment is one of the important such characteristics.

Even though new knowledge of aging is available, stereotyped and traditional notions about the institutionalized elderly still abound. Long-term care facilities tend to create an overprotective atmosphere that results in being both boring and stifling. There is a need to integrate facets of normal community living into all long-term care settings. The presence of children is "normal" in most communities.

WHY INTERGENERATIONAL PROGRAMS?

It is the administrator's responsibility to initiate and support programs that expand interpersonal relationships of clients, especially with persons from the community. One way to do this is through intergenerational programs which can be rewarding to both elderly persons and children. Such programs reintroduce a chance for growth, provide an opportunity for emotional ties and afford a natural exposure to an enriching facet of the real world.

More specifically, what are the goals of a program for intergenerational interaction? First, children are an everyday part of life in the community. Long-term care facilities try to protect residents from unpleasantness, but ideas that children are a bother and that the elders might dislike their noise seem misplaced. By not only permitting but also encouraging intergenerational interactions, at least one area of community life is brought back into the residents' environment.

Second, there can be positive results from the introduction of interaction between the old and the young who may come with innocent perceptions of the very old. Children, especially those of preschool age, do not value a person on the basis of physical or mental perfection. That trait has been saved for those of us who are too old to retain the wonder of life and yet too young to understand it. Young children do not allow wrinkles and infirmities to interfere with their relationships with others.

The third reason focuses on the spontaneous fun and humor that young children can bring to any environment. Children, especially the very young with their curiosity and openness, can change the normally quiet and predictable institution into a vibrant and lively community. Spontaneity and fun are welcomed by residents.

Fourth, many affectional ties of the elderly have been broken by death or separation and they are very difficult to replace, especially in an institution. Children can provide new ties, at least partially filling a void. Finally, a well thought-out program can and should have a positive influence on attitudes toward the aged in future generations.

TYPES OF INTERGENERATIONAL PROGRAMS

Virtually every long-term care facility has some exposure to children. Grandchildren and great-grandchildren are at least occasional visitors to their elderly family members. Not infrequently older grandchildren are employees of the facility where a grandparent lives.

Beyond this, facility programs vary greatly. Children from a local school may have special friends whom they visit weekly during the school year. A nursing home may be associated with a facility for mentally retarded children who are nurtured and helped on a one-to-one basis by frail elderly. A children's day care center may be attached to or associated with a nursing home so that relationships develop over time. Special programs for grandchildren of residents can make such visits "more fun." Grandparents may "baby sit" grandchildren for one or two hours a week. Children may come to the facility for tutoring in special areas.

Foster grandparent programs encourage school-age youngsters to develop a relationship with a resident and hopefully, a friendship. In order for a foster grandparent program to be effective, a great deal of planning and evaluation must be ongoing. Too much structure decreases spontaneity. The mutual needs of two people can be lost within the confines of a pre-established program. The assumption that people respond in a similar manner to a given set of circumstances does not allow for the flexibility needed to make these programs successful.

Lifelink, in Bensenville, Illinois, an organization with both multilevel housing and a nursing facility, started several programs in 1990. About 115 residents participate in on-campus Head Start classes for preschoolers. In addition, they work with three foster-care programs for children from six to 20, helping with homework, crafts, and activities. They even mentor young or troubled parents. Residents have a great sense of purpose.

The Living Center in Berthoud, Colorado, has an on-site child day care center. Like other on-site day care, the groups mix at meal times and for some activities. This facility reports that it has the lowest personnel turnover rate in their company and they do not use nursing pools like most organizations in their area. Employees' children have special rates and even have special discounts when in-service education programs are held.

Jewish Family and Children's Service in San Francisco have both Jewish and nonsectarian programs which include adult volunteers. For two years, a 30 year-old attorney visited two women in their late '90s to discuss politics and current events.

Computers are a part of some programs. In one case, residents are assigned to a pen pal who e-mails messages on a regular basis. When a resident hears "You've got mail," it is a real morale boost. Experience Senior Power of Oak Park, Michigan, is a company created to have older children teach residents of assisted living and retirement communities how to use a computer. It is yet another way to begin intergenerational friendships.

Not all programs have successful outcomes, however. When 86 high school students interested in health careers were exposed to a nursing home, they could not see themselves working there although they found them more pleasant than they had expected (Lawrence et al.). In another study with youth, learning about aging along with exposure to the elderly, the youth ended up having no desire to work with them.

Program success, of course, depends on many variables, such as age, purpose, timeliness, frequency, and access. Another variable is the degree of structure. As structure increases, spontaneity decreases. Relationships develop; they cannot be forced. If either force or too much structure occurs, the program will have limited effectiveness and could even be harmful. Indeed, one study indicates that nursing home residents experienced increased health and more zest for life when they were visited by young people, but these positive factors declined below baseline when the visits stopped. This study seems to imply that starting a program and then stopping it, can be more harmful than not starting it in the first place.

A PIONEER DAY CARE PROGRAM

Most long-term care organizations welcome groups of school children. During the nine-month school year, entire grades often come to visit, to entertain, and hopefully to break the routine of institutional living. But does it? That was the question John Thompson had when he was the administrator of the Retirement Center of Wright County in Buffalo, Minnesota. He thought that watching an amateur performance of a grandchild must be very different from watching young strangers perform. Do these well-meaning events with children, kept at a social distance from residents, serve to frustrate and remind the resident of his or her minimal contacts with others in the community?

And what effect does it have on the children in terms of their feelings about the aged and aging? Does seeing a room full of white-haired strangers in wheelchairs create a fear of the aged and aging? Is it not better to know one person well than to have *no* knowledge of anyone?

These were the questions on Thompson's mind one cool fall afternoon when a school bus unloaded 40 children at the entrance of his skilled nursing facility. This was supposed to be a special day because the second grade of the elementary school was visiting.

The residents waited for them in the large dayroom. Soon the echoes of children's chatter and giggles filled the normally quieter hallways. Then, after a few songs, the teacher ushered the children back to the bus. It was quiet again. There was an empty feeling as the residents slowly returned to their routines: television, games, and naps. The organization had reacquainted the residents with the sight and sound of children, but it seemed more like a parade. The children were to be enjoyed only from a distance as if in a glass case. There was no warmth, no sharing, and no relationship formed. An occasional gnarled hand reached out, but the time was up until the next month.

The administrator thought that if children were there daily and if they were the same children, this kind of frustration would be averted. Coincidentally, the community was discussing the need for a day care center at the same time. Why not in the nursing home? It apparently had not been done before at this time.

There were many considerations in designing and implementing a day care center for children in a long-term care building. Costs, space, staffing, licensing, programming, supplies, and furnishings were all addressed. Through efforts of dedicated volunteers, the necessary funds were raised for initial purchases and start-up costs. A director for the center was hired. The Generations Day Care Center opened its doors in September 1979 with 23 children ages six weeks to twelve years old. The premise was that both residents and children would mutually benefit from the opportunity to interact with each other. This original assumption of benefit was demonstrated over and over again.

For over 15 years the spontaneous interaction of the children's day care program worked its magic. The wheelchair rides, hugs, stories, and occasional tears coupled with the obvious smiles and laughs provided enrichment and growth for both age groups. The halls held evidence of real life . . . a cane propped on the handlebars of a tricycle, mysterious muddy footprints appearing near the kitchen, an occasional "lost" child, usually found later on the lap of a gray-haired storytelling "kidnapper." Even residents who chose not to seek out the children enjoyed their more casual visits when they delivered mail or waved when they passed their rooms. The eventual 40 infants, toddlers, and preschoolers had free access to the nursing home corridors, and the residents had access to the children's play areas in spite of being incorporated and staffed separately.

The community benefited from having a day care center and most certainly, the facility's image in the community changed. No longer was it just a "place for old sick people." Young parents learned that neither the facility nor its residents were depressing as they had once thought. They also found that their children were eager to return to the surroundings because of the genuine appreciation the residents had for the children.

The employees benefited also. The parents of children who were employed in the nursing home found the arrangement secure and loving. They had total access to their children and actually had a part in their lives while carrying out their employment duties. As a bonus, they developed new dimensions in relationships with residents because of their children. Residents and employees had more to share with one another. By the same token, the child and parent had something else to share. As one resident put it, "I can't imagine living in a place where there are no children. You just can't talk to old people every minute of every day."

A number of the same children were at the center for some years. As a result, residents participated daily in their growth, from baby bottles to baseball. The children had an "extra" person who loved them and they had one to love. When a child lost a friend, it was dealt with openly and his or her grief was supported by others who were also saddened. As one parent said, "An introduction to death and grief is a reality with which we all must learn to deal. It is better that their first experience is about a loving friend and with the support of many persons." In one instance the children sorted through pictures of their deceased friend, making a collage which they gave to the family.

The details of this early day care center are presented to show what valuable relationships between children, parent, employees, and older people can develop. Because of changes in ownership and community needs, the day care center, after over 15 years of operation, is no longer a part of the nursing home, but it remains a model for this kind of intergenerational mix.

MAKING LONG-RANGE COMMITMENTS

Many intergenerational programs last only one or two years either because of lost funding or loss of enthusiastic personnel. Since stopping a program may do more harm than never having had a program, it is important to look at some of the programs that strive for permanency. A program started in 1988 in Phoenix, Arizona may provide some insight into a stable ongoing program.

The Community Program began with funding from the local Area Agency on Aging with matching grants from local business and community groups. It began with a part-time coordinator who coordinated weekly or biweekly one-hour visits of five classrooms of children to five nursing homes. Some were four year-olds and some were sixth graders who were studying Social Studies. The developing relationships were videotaped during the first year. They used what they called a Friendship Model.

The initial step was to get school principals and administrators who were "sold" on the idea. They then found enthusiastic teachers and activity directors who usually ran the programs ultimately. For those who worry about the educational value, one only needs to read the children's journals and see some of the newsletters, materials, and written assignments they produced.

The Community Program makes sure that no one goes to a nursing home without some preparation. With grant money, they developed a four-module video training program. It shows how to handle some difficult behaviors and talks about odors. Children look through lenses coated with rubber cement to find out what an older person might see and they listen to tapes with voices. Older children are encouraged to read books about older people and write out, "If I were old I would. . . ."

Residents may be alert or disoriented. Occasionally, a person who is loud or violent is excluded. For residents who do not wish to participate, there is a gallery (a corner of the room where nonparticipants can watch others interact). These residents often join in eventually. At the end of the school year, there is a party to bring closure to the visits for the summer. However, there are often voluntary summer visits. Because children need to be driven to the nursing home, parents get involved also.

Feedback is solicited from all participants. "Over the years, parents have reported two consistent themes: their children develop a greater understanding of aging, death, and the life cycle; and they show increased comfort about being with, ability to communicate with, and empathy for older adults" (Hamilton et al.). Children feel they are doing something that is important to another human being. Residents enjoy being involved in something that is emotionally satisfying.

Because of the fact that there is turnover among teachers and activity directors, it is the commitment of the institutional leadership in both the schools and the nursing homes that keeps the programs going. For readers who wish to emulate this program, the planning manual and video tapes are available from Bifolkal Productions in Madison, Wisconsin.

REFERENCES

Bajoka, K. (2001). Power surge. *Balance,* March/April.

Bonifazi, W. (2001). More than kid stuff. *Contemporary Long Term Care,* January.

Hamilton, G. et al. (1999). Building community for the long term: An intergenerational commitment. *The Gerontologist, 39*(2), 235.

Hook, W. et al. (1982). Frequency of visitation in nursing homes: Patterns of contact across the boundaries of total institutions. *The Gerontologist, 22*(4), 424, August.

Kassab, C., & Vance, L. (1999). An assessment of the effectiveness of an intergenerational program for youth. *Psychology Reports, 84*(1), 198, February.

Lawrence, F. et al. (1999). High school students' perceptions of nursing homes: Before and after experience. *Psychology Reports, 84*(2), 407, April.

Chapter 23

COMPANION ANIMALS IN THE ENVIRONMENT

RUTH STRYKER

Close relationships between people and animals may have existed for as long as people and animals have been on earth. Today, over half of all families in the United States own at least one dog, cat, or both. In addition, families own millions of other animals such as birds, fish, ferrets, rabbits, gerbils, horses, and pot-bellied pigs. A majority of pet owners see their animals as members of their family.

The term "companion animal" can be used in many ways but it usually refers to a dog or a cat and is most commonly referred to as a "pet." In addition to being a pet, dogs can also become a source of assistance for persons with various disabilities. The guide dog is an integral part of the life of many vision-impaired persons, as is the hearing dog for many hearing-impaired persons. The service dog assists the physically disabled. Monkeys have been used to assist quadriplegics while companion animals as well as other animals have been beneficial to the elderly, the mentally disabled, emotionally disturbed, and prison inmates. The "Bird Man of Alcatraz" is an example of the positive effect that birds have on certain prison inmates.

The importance of companion animals is no longer merely a matter of sentimentality. The role of support dogs (guide dogs, hearing dogs, and service dogs) is recognized by law, assuring their entrance to public places and public transportation. In addition, there exists 30 years of research demonstrating the positive effects of companion animals on the physical, psychological, and social health of persons of all ages. Health care practitioners can no longer dismiss the efficacy of a mutually caring interaction with animals on the health of their clients. It has been demonstrated repeatedly that animals can be of therapeutic value both to an individual and the environment.

HEALTH BENEFITS OF COMPANION ANIMALS

Florence Nightingale observed the positive effects of having pets in the care environment and so advocated having them present. In spite of the nearly 30 years of research supporting the beneficial effects of dogs and cats, health care settings, with few exceptions, are still reluctant to include animals in the residential setting.

In many studies, a majority of dog and cat owners consider their pet to be a member of the family (Sable). The emotional depth of these relationships is well-known by veterinarians and grief counselors who deal with people who have lost a pet. They report that grief for a pet often mirrors the grief suffered from the loss of a loved person. Separation from a beloved pet is also traumatic. A person entering senior housing, assisted living, or a nursing home may be suffering from the separation of a much-loved pet as an added sorrow in leaving his or her home.

Aaron Katcher, a psychiatrist who has studied human-pet relationships extensively, holds that pet relationships contribute significantly to the well-being of many people. He further states that the role of pets is closely related to the physiological well-being of humans, especially as related to touch, intimacy and nurturance. They are a part of what he calls a "living" environment which includes plants, fish, birds, animals and people. It is theorized that the strong attachment to pets helps to counter some of the effects of our urbanized and often impersonal surroundings.

The following studies have major applicability to the elderly and long-term care settings. James Lynch noted that blood pressure drops as much as 50 percent when a person pets a dog. Decades ago Harry Reasoner and his "60 Minutes" crew came to Lynch's house to document health benefits of animal companions. The segment continues to be the most frequently rebroadcast in "60 Minutes" history. Besides being effective in reducing blood pressure, pets also influence survival rates in coronary disease (Katcher). A follow-up study of 93 patients a year after a heart attack was conducted. Of those without a pet, 11 had died and 28 were still alive a year later. Of those with a pet, only three had died and 50 were still alive. Four times more people without pets had died. While the researchers took into account many other social relationships, they concluded that pets influenced people quite differently from other human relationships. A Mayo Clinic study showed that owning a pet also stimulated physical exercise, reduced anxiety, and provided an external focus of attention.

Researchers went on to try to discover what caused these major differences. With new technologies, they were able to discover the physiological dynamics that might explain the relationships. They studied 38 children while they were reading aloud and while they were resting. The presence of a dog result-ed in a lowering of blood pressure both at rest and while they read aloud. In a laboratory at Johns Hopkins Medical School, a significant drop in blood pressure occurred when an adult petted a dog. The vascular response also produced relaxation. They conclude that the evidence for greater long-term survival of heart patients with pets is overwhelming.

In addition to physiological changes with the introduction of animals, there are psychological changes also. In a large telephone interview study of Medicare enrollees, elderly pet owners reported less psychological distress and fewer visits to physicians over a one-year period than non-pet owners. This was true of people who lived alone as well as people who lived with oth-ers.

When elderly people were surveyed about the role of pets in their lives, they mentioned the following: dogs and cats give unconditional love and affection, are accepting, and loyal. They increase feelings of happiness, secu-rity, and self-worth. They reduce the feeling of isolation and loneliness and even helped during bereavement of a spouse. Another study of persons over 65 years of age documented the inverse relationship of pet ownership and depression. It certainly seems that pets may be good for both physical and psychological health.

The benefits of pets can be brought to the workplace. A survey by the American Pet Products Manufacturers' Association (APPMA) surveyed com-panies nationwide that permit pets at work. Companies (100%) reported that pets in the workplace relaxed employees and promoted positive work rela-tions. Seventy-five percent reported increased creativity and productivity. No company had increased absenteeism but 27 percent reported a decreased absenteeism. All companies will continue to allow pets in the workplace.

EXPERIENCE IN LONG-TERM CARE

Most long-term care organizations recognize the need for a living environ-ment when they provide living plants, aquariums, and aviaries. While these are important adjuncts to a living environment because they are interesting to watch and may stimulate conversation, they do not interact with humans as cats, dogs, and some other animals do.

Some long-term care facilities have introduced resident dogs and cats. Oth-ers have visiting pets, mostly dogs and cats, brought in by relatives, friends of residents, staff, humane societies, or volunteers. Some Eden Alternative organizations allow residents to bring their pets with them. As a result, there may be many animals and birds in one building and some are allowed free run in the premises.

The benefits from such animal activities and programs have been widely reported in the literature. A common finding is that contacts with animals result in increased sociability and enhanced morale of other residents, staff, and visitors. There are more smiles, more conversations, and greater animation even of the withdrawn. The results have even included a reduction of psychotropic drug use and the opening of a door to communication with the clinically depressed. When animal programs are more formalized, they may be referred to as "pet therapy," "animal facilitated therapy," or "animal assisted therapy." The critical element is that these programs have clinical goals.

Katsinas reports on the use of a canine companion within a rehabilitation model program for nursing home residents with dementia. The program resulted in elimination of some restraints for wanderers, social interaction between the animal and individuals, and between staff and friends about the dog. Her unexpected results included a re-orientation of individuals who were severely withdrawn, and the dog's presence helped in orientation to the day of the week.

In light of the known possibilities for positive physical and psychological changes in elderly persons when animals are introduced into the environment, it almost seems mandatory to allow pets and pet programs in senior housing, assisted living, and nursing homes. Also, because of what is known about the depth of the human/animal bond, it seems important to take a pet history when gathering admission information. It is possible that some residents may be experiencing depression and loneliness due to separation from or bereavement for a pet.

The literature is replete with listings of both potential problems as well as benefits which can be expected with the inclusion of animals in long-term care organizations. Possible disadvantages might be physical harm from zoonotic diseases (diseases transmitted from animal to humans), allergic reactions of staff and residents, or sanitation. Lack of proper facilities for animals, the need for staff involvement, and cost are often a concern also. These concerns were addressed by the Center to Study Human–Animal Relationships and Environments (CENSHARE) at the University of Minnesota.

In the first study, 762 Minnesota long-term care facility administrators were surveyed. Those who had animal programs identified many more advantages than disadvantages while those who did not have animals identified more disadvantages than advantages. In other words, those who had animals were far more positive.

The second study addressed the risks (injuries, allergies, infections) to vulnerable residents as a result of contact with animals. During one year, all mandatory incident reports in 284 Minnesota long-term care facilities were examined. During that period, there were 19 animal-related injuries reported in 18 homes. Seventeen were minor scratches by kittens or puppies and two were serious (one broken wrist and one broken shoulder). The latter two accidents occurred when a pet policy and procedure had been violated. No animal related infections or allergies were reported. Compared to incidents from all causes, there were 4.5 animal-related incidents per 1,000 incidents. The other 995.5 incidents were presumably caused by flawed performance of people or equipment. The researchers concluded that "pets seem to be safer than people."

INTRODUCING COMPANION ANIMALS
TO THE ORGANIZATION

People who work and live in long-term care settings mirror the range of feelings and perceptions of the general population toward animals. Some individuals do not like animals. Others may like dogs but dislike cats. Still others may actually fear a particular species of animal. Others love all animals and still others are neutral in their feelings. These varying perceptions and feelings about animals are especially significant when an organization wishes to introduce animals to achieve therapeutic results.

A visiting animal program may be a wise first step. A knowledgeable person might point out the rationale for using animals as therapeutic adjuncts and note the responses of residents to the visitors. Explaining the concepts of animal-facilitated programs can lay the foundation for further expansion of the program. Administration can lead, but staff and residents need to be involved in the planning and implementation of any animal program (see Chapter 27 for strategies on introducing change).

Personnel may be concerned about having to take on additional duties. These concerns are legitimate and need to be addressed *before an* expanded program begins. If key staff are dubious, a demonstration project in a small area might be initiated. Some organizations have started by having a dog show in the facility. Starting a live-in animal program may not be difficult however, because, like the companies in the APPMA survey discussed earlier, long-term care employees often enjoy the animals as much as, if not more, than the residents.

It is wise to avoid the term "pet therapy" with residents. They think of a pet in terms of companionship, not therapy, but in the end they may well be the same because companionship is often therapeutic. Residents also like to be involved in feeding fish, helping in the aviary, walking a dog, or feeding a cat.

Having responsibility, no matter how small can be important to an individual's self-esteem.

PRACTICAL CONSIDERATIONS

Operational considerations for a live-in pet program include the availability of space, animal behavior, concerns about animal disease, selection, care, and handling of animals. However, attitudinal factors can affect operational factors. For example, the act of defecation by a dog in a common living area is viewed and handled quite differently by a person who does not like dogs than by a person who loves dogs.

The well-being and health of the animal must be considered. A veterinarian is needed to assure that animal programs are in compliance with accepted animal health requirements. A physical examination by a veterinarian needs to certify that there are no signs of infectious disease and that all immunizations have been completed. Licensure and regulatory agencies will be concerned with this aspect of any animal program.

Arrangements for daily care such as feeding, shelter, grooming, training, exercise, and a private place for the animal to rest and sleep are essential. Procedures for care in case of injury or illness as well as annual check-ups and immunizations must be in place. If this does not fit in the budget, it may be possible to raise special funds for such care. If this is impossible, a staff member might bring her or his pet to work each work day rather than have a live-in animal.

In a long-term care setting, there are other considerations for the live-in animal. Residents will need some cautions no matter how enthusiastic they are about a pet. Elderly people tend to enjoy feeding snacks to resident animals. However, too much of this can be detrimental to the animal. At one facility where a German Shepherd quickly gained 35 pounds, the feeding of the dog was then assigned to different residents on a rotating basis.

Regardless of any routine arrangements, all staff should be alert for any mistreatment of an animal by residents, staff, or visitors. Mistreatment could be a matter of malicious intent, on the one hand, or quite innocent differences in appropriate conduct on the other. The animal needs to be protected through staff vigilance.

The behavior of animals plays a key role in the success or failure of animal programs. Long-term care facilities do not want noisy breeds of dogs or animals that are difficult to train. When selecting suitable puppies, it is helpful to include a puppy temperament test as part of the required health examination. Such a behavioral examination, while not definitive, probably will identify animals with obvious inappropriate behavior. To avoid the rigors of training a puppy, it is recommended that adult dogs of known behaviors be used.

Naturally, visiting pets which are usually family pets are another matter. Even when exposure to a resident is a relatively brief visit, the facility needs rules for visiting animals to minimize any problems. Procedures for handling situations of inappropriate visiting animal behavior or inappropriate behavior of the owner or handler need to be established *before* any incident occurs. Indicate that the owner is responsible for pet behavior during the visit and state the policy for violation of the rule. A common procedure is to inform owners and handlers of visiting pets of the guidelines in writing on their first visit.

SUMMARY

Elderly persons are nearly always responsive to animals, especially dogs and cats that interact with wagging tails and purrs when scratched or petted. In rural areas, farm animals stimulate discussion among residents who relive their farming days. Not only do animals bring pleasure and create interest, but research shows that both mental and physical health are improved by their presence. A long-term care setting is humanized and more homelike when thoughtful planning introduces animals to the environment.

REFERENCES

APPMA. (2000). Survey of pets in the workplaces. *Interactions,* Delta Society, *18*(4), 12.

Barnett, J., & Quigley, J. (1984). Animals in long-term care facilities: a framework for program planning. *Journal of Long-Term Care Administration, 12,* 4.

Beale, N. et al. (1986). *Pet-Related Risks in Nursing Homes.* Unpublished MPH thesis, University of Minnesota.

Beck, A.M., & Meyers, N.M. (1996). Health enhancement and companion animal ownership. *Annual Review Public Health, 17,* 247.

Chevremont, N.K., Fuchsburge, A., & Miller, K. *The Eden Alternative.* A Cardinal Stritch University student project August 12, 1999, http://www.edenmidwest .com/edenpaper.html.

Gammonley, J., & Yates, J. (1991). Pet projects: Animal assisted therapy in nursing homes. *Journal of Gerontological Nursing, 17*(1), 12.

Jennings, L.B. (1987). Potential benefits of pet ownership on health promotion. *Journal of Holistic Nursing, 15*(4), 358, December.

Katcher, A.H. (1986). People and companion animal dialogue: Style and physiological response. *Phi Kappa Phi Journal,* Winter.

Katcher, A.H. How pets aid health. *Health and Medical Horizons, 1984 Yearbook.* New York: MacMillan Education Co.

Katsinas, R.P. (2000). The use and implications of a canine companion in a therapeutic day program for nursing home residents with dementia. *Activities, Adaptation & Aging, 1*(13), 132.

Lynch, J.J. (2000). Developing a physiology of inclusion. *Interactions, 18*(4), 4, Delta Society.

McCullock, M.J. (1983). Animal-facilitated therapy: Overview and future direction. In A.M. Katcher & A.H. Beck (Eds.), *New Perspectives on Our Lives with Companion Animals* (pp. 410–426). University of Pennsylvania Press.

Sable, P. (1995). Pets, attachment, and well-being across the life cycle. *Social Work, 40*(3), 95.

Savishinsky, J.S. (1992). Intimacy, domesticity and pet therapy with the elderly: Expectations and experience among nursing home volunteers. *Social Science Medicine, 34*(12), 1325.

Scott, G. (2000). Nursing homes look to playgrounds and pets. *Baltimore Business Journal, 18*(15), 4, September 8.

Chapter 24

END OF LIFE IN A LONG-TERM CARE FACILITY

SHAWN MAI AND RUTH STRYKER

Approximately five percent of all persons over 65 years of age live in a long-term care facility on any given day. However, over 24 percent of those over 85 years of age live in a long-term care facility. With this many institutionalized elderly, it is not surprising that 20 percent of all deaths occur in long-term care facilities, although this percentage varies among states. In addition, the acuity of care in long-term care facilities has risen, making the issue of care practices for a good end of life more important than ever. These facts make it imperative that a long-term care administrator take an active part in seeing that dying residents in his or her facility receive appropriate care in a supportive environment.

A review of the now voluminous literature on death and dying reveals little attention to the specific needs in long-term care organizations except for the need for advance directives. The literature does document that in general, the aged, including those in nursing homes, are less fearful and more accepting of death than the rest of society. But much of the literature relates to issues found in hospitals, and even the nursing literature often leaves the reader to interpret applicability in long-term care settings where so much of the care is provided by inexperienced nursing assistants.

A number of authors have examined how individual long term care facilities, as "communities" and social institutions, have dealt with persons, families, and staff who must deal with death and dying. Findings suggest that facility practices often run counter to support of the dying person, as well as families and staff. Administrative policies and practices need to deal with death as a natural part of life and openly recognize the psychosocial needs of dying persons.

There are other factors that enter into this issue. Many in our society have less involvement in community organizations (churches and others) and become more individualistic. At the same time families have become more dispersed geographically, making support in major life events such as the end of life more dependent on the facility itself. For many, this means physical, emotional, and spiritual support in the dying process becomes dependent on the resources within the facility.

Unfortunately, the literature offers administrators few concrete suggestions to improve care of the terminally ill resident. In one summary of research on attitudes toward death in the long-term care facility, Haber et al. made the following statement:

> Despite the frequency of death, few institutional administrators have given much thought to the special problems of the dying, nor have researchers given much attention to the effects of dying and death on residents and staff in long term care institutions. (p. 25)

Twenty years after Haber's findings, the Minnesota Commission on End of Life Care conducted a 20-month study of deaths in Minnesota in all settings (Harvey). Patients experienced lack of consistent staff, unprepared staff, and lack of use of hospice resources. It is unfortunate that these findings continue in our society because resources are available.

Administrative knowledge of organizational factors that can improve the care and support of dying residents and their families is a first step. One must accept that when the expected outcome is death, it will almost always be an emotional and difficult time for everyone involved. Therefore, the administrator must first focus on goals surrounding death, such as allowing each resident to have a *dignified death* in a setting where family, staff, and other residents have the opportunity to grow and learn from their experience. The administrator should also remember that what constitutes a "dignified death" will ultimately be defined by each resident and family unit. However, the organization lays the foundation for dignity through such objectives as: providing ongoing education on physical, emotional, and spiritual end-of-life issues including effective pain and symptom management and developing relationships with community resources (such as a community hospice) that can help attain the goals of good end-of-life care.

SERVICE GOALS AND OBJECTIVES

Like all services and programs in the organization, care of the dying should relate to the organization's overall mission. In other words, if care at the end of life is not addressed in the mission statement, it will be necessary to review that mission in light of the reality of today's long-term care. Goals and practices can then be established, based on the mission statement.

The organization may have the goal of "restoring or maintaining each resident at the most independent level possible." This goal can also be relevant for a person who may be living in the last hours and days of his or her life. The goal is consistent with developing a plan of care that allows for dignity and independence. Other goals such as the following also need to be included:

- Provide information about Health Care Directives, and related state laws.
- Provide a supportive and accepting environment where death and dying can be discussed openly.
- Allow the person to stay in the facility to die in familiar surroundings if desired and medically feasible.
- Work closely with other community providers to maximize support services available to each dying resident and her/his family.
- Provide access to literature on dying and death from in-house materials, professional schools, local hospice programs, bookstores, or the local library.

Goals and objectives can also serve as a focal point for evaluating the outcomes later. The administrator, working with the DON, medical director, chaplain, and social worker, should evaluate and list the specific needs and issues that will provide a framework for implementing practices, policies, and protocols. This will help department heads to prioritize their efforts, and it also serves as an aid in evaluating progress at some later date.

It is also helpful to evaluate a home's practices after some time has elapsed after a death. For example, a staff member may call a family member to ask what the home did well and what might have been done differently. The death of a parent is a major life event which an organization wants to handle sensitively.

INSERVICE EDUCATION

To achieve the goals of good end-of-life care, the inservice educator is a key person. Since one-third of all long-term care admissions ultimately die at the facility, time spent on this topic is more than justified. To start with, the initial facility orientation needs to raise some level of awareness about the death and dying process. It is important to emphasize a holistic approach to care for all members of the care team, especially nurses and nursing assistants.

Because so much care is provided by nursing assistants, it is important to note that while basic nursing assistant training includes care of the dying person, there is no guarantee that it prepares the trainee to provide emotional support in the actual setting. It is also important to assist these workers to keep from avoiding the dying person by allowing them opportunity to explore their own feelings about death.

Another vital part of the educational process is to provide opportunities for discussion of the emotional and spiritual issues of the dying person. For example, nursing assistants need to be able to recognize or provide access support for those particular issues.

Attention to the greater diversity of both residents and staff is critically important in many settings. This requires that policies and education reflect and promote an understanding of diverse cultural and religious practices associated with death.

Inservice programming will address the special needs of all parties involved:

Resident and Family Needs

- Provide effective pain and symptom management.
- Focus on psychosocial concerns of family and resident.
- Provide privacy and space for family and resident to be together.
- Provide opportunities to address spiritual needs.
- Maintain consistent and well-trained staff.
- Assure the availability of linen and supplies (unique to end-of-life care) in the room for use by family desiring to assist in care.

Staff Needs

- Support staff with opportunities to discuss their feelings when they are experiencing grief.
- Support staff who are experiencing their first death.
- Provide education to deal with the special physical, spiritual, and psychosocial needs of families, residents, and staff.

Needs of Other Residents

- Help other residents to resolve their grief over the loss of a significant friend in the facility.
- Allow other residents to assist and to support friends in their dying.
- Provide information about any death that occurs at the facility.

POLICIES AND PRACTICES

All policies and practices regarding the terminally ill resident are not only affected by federal and state laws but by the customs of a particular national-ity or religion. Organizational policies and practices must conform to federal and state laws. Beyond that, flexibility of policies will also allow for an individual's religious or cultural customs to be practiced.

PATIENT SELF-DETERMINATION ACT OF 1990 AND THE HEALTH CARE DIRECTIVE OF 1998

These two pieces of legislation are intended to allow people to direct their own care by making decisions ahead of time about acceptance or refusal of such issues as life support, resuscitation, nutrition, or aggressive treatments. Ideally, the resident's wishes are made known in writing and on record in the physician's office, in a safe, an attorney's office, or at home. At the time of admission to a facility, it is then brought along and becomes a part of the person's medical record. This advance directive is often called a "living will."

Many elderly persons postpone making a living will and may actually refuse to do so. If the resident does not have some kind of advance directive prior to admission, it is appropriate to suggest that it be done.

An advance directive may also designate a durable power of attorney for health care, also known as a medical durable power of attorney. This document appoints a specific person to represent the patient in making health care decisions if for some reason the patient is unable to do so.

Having two documents (the living will and the durable power of attorney) caused some problems. Therefore, a single document called the Health Care Directive was created. This single document helped to simplify the process for patients making their wishes clear and made the process of following through on those wishes much easier.

Limiting treatment is often seen as antithetical to the basic values and education of health care professionals, especially physicians and nurses. However, the development of medical technology makes it mandatory that health care professionals think through responsible and appropriate applications. It is also important that physicians and nurses keep up with current research. For instance, some recent studies indicate that CPR (cardiopulmonary resuscitation) on the elderly is often futile and may even be harmful (Murphy et al.). This kind of information can be especially helpful to families who feel guilty if they request that a family member not be resuscitated (DNR). Another example is the importance of comfort and pain control in preventing suicide or suicidal wishes (Kastenbaum and other mental health experts). A growing body of research is becoming available to assist people in making decisions about these matters. If the organization has a Biomedical Ethics committee, members of that committee may be asked to talk to families and serve as a resource for staff.

The guiding principle for caregivers in all of these decisions is to have the resident, whenever possible, make the final decision regarding initiation, continuance, withholding, or withdrawal of treatment. This is a major issue in patient's rights cases. The physician's role is to explain medical considerations and the consequences of various decision options. The role of staff is to encourage discussion and assure understanding of options. It is inappropriate for staff to give a personal opinion or judgment about any option.

Supportive Care

A supportive care plan, based on an advance directive, can be initiated by a resident, family member (or guardian), or physician. It should be initiated prior to a crisis event whenever possible. It is suggested that a care conference be arranged with the resident (regardless of competency), family, physician, clergyman, and a representative from the nursing staff.

If a resident's competency is questionable and there is no designated representative, the health care team is obliged to determine in their best judgment what the resident would have wanted as a competent person. Information sources would include the resident, any previously written statements by the resident, the knowledge of family members, friends, and others.

Each organization needs to define "supportive care" as it applies to all residents. Does it mean comfort care? Limited treatment? Then, an individual supportive care plan would address other issues such as:

1. DNR (do not resuscitate)–withholding cardiopulmonary resuscitation. This does not preclude assistance in the event of choking, shock, hemorrhage, etc.,
2. DNI–withholding endotracheal intubation in the event of respiratory failure,
3. avoid hospitalization–a preference for care at home or in the nursing home (except in the event of fracture, uncontrollable bleeding, or uncontrollable pain),
4. the name of the resident's medical durable power of attorney, and
5. list of any treatments that may be unacceptable when restoration of health is impossible and extension of life is of secondary importance.

When a physician writes the orders for a supportive care plan, *all* staff must be informed of the details. A plan might include comfort measures such as relief of pain, good hygiene, skin care, oral hygiene, range of motion exercises, oral and nasal suctioning, maintaining bowel and bladder function, and giving food and fluids by mouth. It also insures dignity and respect including psychosocial support, privacy, and opportunities to visit with family, friends, and clergy.

To develop a policy for a particular nursing home, it is recommended that the home either appoint a Biomedical Ethics Committee of its own or use one already established in the community, possibly at the local hospital. The policy needs to include guidelines for implementation of both federal and state laws. It is also critical to spell out what should be documented, such as: (1) the resident's desires; (2) in the case of incompetence and the absence of written evidence, the basis for determining the person's wishes; (3) the significant persons involved in making the decision (including their relationship to the resident); and (4) the rationale used to determine the supportive care orders.

Special Care Practices and Programs

In consultation with the DON, chaplain, and Medical Director, the administrator should take the time to evaluate the feasibility and appropriateness of special care practices and programs for the dying. In doing this, the administrator needs to weigh the strengths and weaknesses of the organization and realistically assess the feasibility and importance of implementing such practices and programs. Some specific suggestions are:

1. Development of a Hospice Program: This may not be feasible in a typical nursing home. Nevertheless, the administrator should look at what hospice principles can be applied at his/her facility and how the hospice philosophy of care can be integrated into existing practices.

   Hospice is a philosophy of care which attempts to address the total needs of terminally ill persons and their families. Healy's excellent article entitled "Hospice–What is It?" will serve to identify some key elements of hospice care:

   • treatment of the patient and family together as a unit of care;
   • service availability to patients on a home care and inpatient basis, 24 hours a day, seven days a week, with emphasis on medical and nursing skills;
   • care at home is the goal and priority;
   • interdisciplinary care team;
   • physician directed services;
   • central administration and coordination of services, use of volunteers;
   • acceptance to the program based on health needs, not ability to pay;
   • bereavement follow-up service to family.

   Healy also explains as follows:

   > These elements, which may be found in different combinations and concentrations, constitute a philosophy of care more than the

foundation of a specific program. The key to hospice is continuity in the coordination of services. This one consideration tends to place hospice outside the current U.S. health care system, where acute care and long-term care tend to be discrete processes. (p. 51)

This is an important point. The administrator should realize that hospice may refer to a "philosophy" of care, a "program" of care, or a "place" where care is given. One can embrace and practice the *philosophy* of care, implement a full-fledged hospice *program,* or devote beds to the delivery of inpatient hospice care (*place*).

Hospice care can be delivered in any setting, including a person's home. Historically, inpatient hospice programs began with designated beds in acute care hospitals where a high number of nursing hours translated to staffing ratios not generally feasible (for reimbursement reasons) in long-term care facilities. A hospice program also requires special training of staff, providing a continuity of service, obtaining adequate physician support, chaplain involvement, and justifying the additional attention and services for the terminal resident compared with other residents.

Community-based hospice programs have become important partners with long-term care facilities in providing quality end-of-life care. They can provide an enhancement of *services* which include more in-depth and updated coordination of pain and symptom management as well as a greater network of psychospiritual support and bereavement services for staff, residents, and families. They are also a resource for alternative therapies including such things as music and massage.

2. Identify a staff person as an "internal specialist": This person then becomes a known resource for caregivers, residents, and families.
3. Support groups for families of dying residents: This may be feasible for very large homes, but it should be remembered that these groups are difficult to lead and skilled facilitators are necessary. It may be more appropriate to refer families elsewhere if churches or other community groups are available.
4. Interdisciplinary Care Team: Pull together a team of employees representing different disciplines in the facility to develop a program that addresses the holistic needs of the dying resident. This can include drawing support from community resources.

Attention to Surroundings

Physical surroundings provide a context for the dying person. That context needs to be individualized. Special objects, privacy with family, and roommates may be sources of support and comfort. The dying person should not be routinely isolated or moved from their own bed or room. Residents may specifically request not to be removed to a hospital in order to die among friends.

Increased comfort can come from softer linens and specially colored linens (such as a colored pillow case) and can be a visual reminder to staff that special care is required. Providing a comfortable chair or bed in the room can give a family member a place to rest while being present with their family member. A special sign or image placed on the door can be a reminder to all that a resident is having end-of-life care. Lighting and sound are also important to a comfortable environment at this time.

Another context of a dying person's experiences is cultural and spiritual. Being aware of and providing rituals appropriate to the patient's cultural and spiritual background helps to bring continuity with the end-of-life experience.

Residents as Caregivers

Residents live together in community. Part of the experience of living in a long-term care community can be facing the end of one's life. An awareness of and acceptance of this reality can include helping residents care for one another during the dying process. One administrator reports:

> The terminally ill need the comfort and encouragement from our other residents, and by the same token, they are facing their own deaths by teaching others how to die. I have seen our "up and about" residents sitting by the bedside of one who is dying—the relationships are beautiful.

When appropriate and when asked, staff should be honest in telling other residents that someone is dying and needs their support. The long-term care organization is no place for a "conspiracy of silence."

Developing rituals in the long-term care community around recognizing death, such as bedside memorials, can strengthen the bonds of community and enhance an environment of acceptance of death.

Staff Support Mechanisms

Structured support mechanisms can help staff to deal with their own grief over residents' deaths or simply relieve some of the tension and stress that often surrounds care of the terminally ill. Some mechanisms to accomplish this are as follows:

- Hold support group meetings for staff where they can share their feelings regarding the loss of a resident close to them.
- Educate staff around the issues of cumulative grief and how to deal with the long-term effects of multiple losses.

- Use a "buddy" system and assign younger, inexperienced staff to more experienced staff. Older staff can assist their younger counterparts in dealing with death and dying.
- Have a remembrance service for the staff after a death has occurred.
- Provide resources for staff to participate in and lead rituals at the time of death that allow families, residents, and staff to grieve together.
- Invite a consulting chaplain, psychiatrist, psychologist, or psychiatric social worker to assist staff members who need professional help to deal with their grief.

In general, one of the best support "mechanisms" will be a strong orientation and inservice education focus on death, dying, and grief to help prepare staff for the issues surrounding care of the terminally ill. This, in combination with promoting an environment of open communications about death and dying, will serve as a constant support system.

Links with Community Resources

Links and relationships with community resources can assist in improving end-of-life care. Area hospice programs, grief support groups, home health agencies, the local cancer society, and Alzheimer's groups are examples.

Some resources may be able to assist with staff education. Many hospice programs will do inservice programs for long-term care facilities free of charge. At minimum, the administrator, the chaplain, and social worker should compile a list of local resource capabilities and services available for consultation.

Practices and Policies Following a Death

When inquiring about practices and policies following a death, many will quickly refer the inquirer to the policy on "preparation of the body following death" and "notification of family at death" in the nursing policy manual. These policies are obviously necessary, but there need to be policies and practices for the bereaved. Some suggestions follow:

- Assist staff and other residents to attend funerals held outside the facility.
- Hold the funeral or memorial service in the facility to recognize the bereavement needs of other residents and to honor the memory of the deceased.
- Develop rituals around remembering those who have died in the facility. Examples include monthly or quarterly memorial services that might include lighting a candle in remembrance of each person who has died in that time.

- Inviting families of the deceased to such services can be a helpful bereavement tool for both family and the facility.
- Acknowledge that a death has occurred. If other residents ask about a person who has died, give accurate information; this does not mean announcing the death over the public address system, but it does mean allowing natural communications to work. One administrator states, "We have a flower and an easel with a typed sheet describing the resident's life sitting by the front door until after the funeral. This seems to tell the other residents that we will also remember them when they die." Some chaplains pay a special visit to the roommate and close friends.
- Have the administrator write a personal letter to each family following the death of a resident and encourage other staff who were close to the resident to do so also.
- If the facility experiences deaths frequently and is fairly large, it may be feasible to think about a formal bereavement support group for families. Or the administrator may offer a meeting room at the facility for a community-based bereavement group to which families can be referred if the need arises. This is again something that requires trained professionals and should not be done without an accurate assessment of need and community alternatives. At minimum, someone in the facility should be attuned to recognizing pathological grief reactions in families in order to make the proper referrals.

The importance of such practices and policies after a death cannot be stressed enough. It is crucial that other relatives and their families know that death will be handled with dignity and that the lives that were lived will be honored and remembered with respect by staff and the long-term care facility overall. The following "Dying Person's Bill of Rights" can serve as an excellent guide for caregivers.

The Dying Person's Bill of Rights*

I have the right to be treated as a living human being until I die.

I have the right to maintain a sense of hopefulness, however changing its focus may be.

I have the right to be cared for by those who can maintain a sense of hopefulness, however changing this might be.

I have the right to express my feelings and emotions and my approaching death, in my own way.

I have the right to participate in decisions concerning my care.

---

* Copyright © 1975, American Journal of Nursing Company. Reproduced, with permission, from *American Journal of Nursing,* January, Vol. 75, No. 1. "The Dying Person's Bill of Rights," p. 99.

I have the right to expect continuing medical and nursing attention, even though "cure" goals must be changed to "comfort" goals.

I have the right not to die alone.

I have the right to be free from pain.

I have the right to have my questions answered honestly.

I have the right not to be deceived.

I have the right to have help from and for my family in accepting my death.

I have the right to die in peace and dignity.

I have the right to retain my individuality and not be judged for my decisions, which may be contrary to the beliefs of others.

I have the right to discuss and enlarge my religious and/or spiritual experiences, regardless of what they mean to others.

I have the right to expect that the sanctity of the human body will be respected after death.

I have the right to be cared for by caring, sensitive, knowledgeable people who will attempt to understand my needs and will be able to gain some satisfaction in helping me face my death.

REFERENCES

Badzek, L. (1992). What you need to know about advance directives. *Nursing '92,* p. 58.

*Byock, I. (1998). *Dying well: Peace and possibilities at the end of life.* New York: Berkeley Publishing Group.

*Callanan, M., & Kelley, P. (1997). *Final gifts.* New York: Bantam Books.

Haber, D. et al. (1981). Attitudes about death in the nursing home: A research note. *Death Education, 5,* 25.

Hanson, W. (1997). *The next place.* Minneapolis, MN: Waldman House Press.

Harvey, K. 92002). Panel suggests ways to ease death. *St. Paul Pioneer Press,* January 10.

Healy, W. (1980). Hospice . . . What is it? *American Health Care Journal,* p. 51.

Hospice care: Are we shortchanging dying patients? United States Senate Hearing, 106–854, 2001.

*Karnes, B. (1995). *Gone from my sight* (10th ed.), P.O. Box 335, Stilwell, KS.

Kastenbaum, R. (1992). Death, suicide and the older adult. In *Suicide and the Older Adult,* Ed. A. Leenaars et al. New York: Guilford Press.

Minnesota Commission on the End of Life Care Report, 2002. www.minnesotapartnership.org.

Murphy, D. et al. (1989). Outcomes of cardiopulmonary resuscitation in the elderly. *Annals of Internal Medicine, 111,* 199.

---

* Resources for patients and families.

*Norlander, L., & McSteen, K. (2001). Choices at the end of life. Minneapolis, MN: Fairview Press.

Rivera, M. (2001). *Hospice hounds: Animals and healing at the borders of death.* New York: Lantern Books.

Sheehan, D., & Forman, W. (2002). *Hospice and palliative care: Concepts and practice.* Sudbury, MA: Jones and Bartlett.

Thoreen, P. (1981). *Death, dying and terminal care: Issues faced by the long-term care facility.* Minneapolis, MN: Coalition for Terminal Care, Inc.

*Tobin, D. (1999). *Peaceful dying.* Reading, MA: Perseus Books.

---

* Resources for patients and families.

Chapter 25

SPIRITUAL CARE AND THE CHAPLAIN IN THE LONG-TERM CARE FACILITY

MICHELE MICKLEWRIGHT

In the health care industry, there is a growing widespread commitment to holistic care. Over the years there has been a qualitative shift from viewing and treating individuals as physical-psychosocial (body-mind) beings to viewing them as physical-psychosocial-"spiritual" beings. At the same time, numerous studies, research, and long-term quantitative analyses are taking place to understand and uncover the role that faith and spirituality play in the physical and emotional well-being and healing processes of individuals (Dossey, 1993; VandeCreek, et al., 2001; Academic Health Center Task Force on Complementary Care, 1997).

PRIMARY FOCUS AND ROLE

With this recent "scientific" interest in quantifiably understanding and demonstrating the role that spirituality plays in the healing process, medical schools have ventured to develop new curricula in order to expose their students to the art and practice of complementary medicine (Academic Health Center Task Force on Complementary Care, 1997) and to include the spiritual aspects of care in required medical school courses (Moore, 2001). This movement also attests to the growing awareness that the "person" the medical community treats is a much more complex and multilayered individual than

Note: The author is indebted to chaplain colleagues, Alan Hagstrom and Richard Borgstrom for sharing their resources. The insights from our ecumenical dialogues (Methodist, Lutheran, and Catholic) have enriched the content of this chapter.

previously acknowledged. In essence, the medical community is reclaiming some of the ancient understandings of the human being as a "whole" person, i.e., body-mind-community-soul, and is using this reality as a basis to develop its holistic treatment processes.

In the Fall of 2001, in response to the growing interest in understanding the scope and role of chaplaincy in health care institutions, five of the largest health care chaplaincy organizations in North America, representing 10,000 members, jointly prepared and published a white paper entitled, "Professional Chaplaincy: Its Role and Importance in Health Care." As a consensus paper, it presents the perspectives of these bodies on the spiritual care they provide for the benefit of individuals, health care organizations and communities (VandeCreek, 2001). This timely and informative document points to the level of importance to which chaplaincy and spiritual care services in health care institutions have ascended. Long-term care institutions, as total institutions, are invited to take this growing body of knowledge seriously as they strive to provide quality living environments where residents not only live but where they thrive with a sense of meaning that is holistic, purposeful and integrated with an understanding of the "whole" person in mind.

Optimally, pastoral care is coordinated and directed by one or more qualified chaplains who have been trained in the areas of pastoral care and counseling, the theology of aging, spirituality, and/or grief and bereavement processes, and who have the ability to see the larger picture in terms of the unique spiritual dynamics and needs of an individual as they are related to one's health and well-being within a long-term care setting.

Pastoral care is intentionally attuned to and conversant with a myriad of experiences as they relate to spiritual wholeness and well-being. These experiences can include experiences of loss, limitation, dying, fear, hope, guilt, death, change of condition, life-processing, meaning, despair, joy, and family dynamics. Pastoral care moves toward accompanying people in their journeys with the intention of helping them identify, unlock, and draw upon their spiritual and emotional resources so that they may find wholeness, meaning, peace of mind, and sometimes purpose in the midst of an ever-changing and sometimes confusing life situation. This focus of pastoral care assists the individual in the process of healing, promotes peace of mind, and helps to maintain or establish emotional stability.

Finally, in order to accommodate the various faith expressions, pastoral care is intentionally ecumenical and open to all forms of spiritual and cultural expressions. Again, in pastoral care the chaplain assists individuals in uncovering and connecting with their spiritual resources so that these resources may be drawn upon as one moves through the various aspects of their lives in community.

CHAPLAIN'S ROLE

The chaplain assumes primary responsibility to work with other health care staff in an interdisciplinary mode in order to facilitate spiritual support, growth, and development within the total environment as it relates to the spiritual well-being of the residents, family members, and staff. Optimally, the chaplain serves in a managerial role in this capacity.

Attuned to the spiritual well-being of the total environment, the chaplain provides much needed ongoing assessment and quality improvement ideas, dialogue, programs, and processes that can lend themselves to treating the "whole" person as well as creating an environment that is attentive to more than the physical and psychosocial aspects of an individual. In a long-term care setting, this "attunement" to the spiritual aspects of an individual and organization facilitates and contributes to a holistic treatment process.

The chaplain also aids the team in facilitating contacts with residents' own denominations and clergy, if they exist, thereby providing continuity of care connected to the broader community from which residents originated. Secondarily, but importantly, this also strengthens and integrates the facility's ties and bonds with its larger surrounding community.

With these connections in place, the chaplain is able to supplement and enhance the spiritual care of residents on a day-to-day basis. This, too, provides for an overall sense of well-being and peace for residents who may have become distanced from their originating communities by illness or limited mobility.

Specifically, the chaplain is attentive to and assists residents to come to a fuller understanding of life's events and meanings as they relate to spiritual and emotional well-being. The duties of the chaplain fall into several categories. Some of these possibilities are listed in the following pages.

Pastoral Counseling, Pastoral Presence, and Enhancing a Spiritual Environment

The chaplain is trained and versed in an understanding of the physical, psychosocial, and spiritual dynamics that accompany life processes as they relate to change, transition, and inner movements and more specifically as they relate to the aging as well as dying processes. Through a listening pastoral presence and through gentle pastoral counseling, the chaplain accompanies the residents (family members, or staff) and elicits and facilitates their movement toward wholeness, peace, and meaning in the midst of changing circumstances thereby improving their health and adjustment (VandeCreek, 2001, p. 13).

In addition, the chaplain is comfortable with being pastorally present to individuals as they pass through more difficult aspects of their lives. This may include sitting silently with a person who is actively dying, remaining with and supporting an individual who has received an unexpected diagnosis, being spiritually present to and attentive to a person in a coma, sitting with and affirming an individual suffering from Alzheimer's disease, engaging in familiar prayers and hymns to accompany and awaken the memory of someone suffering from dementia. In essence the chaplain is versatile, adaptable, and comfortable with the silences and unknowns of life.

The chaplain, in promoting a spiritual presence and a healing environment, is also intentionally attentive to those residents who are sitting off alone, who may appear isolated or lonely, who may find it hard to engage in community. The chaplain intentionally moves towards these individuals to provide a word of comfort or affirmation, to engage in conversation, to speak their name and to acknowledge them, to sit in silence with them if that seems appropriate, to be a listening and accompanying presence, or, if requested, to whisper a word of prayer so that wholeness and well-being and a sense of belonging can be shared. So too, the chaplain is intentionally attentive to staff and family processes and can recognize when people are experiencing difficulty or are feeling stress. The chaplain can offer a word of comfort, encouragement, a listening presence, or pastoral counseling. In this way the chaplain engages in a process of enhancing the spiritual well-being and environment of the facility as a whole.

Spiritual Assessments

The chaplain is conversant with a number of spiritual assessment tools and uses these tools as a means to assess residents, provide and chart spiritual care plans, and to communicate with staff about significant changes, movements, limitations, and spiritual and emotional strengths that the resident possesses. The chaplain is alert to spiritual issues that arise and provides appropriate interventions to address and work with these issues with the resident, family members, and/or staff. The Association of Professional Chaplains solicits ongoing research and development in the area of appropriate spiritual assessment tools and therefore is a good resource to contact when developing these forms or adopting a form already developed and in use elsewhere.

Administrative

As mentioned above, the chaplain, in an interdisciplinary and dialogical dynamic, has primary responsibility to oversee the overall spiritual well-being of the community and of the individuals participating in the community. This role includes participating in evaluations and assessments of the spiritual care services and programs, setting quality improvement goals, and coordinating efforts to fulfill those goals. In this capacity, the chaplain acts as an agent of change within the long-term care setting.

Closely linked with this responsibility is the relationship the chaplain participates in with the administrator of the facility. The administrator, more than any other, sets the tone, mood, and direction of the facility. It is vitally important that the administrator understand and have an appreciation for a holistic approach to health care and that the administrator promote and foster that understanding within the interdisciplinary team. This sensitivity and relationship to the chaplain will facilitate the work of the spiritual care department and will promote the overall health and well-being of residents, family, and staff.

As a member of the managerial team, the chaplain has primary responsibility to share concerns, ideas, and assessments and to solicit input from staff in order to improve and develop spiritual care services offered to residents, family and staff, and to gather ideas for inservices for staff concerning spiritual care. The chaplain also works closely with the Therapeutic Recreation Department to insure proper screening of volunteers as they relate to spiritual programs and to insure the smooth scheduling of weekly worship services facilitated by local clergy.

Worship Opportunities, Scripture Studies, and Rites

The chaplain is committed to ecumenicity and also appreciative of particular denominational practices, beliefs, spiritualities, and cultural nuances. It is the role of the chaplain to ensure that residents, who are often unable to leave the facility, have community worship services available to them during the week. This can take the form of soliciting and organizing clergy from the community to provide for these services (this is often done in conjunction with the Therapeutic Recreation Department) and/or it can take the form of the chaplain providing weekly ecumenical worship opportunities her/himself so that all residents feel welcomed. These opportunities can also be supplemented with other spiritual opportunities that are community-oriented such as hymn sings, scripture study groups, reading of holy texts, "neighborhood" reflection groups, meditation circles, bedside memorials, monthly memorial services, welcome services for new residents, specialized spiritual services for residents suffering from Alzheimer's disease or other dementia, blessings of rooms with families and residents, sacraments, observing and celebrating holy days, etc.

The chaplain screens and oversees the appropriateness of denominational involvement to ensure that the rights of residents are respected and upheld (COMISS, 1990). Chaplains can reduce and prevent spiritual abuse, acting as gatekeepers to protect residents from unwanted proselytizing. Codes of professional ethics stipulate that chaplains themselves must respect the diverse beliefs and practices of patients and families (VandeCreek, 2001).

Community Involvement

The chaplain maintains open lines of communication with clergy and area congregations and appropriately refers residents to their designated congregations as requested. Chaplains do not replace the local clergy but rather complement these leaders with a special understanding and emphasis on the spiritual dynamics and processes of aging and living within a long-term care setting. Chaplains also network and provide strong links of trust between the long-term care facility and other community stakeholders.

Inservices and Interdisciplinary Education

The chaplain, attentive to the spiritual well-being of the total community, is able to assist in identifying areas that might require ongoing formation or inservices for staff in the area of spirituality, life processes, and health. These inservices, possibly coordinated and/or taught by the chaplain, might include topics such as:

grief and bereavement
spirituality and health care issues
the theology of aging
advance directives
skills in praying with residents
fostering hope in the midst of
    change
interpreting multi-faith/multi-
    cultural traditions
conflict resolution, reconciliation,
    and healing
pastoral care and crisis intervention
prayer as a vehicle to stress
    reduction
health care dialogue on
    body-mind-spirit

death and dying
wholeness and wellness issues
theology of loss and limitation
issues in biomedical ethics
pastoral listening skills
formation of staff as spiritual
    caregivers
guided imagery and relaxation
    technique
screening for pastoral risk
caregiving and theological
    reflection
meditation and self-care
healing touch modalities

Interdisciplinary Staff Member

It is of utmost importance that the chaplain be a member of the interdisciplinary staff. The chaplain receives referrals and passes on referrals to the health care team. Examples of referral forms are readily available through various organizations listed among the "Resources" at the end of this chapter. In order to facilitate a holistic health care process, the health care team including the chaplain must recognize the interdependent nature of the roles of the team members. This requires that the interdisciplinary team be grounded in the understanding of the interdependent nature of body-mind-spirit as it relates to well-being, holistic health, and health care processes. Since, initially, it may be the chaplain who is most attuned to this interdependent dynamic, it is helpful if the chaplain can articulate this understanding and maintain it in the forefront especially in such arenas as daily reports, staff discussions, manager meetings, and staff development opportunities.

Spiritual Care Committee

A growing movement within health care facilities is to organize a Spiritual Care Committee which can provide input, discussion, assessments, ideas, and vision in ways to improve the overall spiritual care programs, services, and spiritual climate in the long-term care setting. The spiritual care committee usually consists of the chaplain and another staff member (possibly the Director of Therapeutic Recreation), two residents, a volunteer, and a family member who meet on a monthly basis. In one long-term care setting, within two years the committee initiated and followed through on the development of a small chapel, a lending library with large print books, and resources on spirituality, prayer, bereavement and aging, a prayer garden, and a series of neighborhood reflection groups where residents from each wing met in a "neighbor's" room to discuss scripture, life stories, and to form community. Committees have found that once the discussions begin, the ideas and enthusiasm for making quality improvements in the area of spiritual care are endless and exciting (St. Croix Chaplaincy Association).

Other Roles

Depending on the identified spiritual and pastoral needs of the long-term care facility and the hours available to the chaplain, the chaplain's role can move in a variety of directions. The list provided is not exhaustive. Other roles can include: participating in patient care conferences and medical rounds; participating in facility or community ethics committees and/or clarifying value issues or end-of-life treatment processes with patients, family, staff, and the organization as they relate to ethical issues; serving as an advocate for residents or family members; participating in critical incident stress debriefing processes with staff; or facilitating or coordinating support groups in conjunction with the Social Services Department, such as cancer groups, Alzheimer's types and family support groups, grief and bereavement groups, etc. In each role, the chaplain's main responsibility is to work with and elucidate the spiritual and pastoral issues that surface within these settings in order to facilitate the process of healing, wholeness, and well-being.

Long-term care administrators attempting to further define the role, scope and recommended outcomes for pastoral caregivers in the long-term care setting may refer to Guidelines for Pastoral Care of Older Persons in Long-Term Care Settings, a project of the Interreligious Liaison Office (American Association of Retired Persons, 1989), as well as to the document *Professional Chaplaincy: Its Role and Importance to Healthcare* (VandeCreek, 2001).

ADDRESSING SPIRITUALITY

As a growing body of research findings demonstrates, the desire to understand the role that spirituality plays in one's life processes is on the rise. Numerous books, periodicals, and research papers are devoted to the topic of spirituality and there is a movement within our culture to reclaim and uncover our own intrinsic spiritual groundedness and rootedness to something greater than ourselves.

The discussion and understanding about what constitutes spirituality is multifaceted. Some discussions are linked strongly to identifying spirituality with one's own denominational faith tradition and lines are clearly demarcated. In some discussions, the understanding of spirituality is more expansive and includes an understanding of a "way of being" in community or in the world or in relationship to a higher power or spirit. In other discussions, "spirituality," rather than being seen as communally-bound is understood as one's "own" journey or stance in the face of the unknown. As the discussion continues, the understanding of what constitutes spirituality will be further debated and nuanced over time.

The recent document, *Professional Chaplaincy: Its Role and Importance in Health Care* begins its reflection on spirituality by stating:

> Spirit is a natural dimension of every person . . . reflecting on the ancient word spirit, May (1982) writes, "Spirit implies energy and power." The word spirituality goes further and describes an awareness of relationships with all creation, an appreciation of presence and purpose that includes a sense of meaning.

Though not true generations ago, a distinction is frequently made today between spirituality and religion, the latter focusing on defined structures, rituals, and doctrines. While religion and medicine were virtually inseparable for thousands of years, the advent of science created a chasm between the two. The term spirituality is a contemporary bridge that renews this relationship . . . in this paper the word spirituality includes religion; spiritual care is inclusive of pastoral care. . . . Spirituality demonstrates that persons are not merely physical bodies that require mechanical care. Persons find that their spirituality helps them maintain health and cope with illnesses, traumas, losses, and life transitions by integrating body, mind and spirit. (VandeCreek, 2001, p. 2)

In addressing and assessing an individual's spirituality, the chaplain seeks to understand the spiritual issues that are at work in a given situation. What underlying emotional, spiritual and theological issues are at play? What are the fundamental questions of meaning and understanding that are being sought? How is the individual coping with or reacting to their current diagnosis, life transition, or change? What spiritual and communal resources have they developed over time that they can call upon as sources of strength at this time? How can the chaplain facilitate this connection in order to elicit a movement toward a sense of wholeness, peace, or calm even in the midst of uncertainty?

Spiritual issues are often seen as polarities. Roy Nash has developed a list of a sampling of some of the polarities that we might find in our lives (see chart). In coping with change, transitions, loss, or even joy in our lives we can often find ourselves at one spiritual polarity or the other. The goal of a pastoral care intervention, therefore, is to facilitate a movement toward balancing these polarities so that one moves toward a sense of calm, wholeness, meaning or well-being even while still experiencing change or uncertainty in one's life.

The Spiritual Issues as Seen as Nineteen Polarities

Dread	*Courage*	*Aloneness*	*Unity*
Helplessness	*Power*	*Bondage*	*Freedom*
Greed	*Charity*	*Brokenness*	*Wholeness*
Curse	*Blessing*	*Foolishness*	*Wisdom*
Guilt	*Grace*	*Injustice*	*Justice*
Despair	*Hope*	*Apathy*	*Compassion*
Revenge	*Mercy*	*War*	*Peace*
Faithlessness	*Faithfulness*	*Misery*	*Joy*
Arrogance	*Humility*	*Ingratitude*	*Gratitude*

Meaninglessness . . . . . . *Fullness of Life (Nash)*

In truth we are always living somewhere along the continuum of these polarities. Major life events (death, loss of mobility, moving from one's home, diagnosis of a debilitating illness, etc.) will move us one way or the other along the continuum. The chaplain's role, therefore, is to provide a pastoral listening presence whereby individuals can talk about their feelings (loss, despair, hopelessness) and be enabled, through connection with their spiritual resources, to move toward a sense of wholeness, peace, or calm even in the midst of the difficulty they are experiencing. This spiritual movement facilitates the overall healing process.

The chaplain's role is not to gloss over the difficulty but rather to uncover and utilize the spiritual resources that individuals have available to them or even to help them "lean into" the feelings of fear, anxiety, helplessness in order to work "through" these feelings so that they can move toward feelings of trust, peace, hopefulness. Most importantly the chaplain's role is "to be with" persons in crises so that they do not feel abandoned. The chaplain offers encouragement and affirmation and a listening, and sometimes silent, healing presence as the individuals sort through their myriad of emotions.

In order to facilitate this movement, the chaplain, through gentle and attentive discussion, will elicit information from the resident. Oftentimes this information will have been gleaned in previous pastoral visits. This information provides a starting ground for understanding an individual's sources of strength and spiritual resources that can be utilized and drawn upon as a person moves through their coping and healing process.

Again, the Association of Professional Chaplains has solicited and compiled ongoing research in the area of spirituality and in the area of developing effective Spiritual Assessment tools for health care settings. One can request these resources by contacting the Association for Professional Chaplains.

RECOMMENDED CRITERIA FOR CHAPLAINS

It is acknowledged that a variety of people may provide residents with basic spiritual care including family members, friends, facility staff, and pastoral caregivers from local congregations. The professional chaplain does not displace these people but rather supplements their spiritual support and counsel on a day-to-day basis. They also complement and augment this care by being specially trained, oriented and focused to deal with spiritual issues that may arise within the context of living within a long-term care facility (Vande-Creek, 2001).

The white paper, "Professional Chaplaincy: Its Role and Importance in Health Care," provides a succinct outline describing who provides spiritual care. This overview is presented in its entirety as its significance is evident.

> Professional chaplains offer spiritual care to all who are in need and have specialized education to mobilize spiritual resources so that patients cope more effectively. They maintain confidentiality and provide a supportive context within which patients can discuss their concerns. They are professionally accountable to their religious faith group, their certifying chaplaincy organization, and the employing institution. Professional chaplains and their certifying organizations demonstrate a deep commitment and sensitivity to diverse ethnic and religious cultures found in North America. An increasing number of professional chaplains are members of non-white, non-Christian communities and traditions.
>
> Professional chaplains are theologically and clinically trained clergy or lay persons whose work reflects:
>
> • Sensitivity to multicultural and multifaith realities
> • Respect for patients' spiritual or religious preferences
> • Understanding of the impact of illness on individuals and their caregivers
> • Knowledge of health care organizational structures and dynamics
> • Accountability as part of a professional patient care team
> • Accountability to their faith groups
>
> In North America, chaplains are certified by at least one of the national organizations that sponsor this paper and are recognized by the Joint Commission for Accreditation of Pastoral Services.
>
> • Association of Clinical Pastoral Education (approximately 1,000 members)
> • Association of Professional Chaplains (approximately 3,706 members)
> • The Canadian Association of Pastoral Practice and Education (approximately 1,000 members)
> • National Association of Catholic Chaplains (approximately 4,000 members)
> • National Association of Jewish Chaplains (approximately 400 members)
>
> Whether in the United States or Canada, acquiring and maintaining certification as a professional chaplain requires:
>
> • Graduate theological education or its equivalency
> • Endorsement by a faith group or a demonstrated connection to a recognized religious community
> • Clinical pastoral education equivalent to one year of postgraduate training in an accredited program recognized by the constituent organizations
> • Demonstrated clinical competency
> • Completing annual continuing education requirements
> • Adherence to a code of professional ethics for health care chaplains
> • Professional growth in competencies demonstrated in peer review.
>
> (VandeCreek, 2001, pp. 6–7)

A set of ecumenical standards developed by the Congress on Ministries in Specialized settings (COMISS) echoes the white paper's report by recommending that the standards for professional chaplaincy staff include:

> Members of the pastoral care staff are professionally trained and maintain or upgrade their skills consistent with other professionals . . . are certified by an appropriate national, pastoral credentialing agency; . . . endorsed ongoing by their religious body; . . . communicates sensitivity to a variety of religious practices and differences through patient or resident interactions; . . . adhere to a professional code of ethics; . . . demonstrates awareness of ethical practices that relate to their area of service; . . . demonstrates the ability to function collegially and professionally in relationship to other disciplines; . . . function as a team intradepartamentally. (COMISS)

PERFORMANCE EVALUATION

The Congress Ministries in Specialized Settings recommends and encourages yearly performance evaluations of chaplaincy and pastoral care services (COMISS). These performance evaluations will ensure quality improvement measures. The evaluations can be structured in order to elicit input from all parties affected by the service provided by the pastoral care department including staff, residents and family members. The evaluations should evaluate their satisfaction with the given spiritual care department and the services they provide and the evaluations should also solicit input and suggestions as to how to improve the spiritual care process and services being offered. Various performance evaluation forms are available from health care facilities that employ chaplains.

Additional sources to contact to request current literature and suggested forms regarding effective up-to-date evaluation processes include: (1) the Association of Professional Chaplains or any other accredited chaplain certifying body (APC); (2) ELCA, Board of social Ministry, which has developed an evaluation process involving focused annual reflections by a five-member committee (ELCA); and (3) the Congress on Ministries in Specialized Settings Standards for Accrediting Pastoral Services in Specialized Settings (Catholic Health Association).

STAFFING AND FUNDING

The development of a benchmark for determining staffing needs for a qualified chaplain in a long-term care facility is in its earliest stages. Because the spiritual aspect of health care has not been fully understood or recognized as it is today, long-term care facilities have historically relied on volunteer pastoral caregivers and sometimes volunteer or retired clergy from the local community. While these services have brought connection, community, and comfort to some residents, they have not always adequately met the needs of the majority of the long-term care community, nor have they addressed the spiritual issues and dimensions of the staff and its environment. It is acknowledged that some churches have traditionally been more responsive to their parishioners who reside in a long-term care setting. But it is also acknowledged that generally residents receive a visit from their pastor perhaps once-a-month and that some residents receive no pastoral visits once they leave their home setting. For others, their only pastoral contact may come by way of a once-a-week worship service that is presided over by a pastor participating in a rotating schedule with pastors from different congregations and denominations. Often the day-to-day individual pastoral needs of the resident traditionally have not been met.

Furthermore, because of the volunteer nature of the program, responsibilities have at times been carried out sporadically and sometimes without a sense of continuity. Volunteers change and commitments vary. When there is no central process available to oversee the day-to-day assessment of spiritual needs of residents, family and staff, then spiritual resources cannot always be coordinated and called upon adequately. Many spiritual needs are therefore not recognized or addressed. Acknowledging that the life situation for a resident in a long-term care setting is often one surrounded by change, loss and transition, this reality is disheartening. Precisely when a resident needs more pastoral support as they search for meaning in attempting to make sense of their changing condition and situation, pastoral care has become constricted and limited (Simsen, 1988).

Traditionally, pastoral care services, including worship services, have been seen as the task and responsibility of the Therapeutic Recreation Department. Spiritual care has been seen as one of many "activities" provided for by the facility. While this relationship between departments is still important, and it has traditionally given pastoral care services and chaplaincy a "nook" in which to rest, it has also tended to hide the important function and role that spiritual care can play in the healing process.

More recently the role and importance of the chaplain in a long-term care facility in helping to create a holistic, healing environment has come to the forefront. With this development has come the desire to determine adequate benchmarks to understand and implement appropriate: chaplain-to-resident ratios; chaplain-to-staff ratios; and chaplain-to-family member ratios. What FTEs (Full Time Equivalents) of staff are needed to adequately address the spiritual needs of the community? Research on these requirements will be forthcoming in the coming years.

Currently, there are some guidelines which can give a sense of direction in this area. It is important to remember that the facility's needs and the level of commitment and desire that the facility has to providing spiritual care services will determine what the facility considers an adequate ratio. The higher the commitment, the more hours that may be required to meet the diverse spiritual roles and duties of the chaplain. The number of hours available to the chaplaincy department will determine, to a large measure, the extent and quality of spiritual care services that can be offered. Some guidelines that are currently available include:

A. The COMISS Standards for Accreditation in Pastoral Care Settings includes a section on staffing which states:
   1. The pastoral care department has a stated personnel ratio sufficient to meet and implement the stated goals and objectives of the pastoral care department.
   2. A formal arrangement is documented when operational needs require pastoral personnel from outside the facility.
   3. The department has identified personnel available to address the linguistic, cultural, and diverse spiritual needs of patients or residents, families, and staff.
   4. The department has support personnel to carry on the duties and programs of the department (COMISS).
B. The ELCA Board of Social Ministry delineates these guidelines for staffing patterns and ratios:
   1. One full-time chaplain is suggested for facilities or campuses that have 200 or more beds/housing units.
   2. A three-quarter time chaplain is suggested for campuses with 125–200 bed/housing units.
   3. A half-time chaplain is suggested for campuses with 50–125 beds/housing units (ELCA).
C. Contacting specific chaplaincy certifying bodies such as the Association of Professional Chaplains, Association of Jewish Chaplains, Association of Catholic Chaplains, etc. and requesting their researched guidelines or suggestions can also yield an understanding of current practices in the health care industry (see recommended resources).

Funding. As with FTEs, understanding options for funding a spiritual care and chaplaincy program is under development. Some guidelines, however, do exist. Appendix E of the Compensation section in ELCA's Board of Social Ministry recommendations states that administrators are encouraged to budget chaplaincy compensation packages based on years of experience, training, long-term care credentials, and job performance. Further it is encouraged that administrators seek guidance from local synod, churches, or district compensation guidelines for clergy and ecclesiastically endorsed or certified pastoral caregiver rostered personnel (ELCA).

Another good source to contact in order to discern a benchmark for an adequate compensation is the Association of Professional Chaplains which bi-annually publishes a scale for salaries of chaplains based upon documented salaries which are delineated by type of facility, education, years of experience, expertise, etc.

Alternative sources for facility reimbursement for chaplaincy programs are varied:

- Some states, such as Minnesota, may reimburse chaplaincy services under Rule 50, other care-related services which states:
  1. Direct costs of other care-related services, such as recreational or religious activities. . . .
  2. The personnel costs of . . . chaplains . . . and other care-related personnel including salaries or fees of professionals performing consultation services in these areas which are not reimbursed separately on a fee for service basis.
- Other facilities may need to build in the salary for a chaplain over a period of time beginning with 10 hours a week the first year and incrementally increasing the hours in consecutive years;
- Some long-term care facilities in a local community may collaborate to jointly hire one chaplain who would divide her/his time between two or three facilities;
- One innovative ecumenical chaplaincy program in Minnesota is directed by, endorsed by and partially funded by a ministerial association representing 26 local churches. Several area health care facilities contract with this association which provides an ecumenical team of chaplains to serve the facilities in the area of spiritual care (see St. Croix Chaplaincy Association). Sources of funding for the services of the chaplains is provided by combining funds from the consortium of churches, the health care facilities, and grants from area foundations.
- Still another model considers the option of a healthcare facility petitioning a local congregation to jointly fund a qualified chaplain to serve dually in the parish and in the health care facility or to assist with start-up funding for a chaplain.
- Local foundations, with a commitment to their community, are also a possible, reliable source of funding for chaplaincy programs (St. Croix Chaplaincy Association).

Methods of funding spiritual care and chaplaincy programs are in development stages. There are various ideas being considered. Creative and innovative thinking as well as dialogue with individuals and organizations who have developed successful programs in this area will provide more options in the future.

As funding is considered, perhaps as added incentive, it is important to keep in mind that there is a cost-benefit to implementing a spiritual care and chaplaincy program in the long-term care setting. As the Association of Professional Chaplains white paper documents, there are studies which demonstrate this overall cost-benefit to health care (VandeCreek, 2001). Furthermore, as the population ages, there will continue to be a growing demand, from consumers of health care, for more complementary, spiritual and culturally-appropriate care. Long-term care facilities, as total environments, are invited to consider this data as they strive to improve quality holistic care that meets these growing needs.

Through professional spiritual care services, overall health, healing and well-being can be enhanced for those touched by these services.

REFERENCES AND RECOMMENDED RESOURCES

Academic Health Center Task Force on Complementary Care. (1997). *Transforming health care: Integrating complementary, spiritual and cross-cultural care.* University of Minnesota, February.

American Association of Retired Person (AARP). (1989). *Guidelines for pastoral care of older persons in long-term care settings.* A project of the Interreligious Liaison Office.

Anderson, H. (2001). Spiritual care: The power of the adjective. *Journal of Pastoral Care, 55*(3), 233–237, Fall.

Association of Professional Chaplains (APC), Spiritual Care Resources, also publishes periodicals with current ongoing research in pastoral care. *Journal of Pastoral Care and Chaplaincy Today,* 1701 E. Woodfield Road, Suite 311, Schaumberg, IL 60173.

Berg, D. (2001). Accessing sacred story: Cultural and spiritual assessment in health care. *Chaplain's Network Link,* pp. 7–14, Winter.

Burgener, S. (1999). Predicting quality of life in caregivers of Alzheimer's patients: The role of support from involvement with religious community. *Journal of Pastoral Care, 53*(4), 433–446.

Coalition of Ministry in Specialized Settings (COMISS). (1997). *Standards for accrediting pastoral services.* Joint Commission for Accreditation of Pastoral Services, P.O. Box 07473, Milwaukee, WI 53207.

Coalition on Ministry in Specialized Settings. *Quality assurance and pastoral care.* Catholic Health Association.

Dossey, L. (1993). *Healing words: The power of prayer and the practice of medicine.* New York: Harper Collins.

Evangelical Lutheran Church of America (ELCA), Board of Social Ministry.

Fitchet, G. (1999). Screening for spiritual risk. *Chaplaincy Today, 15*(1), 2–26.

Fitchett, G. (1993). *Spiritual assessment in pastoral care: A guide to selected resources.* Decatur, GA: JPCP, Inc. Books.

Joint Commission on the Accreditation of Healthcare Organizations (JCAHO), Patient Rights Standard R.1.1.3.5., etc., 1998.

Kimble, M. (ed.). (1995). *Aging, spirituality and religion.* Minneapolis, MN: Augsburg Fortress.

McCullough, M. et al. (2000). Religious involvement and mortality: A meta-analytic review. *Health Psychology, 19*(3), 211–222.

Moore, M. (ed.). (2001). Fairview chaplains and university physicians create award-winning curriculum. *The APC News 4*(4), 11, July/August.

Nash, R. *Highlights from life's major spiritual issues: An emerging framework for spiritual assessment and pastoral diagnosis* (pamphlet).

Newberg, A. et al. (2001). *Why God won't go away: Brain science and the biology of belief.* New York: Ballantine Books.

Pierce, R. (2001). Quality commission task force develops religious/spiritual preference protocol. *The APC News, 4*(4), 10, July/August.

Rause, V. (2001). Searching for the divine. *Los Angeles Times Magazine,* excerpted in *Reader's Digest,* December.

St. Croix Chaplaincy Association, P.O. Box 322, Stillwater, MN 55082.

Shea, J. (2000). *The challenges of aging: Retrieving spiritual traditions.* Chicago: The Park Ridge Center for the Study of Health, Faith and Ethics.

Shea, J. (2000). Spirituality and health care: Reaching toward a holistic future. Chicago: The Park Ridge Center for the Study of Health, Faith and Ethics.

Simsen, B. (1998). Nursing the spirit. *Nursing Times,* September 14.

Spirituality and Healing in Medicine Conference (sponsored by a consortium of healthcare groups), Harvard MED-CME, P.O. Box 825, Boston, MA 02117-0825.

VandeCreek, I. et al. (2001). How many chaplains per 100 inpatients? Benchmark for health care chaplaincy departments. *The Journal of Pastoral Care, 55*(3), 239–300, Fall.

VandeCreek, I., & Burton, L. (eds). (2001). *Professional chaplaincy: Its role and importance in healthcare.* Association of Professional Chaplains.

Part VI

CREATING A BETTER FUTURE

Chapter 26

USING INFORMATION TECHNOLOGY TO IMPROVE QUALITY MEASUREMENT

SANDRA POTTHOFF

The long-term care industry is facing increasing financial constraints as federal and state governments attempt to control expenditures, which accounted for $45.3 billion of the $77.9 billion spent on nursing home care in 1995 (United States Department of Health and Human Services, 1996). Long-term care costs will continue to rise as the proportion of the U.S. population aged 65 and older increases from 13 percent the year 2000 to 41 percent by the year 2040 (Institute for Health and Aging, 1996). These financial constraints occur within the context of a litany of quality problems that have plagued the industry since the passage of Medicare and Medicaid in the sixties (Kane and Kane, 1988). The challenge facing the industry is how to allocate limited financial resources and energies to affect organizational change for quality improvement. Long-term care expenditures, financial constraints, and aging baby boomers are driving the need to align quality management practices with performance outcomes.

This chapter discusses the traditional quality assurance paradigm in long-term care, provides an overview of the quality management paradigm, introduces the concept of a performance measurement system to measure and manage processes, structures, and outcomes, and provides a framework for the role of information technology in automating ongoing measurement for quality monitoring.

QUALITY ASSURANCE

The traditional quality paradigm in nursing homes has been that of Quality Assurance (QA). QA practices in long-term care are similar to those that were found in industry prior to the introduction of quality management principles. Under this paradigm, designated QA staff has responsibility for ensuring quality, and the focus is on studying individuals to compare their performance to specified standards to judge whether the standards have been met. This practice is reinforced by the regulatory environment, with extensive federal and state regulations in place to assure minimum quality standards, making the long-term care industry one of the most highly regulated industries in the U.S. (Castle, Zinn, Brannon, and Mor, 1997). In the regulatory model of quality, state inspectors impose sanctions and cite deficiencies when standards are not met. Landmark federal legislation was passed in 1987 (U.S. Congress, 1987) in response to the indictment of nursing home quality in the 1986 Institute of Medicine report (IOM, 1986). The legislation required minimum training and competency testing for nursing assistants, state-level ombudsman programs to investigate resident and family complaints about nursing homes, equal quality of services to all residents regardless of payment source, and a review of each nursing home resident upon admission and at least annually thereafter using a mandated standardized Resident Assessment Instrument (RAI), resulting in a Minimum Data Set (MDS) of quality of care information collected on each resident that is uniform across nursing homes.

Both the industry and regulators are recognizing the limited usefulness of traditional quality assurance models that rely on inspections by health departments (Hatzell, Halverson, and Kaluzny, 1996). A regulatory approach to quality assurance produces a reactive climate that does not guarantee a change in behavior at the nursing home level: "if regulation is relied on as the sole method for promoting the patients' interest in nursing homes, then the probability of success is not great" (Nyman and Geyer, 1989). Even the Institute of Medicine (1986) acknowledged that regulation alone will not solve quality problems in long-term care. The IOM report recognizes that facility leadership must reinforce and facilitate the front-line nursing assistants' motivation and job performance on a daily basis if high quality care is to be delivered. Because 80 to 90 percent of care provided to nursing home residents is given by nursing assistants (Smyer, Brannon, and Cohn, 1992), the way in which they carry out their duties profoundly impacts the quality of life and clinical care of the residents (Shaughnessy, 1989).

Many nursing homes are trying to move beyond the regulatory quality assurance model of deterrence/compliance toward a proactive framework that incorporates quality management principles. One of the difficulties in moving away from the QA model is that it is much more difficult to define quality in long-term care compared to industries such as manufacturing (Sainfort, Ramsay, Ferreira, and Mezghani, 1994). Its definition is even more difficult compared to the acute care setting in that it encompasses aspects of health, personal, and social care over a long time frame to residents with very different prognoses and physical and mental status (Kane and Kane, 1988). However, there are a growing number of short-term residents in nursing homes who receive rehabilitative or restorative care before returning home. The philosophy of care for these residents may be very different than for those whose functional dependency will slowly deteriorate over time (Shaughnessy, 1989). Definitions of quality are also complicated in nursing homes because of the distinctions between quality of care and quality of life. Because many residents will be in the nursing home the rest of their lives, their quality of life is related to their sense of well-being, satisfaction with life, and feelings of autonomy. Historically, this industry has had few incentives to compete on the basis of providing a higher standard of care any higher than the minimums specified in regulation, since occupancy rates were uniformly high regardless of quality. However, this situation has changed in recent years as substitutes to nursing home care, including assisted living facilities, home health care, and board and care homes, are creating a more competitive environment.

QUALITY MANAGEMENT

Quality management encompasses the intertwining of customer satisfaction, continuous improvement, and an integrated systems perspective that forms a feedback system to understand and improve the link between nursing facility structures, processes, and outcomes (Anderson, Rungtusanatham, and Schroeder, 1994). In long-term care, traditional measures of structure include such things as the quality of the physical plant and environment, available capital, and staff expertise and training. Process measures have typically focused on such measures as staffing levels, while outcomes have tended to focus on financial performance, proxy measures of quality such as citations, and more recently, facility clinical quality as measured by the MDS. In contrast to quality assurance, which focuses on adherence to standards, the goal of quality management is continuous improvement of quality.

Since the early nineties the Malcolm Baldrige Quality Award (Bradley and Thompson, 2000; United States Department of Congress, 2002) has defined a new framework for expanding our thinking about the structures, processes and outcomes of long-term care. Figure 26-1 summarizes the Baldrige Framework for health care. Using this approach, the primary structural input to the nursing facility is the *leadership* of the top management team, generally including the administrator, the director of nursing, and other department directors that may be influential in the facility. Leadership in turn drives the *processes* in the organization, including strategic planning, work processes, human resource practices, the use of information, and the focus on the resident and

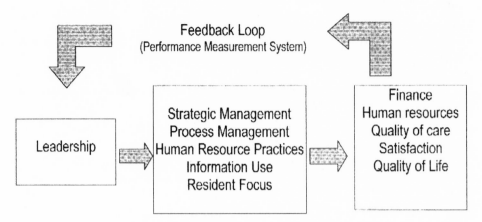

Figure 26-1. Baldrige Award Framework

family as customers. These processes in turn drive facility outcomes, including financial, human resource, clinical quality of care, resident quality of life, and resident and family satisfaction.

The adage that "if you can't measure you, you can't manage it" applies to a quality management framework such as Baldrige. Measures for these areas must be developed and tracked, and the role of information technology becomes key in being able to do this efficiently and effectively. The performance measurement loop shown in Figure 26-1 represents the measurement piece of the process. The measurement system performs the feedback function to inform leadership of how the organization is performing to identify areas in which change is needed.

Data, measurement, and a feedback loop are necessary, but not sufficient, components for quality improvement. A mechanism must be in place to *act* upon the information that is being collected in the quality management process. This mechanism is called the FOCUS-PDSA (Plan-Do-Study-Act) cycle outlined in Figure 26-2 (Bataldan, 1991), which provides a structured continuous improvement process. FOCUS-PDSA is the internal quality management process that drives the improvements. However, it can be seen that the collection and analysis of data in the performance measurement system is crucial to carry out FOCUS-PDSA because it is the information and knowledge created from the data that enable management by fact (Bradley and Thompson, 2000).

PERFORMANCE MEASUREMENT SYSTEMS

Just as advances have been made in quality management, performance measurements systems have also evolved. In the sixties Rockart (1979) intro-

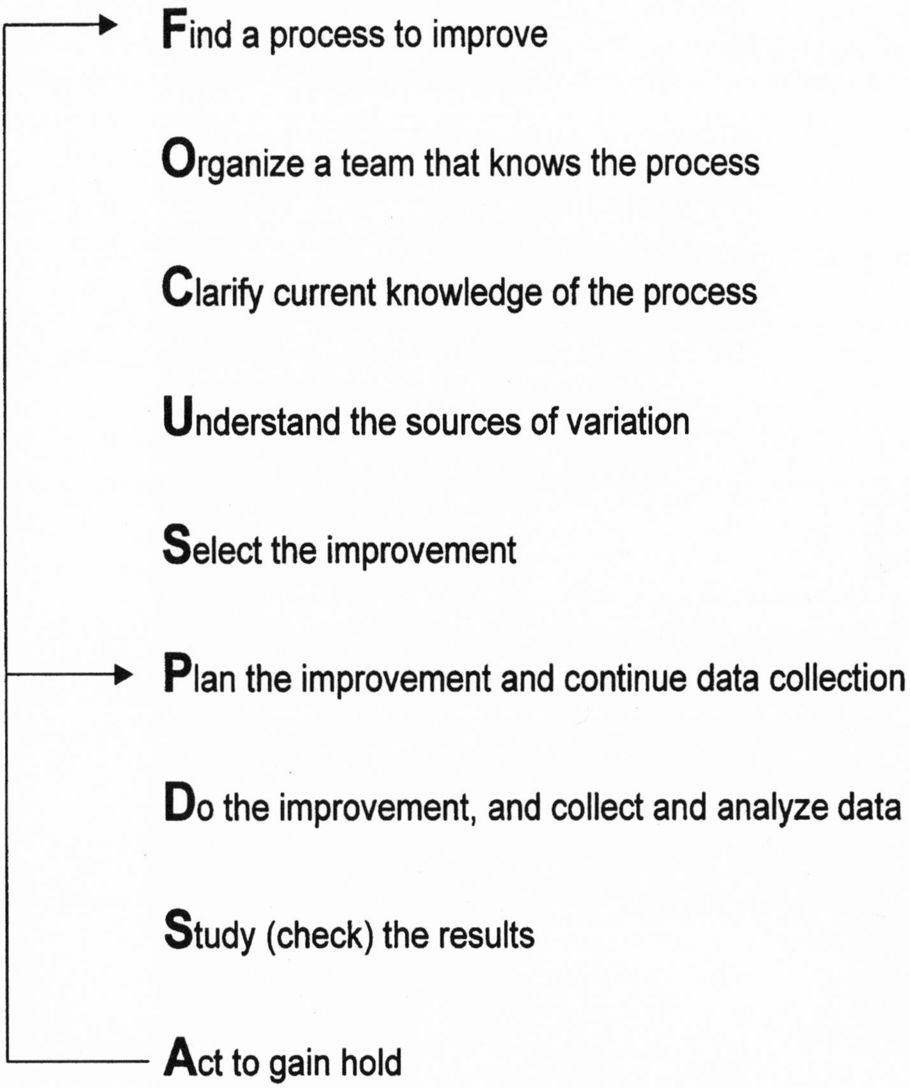

Find a process to improve

Organize a team that knows the process

Clarify current knowledge of the process

Understand the sources of variation

Select the improvement

Plan the improvement and continue data collection

Do the improvement, and collect and analyze data

Study (check) the results

Act to gain hold

Figure 26-2. FOCUS-PSDA Cycle

duced the concept of "critical success factors," the set of performance measures that "must go right" for a company to succeed. In the nineties, the notion of a "balanced scorecard," a limited number of measures that are driven by the company's vision and strategy, has been introduced by Kaplan and Norton (1992, 1993, 1996a, 1996b). The "balanced" concept has two components. First, the set of measures must be tied to the organization's strategic goals, falling into one of four perspectives: financial, customer, internal, and learning and growth. Second, the interrelationships between the measures must be linked in a cause and effect network in order to understand the relationship between performance drivers and outcomes.

The purpose of a balanced scorecard is to articulate corporate strategy in order to make it operational. This should enable its use in linking a company's long-term strategy with its short-term actions: "Lofty vision and strategy statements don't translate easily into action at the local level" (Kaplan and Norton, 1996a, p. 76). But exactly how does an organization ensure this translation occurs? Kaplan and Norton (1996b) cite three mechanisms: communication and education programs to educate all employees about the strategy and required behavior, goal-setting programs to translate the team objectives into personal and team objectives, and reward system linkages to motivate employees through appropriate incentive and reward systems.

Many nursing homes are in the initial stages of developing the technical skills needed for implementing performance measurement systems as part of a broader framework of quality management (McKeon, 1996). For example, trade organizations, such as the American Health Care Association and the American Association of Homes and Services for the Aging, provide computerized data bases for a fee that allow nursing homes to input their own Minimum Data Set (MDS) data and gain access to peer nursing home data to benchmark their quality of care. The MDS has been used to provide data-driven quality of care measures in quality improvement efforts in nursing homes (Zimmerman et al., 1995).

Some long-term care corporations are measuring a variety of indicators in their business units (e.g., assisted living, nursing homes) that are driven by corporate mission, vision, and values, including resident and family satisfaction, resident quality of life and clinical care, human resource indicators, and financial performance. Given that almost half of all nursing homes are part of larger corporate organizations (Strahan, 1987), the potential of a corporate balanced scorecard approach to drive quality within the long-term care industry is substantial.

The key to successful use of the performance measurement system is that it is integrated into the Baldrige or other quality management framework the organization is using to improve quality. For data to be useful, however, they must be reliable. Problems in data reliability arise when different people use different definitions or time frames for measuring a key indicator, such as turnover rates. Without a common definition and time frame for measurement, it is impossible to benchmark the organization to others, or to compare the organization to itself over time. The ability to make sure comparisons is crucial if the organization wishes to implement statistical process control charts (Carey and Lloyd, 2001) as part of its ongoing FOCUS PDSA cycle. Statistical process control charts rely on tracking performance on key indicators over time, including the mean (average) performance and the variability around the mean performance.

Major data reliability problems often arise when an organization requires staff to conduct extensive manual data collection for its ongoing performance measurement system. Collecting data is generally not a core staff function, and it usually falls to the bottom of the priority list of what needs to be done. This results in inaccurate and missing data. Thus, to the extent possible, organizations need to leverage computerized data that are collected as part of routine administrative and clinical activities to minimize the manual data collection burden on employees. Much of administrative data, such as payroll and billing, and increasing amounts of clinical data, including MDS, Admissions/Discharges/Transfers, and incident reports, are now computerized. The next section discusses how to leverage the computerized data for use in a performance measurement system to minimize manual collection.

TURNING DATA INTO INFORMATION AND KNOWLEDGE

Organizations are data rich, but information and knowledge poor. The goal of ongoing performance measurement systems is to transform data from the nursing facility's computerized databases into information and knowledge. As shown in Figure 26-3 computerized data reside in a myriad of databases. However, what is needed from a performance measurement system are data that can be used to benchmark a facility to itself over time, to benchmark its performance to its competitors, to compare itself to other models of care in the long-term care industry, to compare itself to other industries, or to try to predict how it will be performing in the future. Turning data into information and knowledge requires that the data be transformed. This transformation may include merging or linking one data set with another, analyzing the data using statistical methods, graphing the data to determine underlying patterns or trends over time, or using the data to project into the future.

Transforming data into information requires that one determine what key indicators need to be tracked to continuously monitor and improve the organization. Once this has been determined, the next step is to assess whether the indicators can be created by transforming data from existing computerized databases. If computerized data are available, one then needs to determine what transformation needs to be conducted on the data to turn it into the needed key indicator. One also needs to understand how the data becomes computerized to determine whether there are potential problems in that process that create data quality problems. This chapter provides examples of how computerized payroll data can be used to automatically calculate human

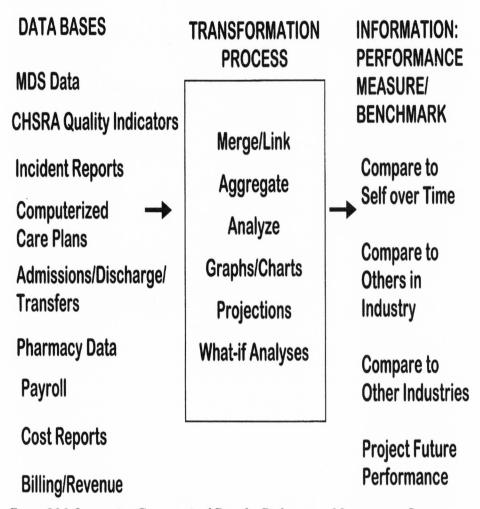

DATA BASES	TRANSFORMATION PROCESS	INFORMATION: PERFORMANCE MEASURE/ BENCHMARK
MDS Data		
CHSRA Quality Indicators	Merge/Link	
Incident Reports	Aggregate	Compare to Self over Time
Computerized Care Plans	Analyze	
Admissions/Discharge/ Transfers	Graphs/Charts	Compare to Others in Industry
	Projections	
Pharmacy Data	What-if Analyses	
Payroll		Compare to Other Industries
Cost Reports		Project Future Performance
Billing/Revenue		

Figure 26-3. Leveraging Computerized Data for Performance Measurement System.

resource outcome indicators of turnover and stability described in Chapter 12 of this book. A second example of using computerized data to track clinical outcomes of hip fracture residents follows.

Human Resource Indicators: Turnover and Stability

Suppose one wishes to calculate the employee turnover rate from October 1 to December 31, 2002. As described in Chapter 12, the turnover rate requires a numerator of how many people left during this time period, while the denominator requires the average number of people on the payroll during this time period. Rather than having to track turnover by hand, how could the computerized personnel data be used to calculate turnover? Most organizations have a computerized personnel file that contains the date each employee started working at the organization, along with the date the employee left the organization. If the data field containing the date of leaving is blank, one would assume the employee is still working at the organization. The goal is to have a computer programmer program an algorithm that could be used over and over again by the computer to calculate the turnover rate for any desired time period. That is, the process of calculating the turnover indicator would become *automated*.

Let's start with the numerator. How many people left the organization during this time period? One would have the computer search the computerized personnel file for the data field containing the date of leaving for each employee record. If the date in that field lies between the start and end date of interest (in our example, October 1 and December 31, 2002, respectively), then the computer would count that employee as having left the organization during that time frame. It is easy for the computer to keep track of how many records it finds that match our date criterion to get a total count for the numerator.

For the denominator, we wouldn't need to calculate the average number of employees over the time frame of interest as is done when calculating by hand, since it is easy for the computer to determine the total number of unique employees in the organization during that time frame. The computer would simply count the total number of employees whose date of leaving is either in our time window of interest (meaning the employee left during that time frame) or blank (meaning the employee is still there).

Rather than tracking quarterly turnover rates by hand, automated computerized calculation enables an organization to calculate ongoing turnover rates easily each pay period. One could use historical data to calculate the average and standard deviation of the turnover rate to develop the appropriate control chart, and plot subsequent pay periods on the control chart to track whether common and special cause variation exists in turnover. See Carey and Lloyd (2001) for more information on constructing control charts and using them to assess variability.

A similar approach can also be used for ongoing tracking of the stability rate of employees. Suppose one defines the stability rate as the number of employees who have been with the organization at least one year (numerator) divided by the number of total number of employees at a given point in time, say December 31, 2002 (denominator) as is done in Chapter 12. In this case, one first needs to have the computer identify all employees who are still at the organization for the end date of interest. Thus, the date of leaving for that employee would either be blank (meaning the employee is still at the organization), or the date would be after December 31, 2002. A count of the number of employees who meet this criterion would constitute the denominator. For that set of employees who are counted in the denominator, the computer would need to subtract the start date of each employee from our date of interest (12/31/02) in order to calculate how long the employee had been employed at the organization. For example, an employee who started work on June 30, 2002 would have worked at the organization for six months by December 31, 2002, while an employee who started on December 15, 2001 would have worked at the organization for a little over one year. The computer would then count the number of employees for whom this length of tenure is at least one year to get the numerator. One can see that with automation, it becomes easy to calculate employee stability on an ongoing rolling basis for each pay period that can then be tracked using a control chart. Similarly, it becomes easy to track average stability simply by automatically calculating the tenure of each employee for the pay period and taking the average.

To calculate turnover and stability rates by employee type (for example, RN, Dietary, CRNA) or age, one would need to identify the data fields that contain these relevant data. One would then simply sort the data by the relevant criterion of interest before calculating turnover or stability.

As stated earlier, one must understand how the data files get created to ensure that the data are accurate. For example, suppose an organization is very lackadaisical about getting the date an employee leaves into the appropriate data field in its computerized personnel records, or it often does not get this piece of data entered at all. If it is simply the case that there is a long time delay, say six months, before one can trust that the data have been entered, then the automated approach to calculating an organization's human resource indicators can be conducted no sooner than the end of the previous six months. If an organization is very sloppy about entering this piece of data into the computerized personnel records, then one either needs to accept that the turnover and stability rates calculated via automated processes may be grossly understated and overstated, respectively, or one must resort to tracking by hand. Although more complicated, the payroll data file could be used as an alternative source by comparing the employee identification numbers that show up each pay period. An advantage of this data file is that because it is used to pay employees, one would expect the data to be more accurate. This approach, however, would assume that if an employee identification number does not show up in a given subsequent pay period, then the employee is no longer with the organization. If this is not the case, for example, an employee would not show up in the pay period if she was on unpaid leave, then the algorithm using payroll data would become even more complicated. However, with a good computer programmer, once the algorithm was programmed, it is usable indefinitely as long as the data file structure does not change.

Tracking Clinical Outcomes: Hip Fracture Residents

As described in Chapter 19, the development of quality indicators by the University of Wisconsin has provided nursing facilities with a wealth of data to track facility and patient level clinical quality. Facilities can access the computerized MDS system to download their facility specific and resident specific information, along with benchmarks to compare themselves to other facilities in their state. Such data can be tracked in control charts to monitor the quality indicators over time (Karon and Zimmerman, 1996).

As facilities become more sophisticated in using their computerized data, they will be able to develop outcomes systems to provide potential consumers of their services with better information to support decision making. Consider the hypothetical case of a family whose cognitively intact 75 year old mother has broken her hip and is in need of rehabilitative care before she can return home after her hospitalization. The woman and her family have every expectation that she will walk again, since she was walking fine prior to breaking her hip. They want data from your facility that show how aggressive your facility is in hip fracture rehabilitation, what the expected trajectory of recovery is that can be expected, and how long they might expect their mother to be in the facility. They will compare your data to that received from other facilities to make their decision about where the woman will likely have the best outcomes. What data will you provide to the family?

As background information, assessing outcomes requires four components: (1) baseline functioning; (2) treatment received from the facility; (3) characteristics of the individual that may affect rehabilitation potential, such as age and presence of dementia; and (4) functioning at discharge. Assessing baseline functioning for hip fracture residents is a bit difficult, since one needs to determine how well they ambulated prior to their hip fractures. However, one can measure ambulatory capabilities at the time the resident was admitted to the facility. Treatment received from the facility includes the types, intensity, and duration of treatment received, for example, number of rehabilitation sessions provided by a physical therapist and walking assistance by nursing aides on the unit. Functioning at discharge includes how well and how far the person could ambulate at discharge.

Although currently time-consuming to merge and analyze because data bases have not been well designed, there are a number of computerized data bases that are available to help address at least some of these data requests. Relevant computerized clinical data files available in most facilities include MDS data, admission/discharge/transfer (ADT) data, and incident report data.

The first step is to identify the relevant comparison group for this family's mother. The relevant comparison group should consist of past and current residents whose characteristics are similar to the woman. The computerized MDS data is a logical data source to use to identify the comparison group, since it contains a data field for age, along with computerized diagnosis codes (called ICD-9 codes). The computer algorithm would need to search all the facility's MDS records for any ICD-9 codes that indicated hip fracture on the admission assessment. To make the data as useful as possible for the family, the ICD-9 codes indicating dementia should also be identified, and any records indicating hip fracture where the resident also had dementia should be excluded from the sample. Depending on how big the size of the comparison group is when this step has been completed, residents whose age is much younger or older than this woman could be excluded from the group. At the end of this step, the comparison group for this woman will have been identified, along with the medical record or patient identification number for each resident in the comparison group.

To calculate the average length of stay for this comparison group requires the ADT file. For this step, the records from the ADT file whose patient identification numbers match those that you identified in your comparison group would be chosen by the computer for further analysis. The discharge status should be checked, and the proportion of those who died should be noted. Now, excluding those who were dead at discharge, a length of stay can be calculated for each person in the comparison group, and an average and range of length of stay determined. Thus, at a minimum, information about the proportion of deaths and the average and range of length of stay for residents with hip fractures similar to this woman who were discharged alive can be provided to the woman and her family.

Without computerized care planning data, providing concrete data about treatment and outcomes becomes more difficult. At a minimum, the computerized incident file can be searched to see if there are any residents in the identified comparison group who experienced falls in the facility, and how their rate of falls compares to the rate of falls of nonhip fracture residents in the facility. However, the meaning of this piece of data is unclear. On the one hand, the presence of falls in residents who were admitted with hip fractures could indicate more aggressive rehabilitation treatment, especially if the falls are occurring in rehabilitation sessions with the physical therapist. On the other hand, it could indicate poor quality.

If the facility has computerized care planning data, the ability to assess the treatment aspect of an outcomes system increases. Many computerized care planning packages contain structured data fields on problems, therapy goals, approaches, rehabilitation potential and discharge date planned. One can search the computerized care data for rehabilitation codes and codes indicating walking on the unit by a nurse aide. If there are dates associated with each of these treatments, then the frequency of treatment can be determined by the computer. Unfortunately, data regarding the progress a resident is making in improving the time and distance walked is generally included in computerized care plans as text in notes fields. This makes it very difficult to have the computer easily analyze such data without a human having to read the notes and enter structured data fields such as distance or time walked on what dates.

Thus, with the current state of computerized clinical data in facilities, it should be possible to identify relevant subgroups of residents using MDS data, determine the average length of stay for each resident subgroup, and assess incidents for these subgroups. If computerized care plans are available, one can determine the approaches and frequency of treatment. As computerized care plans become more sophisticated in tracking structured data on treatment progress, the ability to track resident outcomes will improve.

When attempts are first made to use the various computerized data sources to assess clinical outcomes, many problems in the data should be expected. One may find, for example, that it is difficult to use MDS data to identify residents who were admitted with a hip fracture because of sloppy practices of what ICD-9 codes get identified in the MDS data. There may be many instances of false positives (those who shouldn't be in your sample are identified as belonging in the sample), and false negatives (those who should be in your sample are not because the relevant ICD-9 code was missing). If different patient identification numbers are used for the same patient across the different data files, it will be impossible to merge easily the data needed to calculate the required information. Given the increasing emphasis on data privacy, it is important to avoid using actual patient names to link the data bases. Even when a common patient identifier is used across different clinical data files, it may be impossible for the different data bases to communicate with each other because of different underlying software. If this is the case, relevant information will have to be stripped from the original data files and read and merged into such software programs as Microsoft Access before analysis can be conducted. As organizations become more sophisticated in using their data, however, the mechanisms to ensure more accurate data and ease of merging data should improve.

CONCLUSIONS

Environmental pressures are leading to changes from a quality assurance to a quality management approach to improve long-term care. As facilities have increased the sophistication of their quality management processes, they have implemented performance measurement systems to enable the tracking of key indicators that are strategically and operationally important. Many of these facilities are requiring their staff to manually collect many of the key indicators for their performance measurement systems. As the use of information technology both in administrative and clinical functions increases, facilities have more computerized data at their disposal. Effective leveraging of the computerized data requires transforming the data into information and knowledge through automated generation of key indicators via computer algorithms. As facilities improve in their sophistication in using data, they will be able to better provide information to consumers about the types, outcomes, and quality of care they provide.

REFERENCES

Anderson, J.C., Rungtusanatham, M., & Schroeder, R.G. (1994). A theory of quality management underlying the Deming Management Method. *Academy of Management Review, 19*(3), 472–509.

Batalden, P.B. (1991). Organizationwide quality improvement in health care. *Topics in Health Record Management, 11*(3), 1–12.

Bradley, M.G., & Thompson, N.R. (2000). *Quality management integration in long-term care: Guidelines for excellence.* Baltimore: Health Professions Press.

Carey, R.G., & Lloyd, R.C. (2001). *Measuring quality improvement in healthcare: A guide to statistical process control applications.* Milwaukee: Quality Press.

Castle, N.G., Zinn, J.S. Brannon, D., & Mor, V. (1997). Quality improvement in nursing homes. *Health Care Management: State of the Art Reviews,* pp. 39–54, June.

Hatzell, T.A., Williams, E., Halverson, P., & Kaluzny, A. (1996). Improvement strategy for local health departments. *Quality Management in Health Care, 14*(3), 79–86.

Institute for Health and Aging, University of California, San Francisco. (1996). *Chronic care in America: A 21st century challenge.* Princeton, NJ: Robert Wood Johnson Foundation.

Institute of Medicine, Committee on Nursing Home Regulation. (1986). *Improving the quality of care in nursing homes.* Washington, DC: National Academy Press.

Kane, R.A., & Kane, R.L. (1988). Long-term care: Variations on a quality assurance theme. *Inquiry, 25,* 132–146, Spring.

Karon, S.L., & Zimmerman, D.R. (1996). Using indicators to structure quality improvement initiatives in long-term care. *Quality Management in Health Care, 4*(3), 54–66.

Kaplan, R.S., & Norton, D.P. (1992). The balanced scorecard–Measure that drive performance. *Harvard Business Review,* pp. 71-79, January–February.

Kaplan, R.S., & Norton, D.P. (1993). Putting the balanced scorecard to work. *Harvard Business Review,* pp. 134–147, September–October.

Kaplan, R.S., & Norton, D.P. (1996a). Using the balanced scorecard as a strategic management system. *Harvard Business Review,* pp. 75–85, January–February.

Kaplan, R.S., & Norton, D.P. (1996b). *The balance scorecard.* Boston, MA: Harvard Business School Press.

McKeon, T. (1996). Benchmarks and performance indicators: two tools for evaluating organizational results and continuous quality improvement efforts. *Journal of Nursing Care Quality, 10*(3), 12–17.

National Institute of Standards and Technology, Department of Congress. (2002). Baldrige National Quality Program. www.quality.nist.gov.

Nyman, J.A., & Geyer, C.R. (1989). Promoting the quality of life in nursing homes: can regulation succeed? *Journal of Health Politics, Policy and Law, 14*(4), 797–816.

Rockart, J.F. (1979). Chief executives define their own data needs. *Harvard Business Review,* March–April, 81–93.

Sainfort, F., Ramsay, J.D., Ferreira, P.L., & Lassaad Mezghani. (1994). A first step in total quality management of nursing facility care: Development of an empirical causal model of structure, process and outcome dimensions. *American Journal of Medical Quality, 9*(2), 74–96.

Shaughnessy, P.W. (1989). Quality of nursing home care. *Generations, 8*(1), 17–20.

Smyer, M.., Brannon, D., & Cohn, M. (1992). Improving nursing care through training and job redesign. *Gerontologist, 32,* 327–333.

Strahan, G. (1987). Nursing home characteristics: Preliminary data from the 1985 national nursing home survey. *NCHS Advancedata, 131,* 1–7.

U.S. Congress. (1987). *Omnibus Budget Reconciliation Act of 1987.* Washington, DC: 100th Congress, 1st session, Pub. Law 100-203.

U.S. Department of Health and Human Services, Health Care Financing Administration, Office of Research and Demonstrations, Health Care Financing Review, Statistical Supplement. (1996). Baltimore, MD.

Zimmerman, D.R., Karon, S.L., Arling, G., Clark, B.R., Collins, T., Ross, R., & Sainfort, F. (1995). Development and testing of nursing home quality indicators. *Health Care Financing Review, 16*(4) Summer, 107–127.

Chapter 27

MANAGING CHANGE

Ruth Stryker and George Kenneth Gordon

The field of long-term care has been bombarded with change during the past 25 years. Delivery systems, reimbursement systems, regulations, and survey processes have changed along with increasingly sophisticated needs of its clients. Much of this change has been externally imposed, but creative change, generated internally, has also taken place. Regardless of the source, the administrator must help the organization to initiate change, to be responsive to change, and to adapt to change.

Administrative skill in managing change enables an organization to weather turbulent times and to create much of its own future. This skill is developed through understanding the nature of change, various concepts of change, ways to support people during the change process, and a sensitivity to the timing of initiating change.

Several years ago, long-term care administrators pursuing graduate studies at the University of Minnesota were introduced to systematic mastery of change and required to initiate, conduct, and document outcomes of a planned change project in their own organizations. Their projects revealed the susceptibility to deadly routinization of the daily round of activities and demonstrated the need for adept leadership by the administrator to cultivate and maintain an organization's capacity for progress. These experiences led to the identification of important areas of study regarding change.

THE NATURE OF CHANGE

Change is a dynamic process of transition, alteration, and becoming different. It is not the goal (that was determined in the planning process), it is the "getting there"; it is the trip, if you will, rather than the destination. The trip may be good or bad. Indeed, the same change may be perceived as good by one individual or group and bad by another, so that reactions to change can be expected to vary among individuals and departments. Change is a part of our daily lives. Some is welcome; some is unwelcome; some is unplanned; some we plan and make happen.

Every generation experiences change, but what makes our experience different from that of our ancestors is the rate of change. It is unparalleled in history. New knowledge and technology occurs faster than our ability to apply it. Because both our personal and work lives are affected by rapid changes, it is important to have some understanding of change itself–the kinds, the process, strategies, and how to plan and manage it.

The concept of change must be viewed in the context of the interrelatedness of systems and subsystems. For example, a long-term care organization (a system) interacts with the Medicaid system. It is obvious that change in one affects the other. Making a change in the dietary department (a subsystem of the nursing home) is likely to affect both the nursing and the housekeeping departments (other subsystems).

Two types of change, developmental and revolutionary, each impact people and organizations differently.

> Developmental change tends to be incremental in that the system adapts in bits and pieces as pressures and influences for change are felt. Not that the system moves from one fixed state to the next fixed state, but rather that the system is constantly evolving in a state of "dynamic equilibrium" where its various elements adjust gradually. . . . Revolutionary change is change that upsets the workable balance of a system and throws it out of an established equilibrium. It is change that involves entirely different goals and sets the system off in a new direction. (Taylor)

OBRA '87 made some revolutionary changes in long-term care organizations. Changes in the way of thinking about the use of restraints caused a major shift in goals for caregivers. Similarly, the Balanced Budget Act of 1997 changed the way Medicare charges and payments were made in certain instances.

Change can be planned or unplanned. As we grow older (expected but unplanned), we begin to prepare for retirement income and housing (planned change), just as we plan to wear warmer clothing in the winter than in the summer. An example of unplanned change was the unanticipated effect on the environment from using D.D.T.

What then, do we mean by managing change if so much is either inevitable, uncontrollable, or unpredictable? There are two facets to managing change. First, when unexpected factors affect an organization, we must be prepared to alter our directions and reallocate our resources. Sometimes, one can anticipate the effects of internal or external events and prepare alternatives ahead of time. Second, if an organization is to become dynamic, it must not only incorporate **planned** change, but the *expectation* of planned change if it is to keep pace with new knowledge and the tools to prevent obsolescence and maintain excellence.

Indeed, planned change can also be viewed as organizational development. McGill defines organizational change as ". . . a conscious, planned process of developing an organization's capabilities so that it can attain and sustain an optimum level of performance as measured by efficiency, effectiveness and health. . . ." He also notes that some organizations use a behavioral science consultant when radical changes are planned. While the reader may find that an extravagant idea, it indicates McGill's keen awareness of personnel needs and the need for administrative skills for managing change.

REACTIONS TO CHANGE

A change may represent a challenge or a threat; an opportunity for growth and improved patient satisfaction, or a disruption of accustomed tasks and relationships; a fear of failure or a chance to learn something new. Behaviors such as cooperation, compliance, open hostility, or some type of subversion of the change will reflect an individual's perception of a change.

When instituting change, a manager needs to understand how people change and how differently each of us changes. Each person is a unique mix of genes and experiences which affect the way he or she behaves, thinks, and feels, as well as lifetime patterns of reaction, adaptation, and adjustment to change.

In spite of each person's individuality, there are certain common reasons for resisting change. They are (1) a real **or** perceived threat to one's job or job relationships, (2) an unclear idea of what will be expected, (3) lack of confidence in ability to cope and succeed in the new situation and (4) loss of sense of worth. Even a desired change, such as accepting a new job promotion, can raise these specters and make us want to cling to our status quo and the known.

In an organization, such fears of the unknown will lurk to some degree in everyone, including the administrator. Stress reactions may include anger, disorganization, reduced productivity, outright refusal, and illness. Other persons will turn their energies to planning, preparing themselves, finding satisfactions outside of work, physical exercise, and maintaining their sense of personal worth in spite of defeats or change.

The administrator's response to staff reactions can alter the degree of resistance, negatively or positively. It can generate more resistance if there is no self-understanding or a lack of comprehension of what employees are feeling and thinking. On the other hand, if the administrator understands the dynamics involved in change, he or she can proceed with planning not just what will be changed, but how the process of change itself will take place.

Individual responses to change may also affect organizational responses. Moore and Gergen point out the difference between organizational responses based on the kinds of employees as well as their experience with change. ". . . organizations with a history of little change probably maintain a work force of low to moderate risk takers. High risk takers would not find such an environment stimulating." They go on to say that such organizations have greater difficulty with change because greater effort must go into creating a supportive environment for the staff.

CHANGE STRATEGIES

The administrator needs to assess the degree of potential impact on each part of the organization, recognizing that the change process can become emotionally charged. Then, he or she can prepare strategies for assisting individuals and groups to accommodate according to the degree of impact. While managing the change, Robert Taylor recommends that administrators begin with conceptual strategies to formulate a management approach to specific situations. A review of such strategies will make his statement more applicable.

The Empirical-Rational Strategies (described by Bennis et al. in *The Planning of Change*). These assume that people are guided by reason and self-interest. This approach suggests that giving useful information and knowledge will provide the wisdom to stimulate doing the right things. One problem with this approach is its failure to consider nonrational aspects of behavior. It is exemplified in the nursing home when we find little behavior change resulting from an inservice program. The narrowness of this approach has also been criticized in recent years because it does not adequately take into account the effect of one thing on other things (the systems approach). For instance, damming rivers on the North Pacific coast for hydroelectric power caused a deterioration of the salmon fishing industry in the Pacific Ocean. Similarly, when there was a shortage of water in San Francisco, residents were asked to conserve water; but when they used less water, the unit price to consumers went up. Thus, a rational change will first require an exploration of its possible effects on other parts of the system even though they do not appear to be affected at the time of initial consideration.

Normative Re-education Strategies (also described by Bennis et al.). These build upon assumptions about human motivation. They relate to the attitudes, values, and beliefs that support patterns of action and practice.

While rationality and intelligence are not denied in this approach, it emphasizes that changes in practice or behavior occur when persons change their value orientations and become committed to new ones. This requires that persons participate in the change process, that unconscious resistance be brought out in the open for examination, and that the concepts of the behavioral sciences be used to deal with change effectively.

Power-Coercive Strategies. These are a third approach to change. They are based on the use of power to effect change which may stem from the law or an influential group. Power and authority are used to gain compliance in these strategies. This is familiar to long-term care administrators. Regulatory agencies and Medicaid reimbursement systems are a part of the administrator's daily life. Medicaid legislation in the sixties, changed nursing homes in radical ways for decades to come. This approach, however, can be identified in other more subtle and not so subtle situations. Power can emanate from a position, a group, a personality or by virtue of knowledge and may or may not be used appropriately. This approach may be needed when a change is selected, sanctioned, opposed or modified. It does not, however, speak to the dynamics of implementing and managing a change within an organization unless it is used as a backup when combined with a behavioral approach.

Havelock and Havelock describe the **social-interactive approach** to change. This approach takes into account that people influence change according to their degree of social affiliations, their influence on views held by opinion leaders and informal personal contacts. This approach might describe the political process. An administrator uses this approach when preparing for a major expansion, raising funds, or speaking before community groups. It begins with opinion leaders who work through networks of influence.

PLANNING CHANGE

Force Field Analysis, a method of analysis developed by Kurt Lewin, makes an excellent administrative tool when initiating a change. This method identifies three operating forces in a change situation: driving, resistance, and interference. Driving forces work toward a change. Certain people, a desire for progress, or dissatisfaction with the present situation would be examples of forces positively disposed to a proposed change. Resistance forces work against a change. Disagreement, fear, a desire to maintain the status quo are examples of resistance forces working against a proposed change. Interference forces are ones that divert energies away from a change. They are not necessarily opposed, but a shortage of time, energy, and money would be considered interference forces. The administrator can use Force Field Analysis when he or she is preparing for a change. Identifying the driving, resistance, and interference forces provides insight into some of the strategies necessary to initiate a change. One can increase driving forces while looking for ways to decrease both the resistance and interference forces.

Kurt Lewin's view of the change *process* provides some rather specific guidelines for the administrator. His views account for the need to plan and develop change. It avoids the unwise use of power, takes time into consideration, and seems to integrate the normative re-education and social-interactive approaches. He describes three phases of the change process.

Lewin's first phase, **unfreezing,** aims to prepare and motivate an individual or group for change. During this phase, the objective is to induce dissatisfaction with established practice, apply pressure for change, and to neutralize resisting forces while avoiding polarization. Activities during this period might include (1) circulation of pertinent readings, (2) inservice education, (3) continuing education for a few key persons responsible for the change, (4) demonstration of change in one area or with a few residents, (5) reward of voluntary new behaviors, (6) disciplined elimination of reward for old behaviors and (7) participation of staff in determining ways of achieving the goals.

Lewin's second phase is **changing or moving** to new behaviors. It occurs when there is further examination, and trying a new behavior or procedure by all parts of the system involved. First, identification of reasons for change can be focused by (1) providing a model to emulate (for example, the effect on residents), (2) setting high expectations, (3) helping people to feel safe by showing them they can succeed, and (4) increasing the attractiveness of the change. Gradually, new behaviors will become internalized and the only acceptable ones. They need to be reinforced continuously by incorporating the concepts in care plans, performance appraisal systems, and informal support.

Lewin's final phase, **refreezing,** occurs when the new behavior becomes constant. It involves integration into the system, prevention of backsliding, and follow-up. During this time, reinforcement should move from continuous to intermittent, policies should reflect the change, and it should be included in the orientation of personnel, families and residents. This phase culminates in a new sense of self-worth and achievement.

Dorothy Coons states that "staff will change when they have a sense of self-worth." When the Geriatric wards of Michigan's Ypsilanti State Hospital were changed from a custodial to a therapeutic focus, staff had to (1) realize that their usual and established practices were obsolete, (2) learn new skills that would not reinforce long-term illness, and (3) develop new attitudes and expectations that would allow patients to improve. Coons' problems parallel those in many nursing homes. Her experience and success are applicable and instructive to long-term care administrators.

Five Principles of Helping Staff–Coons

1. Direct service staff should be involved in developing plans for change. Note, they did not decide if there would be a change, but they decided some of the "hows." Such participation prevents problems that could not be anticipated by persons removed from the immediate work situation. The staff immediately affected are best able to anticipate problems and suggest solutions.
2. "Staff must have time." They need to have time to read about new ideas, understand them, consider their effects, and get used to them. This assimilation time can be likened to that needed for a person in psychotherapy or dealing with a death. It is necessary for successful adaptation.
3. Everyone involved in an implementation plan must have a clear understanding of what it is and the steps needed to carry it out. Decisions made in meetings can be put in writing and distributed in order to clarify any misunderstandings.
4. Staff should focus on developing one phase of the change at a time. This reduces disorganization from possible "overload" as described in Toffler's *Future Shock*.
5. "Staff must have opportunity to report on successes or problems." This sharing with one another can increase successes and help to resolve any new problems more quickly than if this step does not occur.

THE ADMINISTRATOR'S ROLE

Creative long-term care requires an administrator who will assume the role of change agent as a primary responsibility. Not everyone is suited to this role because it requires an open personality, knowledge and skill in human relations, the willingness to take calculated risks, flexibility, and a sense of personal worth and confidence that is not dissipated with a failure.

Personal Qualities

The administrator who takes the change agent role seriously will select future-thinking personnel, will listen to and be influenced by those in the organization, have a natural inclination to reach out for new ideas, and realize that innovation is not the prerogative of only one person. Openness to new ideas and the ability to imagine the future also comes from exposure to a broader life–travel, history, philosophy and social activities.

Because change may produce conflict, the administrator must be knowledgeable about conflict resolution and possess negotiating skills. Thus, the administrator will be flexible in equalizing power relationships and in assigning authority and responsibility in order to produce win-win rather than win-lose results. This capacity requires well-founded trust in the character of the administrator which will be demonstrated by avoidance of coercive or devious manipulation of people.

The change agent will be committed to the need for change, comfortable with obtaining satisfaction from the successes of others, and provide staff support throughout the change process. Each planned change will lay the groundwork for the next, and eventually more and more staff will begin to view change as an opportunity for personal growth and greater contribution to resident care.

Administrator Tasks in the Change Process

When an organizational change has been decided upon, the administrator needs to reflect upon the change process before implementation begins. This is necessary regardless of who initiated the idea for change and for many seemingly small as well as large changes. The following guidelines are suggested:

1. Planning
   a. Clearly state objectives in writing so that others understand where they are going.
   b. Assign resources (time, dollars, materials, personnel, etc.).
2. Assessing
   a. Who will be affected (departments, personnel, residents, families, others)?
   b. What variety of responses might be anticipated and why?
   c. Who will be supportive? Who will be unsupportive?
   d. What can be done to assist those involved during the change process?
3. Communicating
   a. Share objectives and discuss plans.
   b. Encourage suggestions and modifications by those involved.
   c. Involve inservice personnel if new knowledge, skills, or roles are required.

4. Monitoring
   a. Assess any new or continued problems.
   b. Work with others to deal with daily changes.
   c. Prepare alternative strategies for timing and methods of implementation.

The more rigid the organization, of course, the greater the likelihood of resistance to new ideas. Creative organizations are more flexible and embrace a greater range of internal diversity. Indeed, diversity is a critical resource of creative organizations, but the administrator must learn how to use it so that it does not result in polarization of individuals and groups. Creative organizations have special characteristics (Schaller). They include the following:

1. The administrator recognizes that conflict is a part of the creative change process, but that polarization can be a barrier to planned change. Thus the administrator:
   a. Keeps communication channels open.
   b. Attempts to depersonalize dissent.
   c. Attempts to identify the needs and fears of others.
   d. Encourages meaningful participation in planning by every person involved.
   e. Begins by seeking agreement on short-term or intermediate goals.
   f. Builds a sense of trust throughout the organization.
2. The primary organizational focus is on contemporary practice, not that of yesterday or perpetuation of the organization.
3. There is constant awareness that problems do exist.
4. The emphasis is on problem solving.
5. There is emphasis on locating important and relevant knowledge from a variety of disciplines and "an unusual flare for utilizing and applying the knowledge, wisdom, and insights of other disciplines."
6. Continuous monitoring of the benefits and pace of change prevent the possibility of too much disruption.
7. When new ideas are proposed, the leader knows the most receptive points of intervention.

In summary, the administrator needs to continually monitor the pulse of the change process. Is it too fast? Can it be speeded up? Do certain individuals require special attention (counseling, reassurance, education, etc.)? What can be done to maintain participation, maintain movement toward the new goals, and support those involved during the process?

If long-term care organizations are to develop their capabilities, and at the same time maintain their missions and services, organizational viability and productivity, the administrator must become a change agent. Changes can be successful and foster growth in organizational outcomes if the administrator understands not just the goals and mechanics of a change but management of the change process itself.

REFERENCES AND RESOURCES

Bennis, W.G. et al. (1976). *The planning of change* (3rd ed.). New York: Holt, Rinehart, and Winston.

Coons, D. (1973). *The process of change*. Ann Arbor: Institute of Gerontology, University of Michigan.

Covey, S.T. (1989). *The seven habits of highly effective people: Lessons in personal change*. New York: Simon Schuster.

Gergen, P., & Moore, M. (1985). Risk taking and organizational change. *Training and Development Journal, 39*(3), 284, June.

Greiner, L.E. (1998). Evolution and revolution as organizations grow. *Harvard Business Review,* May–June.

Hallett, J. (1985). Today's trends suggest revolutionary changes for business in the future. *Personal Administrator, 30*(2), 64–74.

Havelock, R.G., & Havelock, M.C. (1973). *Training for change agents*. Ann Arbor: Institute for Social Research.

Kanter, R.M. (1983). *The change masters: Innovating for productivity in the American corporation*. New York: Simon and Schuster.

———. *Men and women of the corporation* (2nd ed.). New York: Basic Books.

Kotter, J.P. (1996). *Leading change*. Boston: Harvard Business School.

McGill, M.E. (1977). *Organizational development for operating managers*. New York: AMACOM.

Pascale, R. et al. (1997). Changing the way we change. *Harvard Business Review,* November–December.

Peters, J.P., & Tseng, S. (1984). Managing strategic change: Moving others from awareness to action. *Hospital and Health Services Administration,* July–August.

Schaller, L.E. (1972). *The change agent*. Nashville: Abington Press.

Senge, P.M. (1995). *The fifth discipline: The art and practice of the learning organization*. New York: Doubleday.

Taylor, R. (1992). The management of change. Monograph. Division of Health Services Administration, University of Minnesota, Minneapolis.

Tichy, N. (1983). *Managing strategic change: Technical, political and cultural dynamics*. New York: John Wiley.

Tofler, A. (1970). *Future shock*. New York: Random House.

Appendix A

COMPETENCIES OF DIRECTORS OF NURSING/NURSE ADMINISTRATORS IN LONG-TERM CARE FACILITIES[1]

Organization Management:

Serves as a member of the executive staff of the organization and develops effective working relationships with the chief executive officer and the medical director.

Participates in the development of institutional policies.

Shares in development of long-range plans for the institution.

Participates in development and administration of an evaluation plan for the institution based on institutional goals and objectives on nursing standards.

Works in establishing and facilitating effective employer-employee relations.

Minimizes legal risks.

Participates in establishing and maintaining management information systems to facilitate administration of the institutions nursing department.

Designs and implements organizational structure for the nursing department.

Formulates and administers policies and procedures for the nursing department.

Implements federal, state, and local regulations pertaining to nursing service.

Develops long-range plans for the nursing department.

Formulates and administers the departmental budget based on nursing department goals and projected revenue.

---

[1] *Professional Practice for Nurse Administrators in Long-term Care Facilities* (1984) document developed through a project jointly sponsored by the American Nurses Foundation and the Foundation of the American College of Health Care Administrators.

Participates in establishing a competitive wage, salary, and benefit plan for nursing services staff.

Operates the department in a cost-effective manner.

Designs and implements a quality assurance plan for nursing care.

Formulates and administers an evaluation plan for nursing services in relation to the departments' established goals, objectives, and standards.

Raises consciousness, educates, and participates in formulating policy relative to bioethical issues.

Initiates research projects that address problems and issues specific to the nursing department.

Human Resources Management in Nursing:

Recruits, selects, and retains qualified nursing staff.

Develops and implements a master staffing plan based on client needs and nursing service goals and standards.

Initiates and approves position descriptions for nursing personnel.

Promotes a scheduling system that balances employee and client needs.

Formulates, implements and evaluates a departmental plan for orientation and staff development.

Assists individual staff members in development of career plans.

Designs and implements a performance appraisal system for nursing.

Promotes resolution of conflicts.

Promotes and implements personnel policies.

Creates a work climate that promotes a high-quality work life.

Nursing/Health Service Management:

Develops philosophy, goals, and objectives for the department of nursing.

Assesses the implementation of effective strategies and methods for delivery of nursing care.

Implements actions to meet and maintain nursing care standards.

Cooperates in developing and implementing a process for an interdisciplinary approach to health care services.

Facilitates creative use of community resources.

Ensures that clients' rights are protected.

Encourages independence of clients through use of self-care and rehabilitation concepts.

Initiates formal or informal testing of nursing interventions.

Evaluates the organization of nursing care.

Evaluates plans of nursing care.

Professional Nursing and Long-Term Care Leadership:

Plans for future health and nursing care actions based on social, economic, political, and technological changes.

Promotes changes in community health care systems based on social, economic, political and technological changes.

Encourages innovative methods for delivery of long-term care.

Encourages entrepreneurial activities associated with development of nursing models for health care delivery focusing on health promotion, health education, and direct services.

Establishes linkages with existing community resources.

Influences public policy affecting long-term care and nursing.

Establishes relationships with colleges and universities to promote formal educational opportunities for nursing staff, faculty practice, student learning experiences and research.

Promotes a positive image of long-term care, nursing in long-term care and long-term care institutions.

Seeks opportunities for personal and professional growth.

Appendix B

DETERMINATION OF STAFFING USING THE RUG-III CASE-MIX CLASSIFICATION SYSTEM FOR NURSING TIME

RUG-III Groups	Number Residents	RN Minutes	Subtotal	LV/PN Minutes	Subtotal	CNA Minutes	Subtotal	Total Minutes
RUC	4	112.7	450.8	53.8	215.2	180.1	720.4	1386.4
RUB	4	87.7	351	37.4	150	123.8	495	995.6
RUA	3	64.5	194	40.4	121	98.4	295	609.9
RVC	3	90.9	273	50.7	152	164.9	495	919.5
RVB	2	94.7	189.4	41.6	83.2	136.3	272.6	545.2
RVA	4	75.6	302	30.0	120	106.8	427	849.6
RHC	3	110.6	331.8	53.5	160.5	167.0	501.0	993.3
RHB	2	102.3	204.6	39.9	79.8	129.9	259.8	544.2
RHA	2	89.7	179	27.6	55	102.6	205	439.8
RMC	2	111.2	222.4	66.8	133.6	180.0	360.0	716.0
RMB	3	101.2	303.6	42.4	127.2	141.8	425.4	856.2
RMA	3	95.0	285	33.9	102	117.3	352	738.6
RLB	4	79.0	316	48.9	196	191.3	765	1276.8
RLA	3	64.5	194	32.0	96	122.8	368	657.9
SE3	1	140.7	140.7	101.5	101.5	191.3	191.3	433.5
SE2	2	110.4	220.8	85.4	170.8	163.2	326.4	718.0
SE1	4	77.9	312	60.1	240	195.3	781	1333.2
SSC	4	72.9	291.6	64.3	257.2	184.1	736.4	1285.2
SSB	3	70.9	213	55.0	165	172.4	517	894.9
SSA	2	91.7	183.4	41.8	83.5	130.4	260.8	527.7
CC2	1	85.2	85.2	42.5	42.5	191.1	191.1	318.8

Appendix B (continued)

RUG-III Groups	Number Residents	RN Minutes	Subtotal	LV/PN Minutes	Subtotal	CNA Minutes	Subtotal	Total Minutes
CC1	1	55.7	56	57.7	58	176.9	177	290.3
CB2	2	61.5	123.0	41.9	83.8	159.0	318.0	524.8
CB1	1	59.0	59	36.2	36	147.3	147	242.5
CA2	1	58.8	59	43.3	43	130.3	130	232.4
CA1	1	59.7	59.7	37.6	37.6	103.3	103.3	200.6
Totals	65		5598.1		3110.4		9822.4	18530.9

	RN			LVN			CNA			Total Staff	
	Min/ 24 hrs	Hrs/ 24 hrs	No. Staff	Min/ 24 hrs	Hrs/ 24 hrs	No. Staff	Min/ 24 hrs	Hrs/ 24 hrs	No. Staff	Hrs/ 24 hrs	No. Staff
Days %	2239.2	37.32	4.67	1244.2	20.74	2.59	3929.0	65.48	8.19	123.54	15.44
PM %	1959.3	32.66	4.08	1088.6	18.14	2.27	3437.8	57.30	7.16	108.10	13.51
Noc %	1399.5	23.33	2.92	777.6	12.96	1.62	2455.6	40.93	5.12	77.21	9.65
Totals	5598.1	93.30	11.66	3110.4	51.84	6.48	9822.4	163.71	20.46	308.85	38.61

Appendix C

TWO-WEEK BLOCKS FOR NURSING STAFF SCHEDULE

Complex Medical (24 Beds/Census: 23)

RN Staff 6a–6p	Sun	Mon	Tue	Wed	Thu	Fri	Sat	Sun	Mon	Tue	Wed	Thu	Fri	Sat	FTEs
RN 1	12	12	x	x	x	12	x	x	12	12	x	x	x	12	0.9
RN 2	x	x	12	12	x	x	12	12	x	x	12	12	x	x	0.9
RN 3	x	x	x	x	12	12	x	x	x	x	x	x	12	x	0.3
RN 4	x	x	x	12	x	12	12	12	x	x	x	x	12	12	0.9
RN 5	12	12	12	x	x	x	12	x	12	12	x	x	x	12	0.9
RN 6	x	x	x	x	12	12	x	x	x	12	12	12	x	x	0.3
Total Hours	48	48	48	48	48	48	48	48	48	48	48	48	48	48	
6p–6a															
RN 1	12	12	x	x	x	12	x	x	12	12	x	x	x	12	0.9
RN 2	x	x	12	12	x	x	12	12	x	x	12	12	x	x	0.9
RN 3	x	x	x	x	12	12	x	x	x	x	x	x	12	x	0.3
RN 4	x	x	x	12	x	12	12	12	x	x	x	x	12	12	0.9
RN 5	12	12	12	x	x	x	12	x	12	12	x	x	x	12	0.9
RN 6	x	x	x	x	12	12	x	x	x	12	12	12	x	x	0.3
Total Hours	48	48	48	48	48	48	48	48	48	48	48	48	48	48	8.4

Appendix C (continued)

LPN Staff

10a–6p	Sun	Mon	Tue	Wed	Thu	Fri	Sat	Sun	Mon	Tue	Wed	Thu	Fri	Sat	FTEs
LPN 1	8	x	8	8	8	8	x	x	8	8	8	8	x	8	1
LPN 2	x	8	x	x	x	x	8	8	x	x	x	x	8	x	0.4
Total Hours	8	8	8	8	8	8	8	8	8	8	8	8	8	8	1.4

CNA Staff

6a–6p	Sun	Mon	Tue	Wed	Thu	Fri	Sat	Sun	Mon	Tue	Wed	Thu	Fri	Sat	FTEs
CNA 1	12	12	x	x	x	12	x	x	12	12	x	x	x	12	0.9
CNA 2	x	x	12	12	x	x	12	12	x	x	12	12	x	x	0.9
CNA 3	12	x	12	12	x	x	x	x	12	12	x	x	x	12	0.9
CNA 4	x	12	x	x	12	12	x	12	x	x	x	12	12	x	0.9
CNA 5	12	x	x	x	12	x	x	x	x	x	12	x	12	x	0.6
CNA 6	x	12	x	12	x	12	12	12	x	12	x	12	x	x	1.0
CNA 7	x	x	12	x	x	x	12	x	x	x	x	x	12	x	0.4

6p–6a	Sun	Mon	Tue	Wed	Thu	Fri	Sat	Sun	Mon	Tue	Wed	Thu	Fri	Sat	FTEs
CNA 1	12	12	x	x	12	x	x	x	12	12	x	x	x	12	0.9
CNA 2	x	x	12	12	x	x	12	12	x	x	12	12	x	x	0.9
CNA 3	12	x	12	12	x	12	x	x	12	12	x	12	12	12	0.9
CNA 4	x	12	x	x	12	12	12	12	x	x	12	12	12	x	0.9
CNA 5	x	x	x	x	x	12	12	x	x	x	x	x	12	x	0.6
Total Hours	60	60	60	60	60	60	60	60	60	60	60	60	60	60	9.8

Hours per Resident Day

6a–6p	3.0
6p–6a	2.1
Total	5.1

	Total FTEs	Number of Staff Needed on a Daily Basis
6a–6p	12.0	11
6p–6a	8.4	4
Total	20.4	15

Appendix C (continued)

2-Week Block Schedule

Special Care Dementia Unit

DAYS	Sun	Mon	Tue	Wed	Thu	Fri	Sat	Sun	Mon	Tue	Wed	Thu	Fri	Sat	FTEs
RN 1	x	8	8	8	x	8	8	8	8	x	8	8	8	x	1.0
RN 2*	8	x	8	x	8	8	x	x	8	8	x	x	x	8	0.2
RN 3	8	x	x	x	x	x	x	x	x	x	x	x	x	8	0.2
Total Hours	8	8	8	8	8	8	8	8	8	8	8	8	8	8	

* Also works on Unit B

	Sun	Mon	Tue	Wed	Thu	Fri	Sat	Sun	Mon	Tue	Wed	Thu	Fri	Sat	FTEs
CNA 1	x	8	8	8	x	8	8	8	x	8	8	8	8	x	1.0
CNA 2	8	x	8	8	8	8	x	x	8	8	8	8	x	8	1.0
CNA 3	8	8	x	x	8	x	x	x	8	8	x	x	8	8	0.6
CNA 4	x	x	x	x	x	x	8	8	x	x	x	x	x	x	0.2
Total Hours	16	16	16	16	16	16	16	16	16	16	16	16	16	16	4.2
Total Day Hrs	24	24	24	24	24	24	24	24	24	24	24	24	24	24	

EVES	Sun	Mon	Tue	Wed	Thu	Fri	Sat	FTEs
RN 1	x	8	8	8	8	8	x	1.0
RN 2*	8	x	x	x	x	x	x	0.2
RN 3	x	x	x	x	x	x	8	0.2
Total Hours	8	8	8	8	8	8	8	
*Also works on Unit B								
CNA 1	x	x	8	8	8	8	8	1.0
CNA 2	8	8	6	6	6	x	x	0.85
CNA 3	6	6	x	x	x	6	x	0.45
CNA 4	x	x	x	x	x	x	6	0.15
Total Hours	14	14	14	14	14	14	14	3.85
Total Eve Hrs	22	22	22	22	22	22	22	

NOCS	Sun	Mon	Tue	Wed	Thu	Fri	Sat	FTEs
RN 1	x	8	8	8	8	8	x	1.0
RN 2	8	x	x	x	x	x	8	0.4
Total Hours	8	8	8	8	8	8	8	
CNA 1	x	8	8	8	8	8	x	1.0
CNA 2	8	x	x	x	x	x	8	0.4
Total Hours	8	8	8	8	8	8	8	2.8
Total Noc Hrs	16	16	16	16	16	16	16	

Appendix C (continued)

Hours per Resident Day

Days	1.2
Eves	1.1
Nocs	0.8
Total	3.1

	Total FTEs	Number of Staff Needed on a Daily Basis
Days	4.2	3.0
Eves	3.9	2.8
Nocs	2.8	2.0
Total	10.9	7.8

Mueller, C. (2001). *Developing a Comprehensive Staffing Program.* University of Minnesota, School of Nursing. (http://ltcnurseleader.umn.edu)

AUTHOR INDEX

SUBJECT INDEX